Forced Migration and Health Justice

Forced Migration and Health Justice

Edited by LISA A. ECKENWILER,

VERINA WILD,

ANNA GOTLIB,

RYOA CHUNG,

and

DEBORAH ZION

Managing Editor JAKE SCHROEDER

OXFORD
UNIVERSITY PRESS

OXFORD
UNIVERSITY PRESS

Oxford University Press is a department of the University of Oxford.
It furthers the University's objective of excellence in research, scholarship,
and education by publishing worldwide. Oxford is a registered trade mark of
Oxford University Press in the UK and in certain other countries.

Published in the United States of America by Oxford University Press
198 Madison Avenue, New York, NY 10016, United States of America.

CIP data is on file at the Library of Congress

ISBN 9780197795491

DOI: 10.1093/oso/9780197795491.001.0001

The manufacturer's authorized representative in the EU for product safety is
Oxford University Press España S.A. of Parque Empresarial San Fernando de Henares,
Avenida de Castilla, 2 – 28830 Madrid (www.oup.es/en or product.safety@oup.com).
OUP España S.A. also acts as importer into Spain of products made by the manufacturer.

We dedicate this book to our beautiful families, especially Emmanuel, Felix, Rasmus, Jeff, Hwayap, Chan, Felix-Yujin, Paul, Benjamin, and Rafael, and to the journalist and poet Behrouz Boochani for reminding us that we all look up at the same moon.

CONTENTS

ACKNOWLEDGMENTS

We want to express our most heartfelt appreciation to everyone at Oxford University Press who has supported this project from the start, especially Sarah Humphreville, Mary Funchion, Devasree Vasudevan, and the design team. We also owe our deepest thanks to the graduate students who assisted us along the way: Allie Edwards, a former MA student in George Mason's Philosophy Department, helped with the early communications and organization of papers; Isabel Fernandez Mayor and Juenna Fiola, both students at the University of Augsburg, assisted with endless patience, friendliness, and skill with editing, formatting, and references. Then there is our managing editor, Jake Schroeder, another MA student from Mason's Philosophy Department. His abilities at communicating, organizing, editing, and serving as an overall font of thoughtfulness, joy, and dependability are unmatched. It has been our great honor to work with him throughout these many months. Thanks are due to the College of Humanities and Social Sciences at George Mason for their support of these students. We express our appreciation to Verena Lippert from the University of Augsburg, who assisted us over some administrative hurdles. We also wish to thank Marianne Saillant-Sylvain from the Université de Montréal for her invaluable assistance on the Index. In addition, we want to thank the Montréal-based designer-artist Layla Chergui for introducing us to Aya Haidar and her work. Last, we are grateful to our family members and to many people who brought us inspiration—especially the students whose families or who themselves have experience with forced migration.

EDITOR BIOS

Lisa Eckenwiler, PhD, is a full professor in the Department of Philosophy at George Mason University, Virginia, United States, where she teaches courses in bioethics and global justice and on a range of topics in global health ethics. Her research centers on vulnerability and structural health injustice, and she has published widely on migration and health justice, humanitarian health ethics, and placemaking and health justice. She is at work on a book titled *Placemaking for Health Justice*, and another project on humanitarian ethics. Her previous books include *Long-Term Care, Globalization and Justice* (2012) and *The Ethics of Bioethics: Mapping the Moral Landscape*, co-edited with Felicia Cohn (2007). Professor Eckenwiler is a fellow of the Hastings Center and served as vice president of the International Association of Bioethics. She is also founder and current chair of the Migrant Health and Ethics Network (within the International Association of Bioethics) and a founding member of the Independent Resource Group for Global Health Justice.

Verina Wild is a professor of medical ethics and director of the Institute for Ethics and History of Health in Society at the University of Augsburg, Germany. She has a research focus on public health ethics, health justice, and vulnerabilities. In her work she explores the relation between the individual, the population, and social and environmental structures. She discusses this relation in various areas, such as migrant health and climate/environmental health impact. She is the co-founder of the international public health ethics working group, which is associated to the German Academy for Ethics in Medicine and the German Public Health Association, and she is associate editor at the journal *Public Health Ethics*. She is or has been an advisory member of various institutional and governmental bodies, such as the German Medical Association and WHO.

Anna Gotlib is an associate professor of philosophy at Brooklyn College CUNY, New York, United States, specializing in feminist bioethics/medical ethics, moral psychology, and philosophy of law. She received her PhD in philosophy from Michigan State University and a JD from Cornell Law School. Anna is the current editor-in-chief of the *International Journal of Feminist Approaches to Bioethics*. Her work has appeared in the *Kennedy Institute of Ethics Journal, Journal of Bioethical Inquiry, Journal of Medical Humanities, Hypatia, Teaching Philosophy, Aeon/Psyche*, and other publications. She also edited two volumes on moral psychology—*The Moral Psychology of Sadness* (2017) and *The Moral Psychology of Regret* (2019). Her most recent edited collection is *Responses to a Pandemic: Philosophical and Political Reflections* (2022). Currently she is completing a co-edited collection on Barbie as a feminist phenomenon, as well as working on a monograph on identity, memory, and trauma. In 2020 and 2022, she was a Fulbright specialist scholar at the University of Iceland. She is also a member of a team of colleagues from Iceland (and elsewhere) which received the Ethics in Motion: Feminist Ethics and #MeToo (EMFEM) grant from the Icelandic Research Fund.

Ryoa Chung is a full professor in the Department of Philosophy and also teaches in the Faculty of Medicine at University of Montréal, Quebec, Canada. She was trained at University of Montréal, École Normale Supérieure de Fontenay St-Cloud in Paris, was visiting scholar at Columbia University and the Harvard School of Public Health, was visiting professor at Université de Lyon III and Paris Science Po. She is also co-director of the Center for Research in Ethics and president of the Canadian Association of Philosophy (2024–2025). Chung was awarded a Research Prize from the Fondation de la Croix Rouge Française in 2023. Her fields of research are international ethics and health inequalities. Her work has been funded by the Canadian Institutes of Health Research and the Social Sciences and Humanities Research Council of Canada.

Deborah Zion is an associate professor. She has been investigating the ethics of healthcare for asylum seekers for 20 years. She is a bioethicist and chairs the Human Research Ethics Committee at Victoria University, Australia. She has published widely on issues related to research with vulnerable populations and issues related to ethics and human rights for Aboriginal and Torres Strait Islander populations.

LIST OF CONTRIBUTORS

Thalia Arawi Co-Founder and CEO, T2P Center for Health Ethics Training and Consultancy, Beirut, Lebanon

Y. Y. Brandon Chen Associate professor, University of Ottawa's Faculty of Law, Common Law Section, Ontario, Canada

Ryoa Chung Professor of philosophy, Université de Montréal, co-director of the Center for Research in Ethics, Québec, Canada

James Dwyer Professor Emeritus, State University of New York Upstate Medical University, Syracuse, New York, USA

Lisa Eckenwiler Professor of philosophy, George Mason University, Fairfax, Virginia, USA

Catherine El Ashkar Department of Health Promotion and Community Health, Faculty of Health Sciences, American University of Beirut, Lebanon

Anas El Zouhbi Faculty of Medicine, American University of Beirut, Lebanon

Ryan Essex Research Fellow, The George Institute for Global Health, Sydney, Australia, and Conjoint Senior Lecturer, University of New South Wales, Sydney, Australia

Juenna Fiola Student in English and American Studies, Student assistant at Institute for Ethics and History of Health in Society, University of Augsburg, Germany

Mike Frick Co-director of the Treatment Action Group tuberculosis program, New York City, New York, USA

Shannon Fyfe Assistant professor of law, assistant professor of philosophy (by courtesy), Washington & Lee University, Lexington, Virginia, USA

Anna Gotlib Associate professor of philosophy, Brooklyn College, City University of New York, USA

Debbie C. Hocking Adjunct research fellow, Monash University, Department of Psychiatry; clinical psychologist and mental health researcher at Cabrini Outreach, Melbourne, Australia

Matthew Hunt Professor, School of Physical and Occupational Therapy, McGill University; researcher, Centre for Interdisciplinary Research on Rehabilitation, Montréal, Québec, Canada

Dilshad Jaff Clinical associate professor, Public Health Leadership and Practice Department, Gillings School of Global Public Health, University of North Carolina, USA

Fabian Linder Master of Arts in European Studies / Political Science, Institute for Ethics and History of Health in Society, University of Augsburg, Germany

Joanne Liu Pediatric emergency physician at University of Montréal and professor at the School of Population & Global Health, McGill University, Québec, Canada

Jihad Makhoul Professor, Department of Health Promotion and Community Health, American University of Beirut, Lebanon

Robyn Mellett Medical student, Cumming School of Medicine, University of Calgary, Alberta, Canada

Thierry Ngosso Lecturer, Department of Philosophy and Psychology, University of Maroua, Cameroon; Institute for Business Ethics, University of St. Gallen, Switzerland; Faculty of Philosophy, Catholic University of Central Africa, Yaoundé, Cameroon

Monika Noble Physician, Family Medicine Residency Program, Memorial University of Newfoundland and Labrador, Canada

Sandra Passardi Psychologist, Department of Consultation–Liaison Psychiatry and Psychosomatic Medicine, University of Zurich Hospital, Switzerland

Amy Reed-Sandoval Associate professor of philosophy and participating faculty, Latinx and Latin American Studies Program, University of Nevada, Las Vegas, USA

N. Sarita Shah Professor, Faculty of Epidemiology and Global Health, Rollins School of Public Health, Emory University, Atlanta, Georgia, USA

Mathieu Simard PhD candidate and course coordinator and lecturer, rehabilitation sciences, School of Physical and Occupational Therapy, McGill University, Montréal, Québec, Canada

Suresh Sundram Department of Psychiatry, School of Clinical Sciences, Monash University, and director of research, Mental Health Program, Monash Health, Melbourne, Australia

Peter West-Oram Senior lecturer in bioethics, University of Sussex, Brighton, and Sussex Medical School, UK

Verina Wild Professor of medical ethics and director, Institute for Ethics and History of Health in Society, University of Augsburg, Germany

Allison B. Wolf Associate professor of philosophy, Universidad de los Andes, Bogotá, Colombia

Deborah Zion Associate professor, chair of Human Research Ethics Committee, Victoria University, Australia

BIOS FOR POETS AND COVER ARTIST

Dr. Sylvia Agbih is a qualified nurse, holds a doctorate in philosophy, and worked on refugee migration and health for her dissertation at the interdisciplinary graduate school FlüGe at Bielefeld University, Germany. Since 2021, Sylvia has been a research associate at the Institute for Ethics and History of Health in Society at the University of Augsburg. Sylvia loves creative teaching and is trained in scenic role-play for nursing education.

Dr. Ayesha Ahmad is a reader in global health humanities at City St. George's University of London, UK. She holds a PhD in medical ethics as well as a postgraduate qualification in psychoanalysis, specializing in trauma. Her research expertise is in transcultural psychiatry and refugee mental health, with a particular focus on people affected by violence, humanitarian crises, and displacement. In her work, Ahmad critically explores the biomedical paradigm of trauma and prevailing methods for care. Ahmad also works as an expert witness providing academic reports on asylum-seeker cases related to war, mental health, and gender-based violence. She writes poetry to reflect on the stories she receives.

Anna Dziuban is a doctoral candidate in comparative literature at Ludwig Maximilian University of Munich, Germany, under the supervision of Prof. Dr. Juliane Prade-Weiss. Her dissertation project, preliminarily titled "Food for Thought or Water Under the Bridge: Representations of Porous Memory in Irish and Ukrainian Post-Famine Literature," explores the lingering impact of traumatic past and history of cultural subjugation on collective memory and familial narratives. Anna moved to Germany from Ukraine in 2016 to pursue a bachelor's degree in philosophy and holds an MA in comparative literature and an MA in philosophy from LMU Munich. Her research interests include memory politics, postcolonial studies, political philosophy, and the philosophy of emotions.

Aya Haidar graduated with a BA in Fine Art from the Slade School of Fine Art and holds an MSc in NGOs and Development from the London School of Economics and Political Science. Based in London, UK, she has had numerous international solo and group exhibitions and has been involved in a wide range of social engagement projects. Aya's work has been featured in *Hole & Corner*, *De Fil En Aiguille* by Charlotte Vannier, *Tribe* magazine, *Art of the Middle East, Modern and Contemporary Art from the Middle East and Iran* by Saeb Eigner, *Canvas, Harper's Bazaar Art Arabia, The National, Contemporary Practices*, and *Elle* magazine. The Victoria and Albert Museum (UK), Jameel Collection (Dubai), and the Guggenheim (Abu Dhabi) are among the major art institutions that have acquired her pieces.

Prof. Alison Phipps is UNESCO chair in Refugee Integration through Education, Languages and the Arts at the University of Glasgow, Scotland, and professor of languages and intercultural studies. She was De Carle Distinguished Visiting Professor at Otago University, Aotearoa 2019–2020. She was a Thinker in Residence at the EU Hawke Centre, University of South Australia in 2016, visiting professor at Auckland University of Technology, and principal investigator for AHRC Large Grant "Researching Multilingually at the Borders of Language, the Body, Law and the State". She was also a Principal Investigator for Cultures of Sustainable and Inclusive Peace; for Cultures of Sustainable and Inclusive Peace; and was co-director of the Global Challenge Research Fund South Migration Hub 2019–2024. She is an ambassador for the Scottish Refugee Council. She received an OBE in 2012 and honorary doctorates from the University of Edinburgh and the University of Waterloo, Canada, in 2023. She is an academic, activist, educator, and published poet and a member of the Iona Community.

INTRODUCTION
LISA A. ECKENWILER

We live in an age of extreme mobility. While migration has been a human constant and so is not "exceptional," the past decade has brought an unprecedented number of migrants fleeing uninhabitable conditions in the countries or regions where they have been living. These people, displaced by famine, drought, disease, armed conflict, persecution, or some layered combination, often endure these conditions only to find themselves in another set of hostile circumstances as they try to find their way toward safety, at least, and a life of thriving at best. A great deal has been written about migration, including forced migration, and there is a rich literature on migration and health. Absent, until now, though, has been a book that focuses directly on forced migration, health, ethics, and justice.

In truth, this book started with our students. As scholars from varied disciplines but grounded in moral philosophy and health ethics who do research and write on migration, heath, and ethics, and especially justice, we felt it was urgent to bring these issues to our teaching in bioethics, public health, and global ethics. Seeing both opportunity and relief (at last something we can use for classes!), we banded together to create this volume. It is our offering to students, both advanced undergraduates and graduates in health ethics, the humanities, social sciences, and health sciences (e.g., bioethics, public health ethics and global health ethics, moral and political philosophy, migration studies, migrant health, and health policy); to scholars seeking a high-level introduction to the intersection of health, migration, and justice; to non-academics with related interests; to other professionals engaged in work with migrants, in the public health sector, and in international law or health policy, such as people working in humanitarian assistance or government in the health services and health policy domain; and, we hope to all concerned with displacement and its myriad injustices. The book should, as well, serve as an inspiration for the field of bioethics, which has not for the most part taken migration to be a central concern. In our vision, all work around bioethics and health justice should start from an understanding of the world as a migrating and radically inequitable world, a conception of people (and indeed, histories) as interdependent, and a view of health—individual, public, and global—as profoundly relational.

Before going further, a note on terminology. In using the term "forced," we mean to include people who have had to leave their place of birth, or a place they considered their proper home, for reasons that are not a matter of choice, such as in (many) cases of immigration. In other words, we are focusing on those migrants who have had to flee, either by force or for reasons that made remaining in their original home impossible or existentially threatening, such as persecution or the fear of it, conflict, famine, or social and environmental conditions that render it nearly impossible to sustain life. One of the main themes in these essays, indeed, is that the complexities involved in decisions to migrate make sharp distinctions, for example, between forced and voluntary migrants, undocumented migrants and refugees, inadequate for capturing the range of people's experiences. Legal and other instruments that make use of rigid distinctions are morally suspect under current conditions. Readers will find that the authors here describe forced migrants in different ways, often resisting official categorizations.

With respect to our theoretical lens for the project, we draw on the conception of structural injustice articulated by Iris Marion Young, which argues that it "exists when social processes put large categories of persons under a systematic threat of domination or deprivation of the means to develop and exercise their capacities, at the same time as these processes enable others to dominate or have a wider range of opportunities for developing and exercising their capacities" (2011, 52). We see this as a potent analytical framework for understanding how health justice is threatened by social and institutional norms, stereotypes, health policies and practices, legal structures like immigration policies, and transnational economic processes (Chung 2021; Ahmad et al. 2022; Eckenwiler 2012, 2022). These social structures function as an apparatus that makes it hard, if not impossible, for forced migrants to be healthy, to live a life of flourishing. We recognize that there are alternative conceptions of "health justice" (Powers and Faden 2008; Venkatapuram 2011), but for our purposes what we mean is that people should be living amid social structures and environmental conditions that allow for humans to be healthy and do things they value over the course of a normal lifespan. Global health justice calls for everyone to experience this—and certainly the world's most vulnerable.

We believed it was crucial to organize the book in a way that helps to capture the movement of forced migrants from countries of origin, across diverse and often dangerous terrains, toward destination countries, with varying results, and to highlight the ways in which structural injustice is central to what threatens health and health justice for migrants. We have therefore taken a journey approach in our project, in appreciation of the fact that health injustice arises before people decide to migrate—and may well be implicated in their decision—and all along the way, including in destination countries should they reach them. The essays start with departure and follow the route of the forcibly displaced, analyzing the cultural norms; political, economic, and social policies; and institutional structures encountered along the way that thwart health justice for forced migrants. These structural barriers may be present in people's home countries; confronted in transit, even in ostensibly caring environs like humanitarian settings; and, for those who make it, in destination countries, both during and after the asylum process, even when it is successful.

We have divided the book into four parts: "Forced to Flee," "Detention and Encampment," "'Host' Countries," and "Responsibilities for Justice," where contributors offer arguments on the responsibilities of governments and government personnel, international humanitarian organizations and their staff, health professionals, civil society, and more concerning structural health injustice. Included, as well, is an appendix containing a table of compacts and conventions related to the health of migrants.

We wanted this collection to be more than a set of academic essays and, instead, something closer to a curation. Readers will find here a range of writing styles and tones. There is also poetry in these pages. We are honored to include a poem, "Map of the World," written by one of our editors, Anna Gotlib. Readers will also see poems from Alison Phipps ("Crossing the Volta" and "The Waiting Word") and from Anna Dziuban ("The Wait"). Interspersed are fragments authored by Sylvia Agbih: "Place?," "Hosts?," and "Refuge?"

It is our great privilege to adorn the cover and back with the art of London-based artist Aya Haidar. The front cover includes a work from her series, *Battlegrounds*; the back comes from her series, *Soleless*, which feature embroidered stories of people—especially women and children—in flight from their homelands on shoes worn by fellow forced migrants. Her woven wonders are more evocative than any statistic, or maybe even philosophical paper, could be. We are so grateful to include the work of these contributors who have helped to bring alternative text/textures, love, and living color to this project.

PART I: FORCED TO FLEE

Tracing the path of Oliver, a migrant with tuberculosis, co-editor Verina Wild, along with Dilshad Jaff, N. Sarita Shah, and Mike Frick chart the barriers and deterrents to care he confronts which threaten his health specifically, and health justice more generally. In the opening essay, "Tuberculosis, Human Rights, and Ethics Considerations Along the Route of a Highly Vulnerable Migrant from Sub-Saharan Africa to Europe," the authors aim to "show how all steps [of the journey] are connected and . . . [to] identify crucial points at which human rights principles and ethical values such as non-discrimination . . . and health justice are relevant for implementing public health policy and practice." They raise crucial questions about the relationship between public health ethics and global health justice and underscore the benefits of a human rights approach in addition to cosmopolitan theories of justice in analyzing obligations concerning the health of forced migrants. They also highlight the significance of stigma in health justice, a theme that recurs across several essays.

The next contribution comes from James Dwyer and considers the plight of climate refugees, people displaced due to changing environmental conditions. In "Environmental Migrants, Structural Injustice, and Moral Responsibility," an essay greatly inspired by Iris Marion Young's work, Dwyer highlights the "diversity and complexity" of environmental migration and argues that we should understand it as raising issues of structural injustice. It is hard to overstate the health and health justice implications of climate change, ranging from displacement-induced trauma to drought and heat-related illnesses among the world's most vulnerable populations, deepening global health inequities (Ahmad et al. 2023). Dwyer points out that the risks of becoming an environmental migrant are not equitably distributed. There is also an incongruity between *who* faces the greatest risk from climate change–related displacement, *who* contributes the most to changing environmental conditions via global structural processes, and *who* is best provisioned for protection from its consequences, including its many health effects. In assessing, again, what should be seen as structural injustices, Dwyer points to decision-making processes concerning environmental policy: whose knowledge and whose voices are present and part of agenda-setting, organizing decision-making processes and formulating plans for moving forward? He also underscores the significance of respect and equitable participation. Responding to the question of why we might have responsibilities for responding to environmental migration, the author outlines three different lines of argument: concern for humanity, liability, and a relational conception of responsibility that highlights our contributions to this global structural injustice. Dwyer closes with a helpful set of considerations for how to think about assigning responsibilities to a wide range of agents who contribute to environmental migration. A central point in his piece is that distinctions between forced and voluntary migrants, environmental and economic migrants, and migrants fleeing conflict and those displaced for environmental reasons obscure realities and lead to failures in meeting moral and political obligations. This is another theme that surfaces in several essays.

Thierry Ngosso's chapter, "Health Challenges and the 'Forced' Migration of the Cameroonian Middle Class," shines a light on the migration of families with children who suffer from mental health conditions that are ignored and untreated in a broader context of health institution failure. Examining the structural conditions that lead, indeed "coerce" many middle-class Cameroonians who have children with conditions like autism to move, he calls for abandoning distinctions between "forced" political and economic and other migrants who, it is assumed, choose to migrate. Ngosso, too, insists on rejecting and reimagining current categorizations for their grave inefficacy in responding to people's lived experiences and enabling justice for migrants facing conditions that leave them no meaningful choice but to depart and confront another set of risks. Ngosso maintains that structural global inequality is a crucial reason for the diminished state of the Cameroonian health (and educational) system, especially when it comes to support for children and others with serious mental health challenges.

Not only does this deepen health inequities within Cameroon (and many other countries), Ngosso argues; it also contributes to stigmatization, a grave threat to health justice highlighted by other authors here. With a feminist lens, Ngosso helps to reveal how the inadequacy of care services disproportionately harms the health of caregivers, who are almost always women and girls. In another poignant line of argument, he suggests that when people feel forced to migrate, it undermines solidarity with other families in Cameroon facing similar circumstances who cannot leave. This fraying of social relations, he laments, also thwarts social and structural change that could advance health justice for these children and their families; the departure of middle-class families contributes to "the neutralization of any catalyst for the convergence of social and political struggles, which could lead to substantial improvements in the health system and post-medical support for the mentally disabled."

Allison Wolf writes about the experience of pregnant women migrating from Venezuela to Colombia through the story of a young Afro-Venezuelan woman, Acacio. With a vivid portrayal of the many barriers to reproductive health services, such as lack of information, denial of care, financial barriers, and racism (despite formal access) that Acacio confronts, Wolf centers on the obstetric violence Acacio and women like her are routinely subjected to: verbal abuses, assaults, and what the author calls "metaphysical violence." In "'You Venezuelans Are Shameless!' Connecting Reproductive and Immigration (in)Justice," she argues that immigration injustice and reproductive injustice are intersecting forms of oppression and must be addressed as such to protect and promote health justice. Wolf outlines a helpful set of recommendations aimed at different responsible agents—governments separately and in collaboration, healthcare providers and staff, public health officials—for improving prospects for health justice. She is another contributor whose work, specifically her analysis of *why* pregnant Venezuelans migrate to Colombia, reveals the need to rethink purported divisions between forced and voluntary migrants. Wolf's chapter might fit well in Parts III or even IV, but we include it here for its moving portrayal of what can motivate people to flee.

PART II: DETENTION AND ENCAMPMENT

As states increasingly treat asylum as a privilege rather than an entitlement, rapidly rising numbers of people dwell in detention facilities or encampments of some sort—transit camps at borders, IDP (internally displaced person) camps, urban settlements, refugee camps run by international humanitarian organizations—typically isolated and suffering severe deprivation. While many people forced into displacement are in some sense on the move until—that is, if—they find a new home, part of the time in transit is likely spent living in conditions that allow for little if any mobility. A great number of forced migrants live hiding in fear, and others find themselves in what feel like, and often intentionally are, carceral confines (Oliver 2017). The chapters in Part II speak to this liminal space "inhabited" by so many forced migrants. This neither-here-nor-there part of the journey may be brief or, as is more common now, span decades (Fiddian-Qasmiyeh et al. 2014; UN Office for the Coordination of Humanitarian Affairs 2019). Whether short-lived or protracted, this threatens not only the agency and identity of forced migrants but also their political community, raising further concerns about structural health justice.

People in such settings suffer from a range of health conditions (Tufan et al. 2013; World Health Organization 2022). Many have faced food insecurity, violence, fear, torture, loss of loved ones, and other psychological, social, and economic circumstances that undermine health and deepen health inequities (Alpak et al. 2015; Wild et al. 2017; Acarturk 2018). PTSD, boredom, and agitation abound. If there is access to health services where people "reside," it is often restricted to acute medical care; there is rarely care for chronic illnesses. People living in these conditions are denied the opportunity to be and remain healthy, which, in turn, profoundly diminishes their opportunity for a flourishing life and prospects for health equity (Wild 2013; Eckenwiler and Wild 2021).

Australia, without question, has one of the world's most restrictive and, indeed, controversial set of policies concerning asylum seekers who arrive by boat. In "Immigration Detention and Health in Australia: A Structural Perspective," Ryan Essex calls for using a structural injustice lens to help explain that country's policy of mandatory detention for unauthorized maritime arrivals and the inhumane treatment to which they are systematically subjected. Australia is not alone in this—the US, to take another example, has its own policy of intercepting migrants at sea and placing them in carceral settings without access to services of nearly any kind, including health-related, and often for prolonged periods. Cuban migrants, for instance, are often picked up by and sent to Guantanamo Bay, Cuba, a US military installation. Essex explains why calls for at least meeting acute health needs are inadequate if responsibilities for health justice are to be realized. Instead, Essex argues, the abolition of detention as a response to asylum seeking and reforming the background conditions that generate and sustain these policies (assumptions regarding deterrence, or racism and xenophobia, for example) are required by justice.

Suresh Sundram, Debbie C. Hocking, and Sandra Passardi focus on detainees' mental health, once again centering on Australia. In "The Health Impacts of Immigration Detention: Examining Moral Injury," the authors examine the conditions of Australia's detention settings and argue that they create "a constellation of psychological harms"—a sense of betrayal and loss of trust in others, an altered sense of identity and more—that are analogous to moral injury. For the sake of health justice (and many other ethical ideals) these authors call on policymakers to prioritize reforming the country's immigration policies, including its provisions for caring for newly arriving asylum seekers who may already be enduring trauma when they find themselves in settings that exacerbate it. The essay by Sundram and colleagues introduces another key theme in this collection: migrants can confront as much peril in destination countries as in the ones they have left, or even more, compounding traumas and posing lethal threats to health and health justice.

From Lebanon, the country where currently the largest number of refugees reside per capita, including people from Syria, Iraq, Sudan, and the Occupied Palestinian Territory, Thalia Arawi and Anas El Zouhbi draw on the rich conceptual resources of Michel Foucault and Achille Mbembe to analyze the plight of people ensconced in humanitarian and other settings, rendered immobile by immigration policies that exclude them from membership in the citizenry and, simultaneously, threatened by the health systems of so-called host countries that see them as undeserving. Their chapter, "Toward a Pragmatic Solidarity with Refugees," invokes Foucault's notion of "biopolitics" and Mbembe's "necropolitics" as analytical lenses that help make sense of the ironies and often the horrors in the lived experiences of forcibly displaced people. The authors' depiction of how access to healthcare is denied, diminished, even harrowing for refugees makes it abundantly clear what is at stake.

Jihad Makhoul and Catherine El Ashkar, also from Lebanon, illuminate ethical concerns involved in the growing "corporatization" of humanitarian aid, that is, the provision of financing, expertise, food, and more in settings where displaced people dwell. Their essay, "The Double-Edged Sword of Corporate Assistance to Humanitarian Work: The Case of Lebanon," examines the ethical implications of this assistance from the for-profit sector and raises concerns about the potential compromises to key humanitarian principles, such as the principles of humanity and independence. Humanitarian organizations, they argue, are responsible for more carefully scrutinizing their relationships with corporations and standing firm on their ethical commitments.

PART III: "HOST" COUNTRIES

In this part, the collection turns to destination countries and their treatment of the forcibly displaced in the context of healthcare. Even when people are granted asylum and/or make their way to a new country, they confront structural barriers to healthcare or unethical treatment.

The first essay in this section comes from co-editor Anna Gotlib. In "Phenomenologies of 'Successful' Exile: Narratives of Displacement and Disorientation," Gotlib offers a "phenomenology of displacement." Citing research along with her own experience, Gotlib argues that the perils faced by refugees—to their identities and often also their lives—start before they leave and persist even once they arrive in (allegedly) "safer" environs. With a rich philosophical analysis one might categorize as a contribution to epistemic justice, she furthers an important line of investigation started with authors like Dina Nayeri (2017) and her autobiographical analysis of the "Ungrateful Refugee" and highlights the threat to well-being that comes from "how they are storied via master narratives"—prominent portrayals of refugees based on stereotypes of them as "good" or "bad" or broken or resilient, for example—in their new home. Another threat stems from refugees' "internal monologues" and concerns the disorientation (which begins before departure) endured when connections are cut and a sense of belonging somewhere is persistently and painfully absent. As Gotlib underscores, this suffering, or rather "existential despair," "is not only a moral concern for all those engaged in the work of refugee justice but also a matter of refugee well-being and psychological health. Invoking Maria Lugones's

(1987) "world traveler," her conclusion points toward a sort of process ontology and calls for a more fluid and hybrid conception of the self, indeed "of the various selves that constitute her," than many experience or imagine. Like Wild et al., Gotlib underscores the importance of taking account of all phases of forced migrants' experiences in the effort to advance health justice, and with Sundram et al., Wolf, and others, the need to not take for granted that all is well when people forced to relocate find their new "home."

Y. Y. Chen, in his essay, "Disqualify, Disincentivize, and Dissonate: Immigration Law as a Barrier to Migrants' Healthcare Access," analyzes the ways in which Canadian immigration law, specifically, creates barriers—via disqualification, deterrence, and stigmatization—to healthcare for migrants, including refugees. The law, indeed, is a prime example of a social structure that can generate and maintain injustice, including health injustice. Chen underscores the importance of healthcare access to migrants' integration in newfound communities and offers ideas on reforms that would help to advance health justice.

In their essay, co-editor Ryoa Chung and colleague Joanne Liu begin by pointing to the proclaimed universality of the human right to help and the reality that citizenship is, to a great extent, a prerequisite for access to healthcare around the world. While citizens may struggle, they are taken to be entitled in most countries; noncitizens, on the other hand, almost always have it worse when it comes to reliably securing needed health services. Their essay, "The Securitization of Migrants' Health and the Medicalization of Citizenship," takes issue with the fact that forced migrants all too often depend on humanitarian organizations to meet their basic healthcare needs. Contributing to this is the "medicalization of citizenship," which refers to the phenomenon whereby health considerations serve as a barrier to the admission of asylum seekers. Displaced people and asylum seekers, indeed, are often suspected to represent a public burden to the health systems of destination countries. In Canada and the US, for example, selection criteria for new migrants or refugees include questions concerning whether the person is likely to represent a "reasonable public charge to the health system." Chung and Liu reject such barriers as a violation of the human right to health and an unconscionable assault to health justice for forcibly displaced people. On their account, also inspired by Iris Marion Young's conception of global structural injustice, wealthier countries have an obligation to welcome displaced people to the best of their ability without discriminating against them based on their health status. This is a matter of justice for asylum seekers and other forced migrants, and also holds import for international humanitarian organizations that have been going far beyond their mandate whenever possible, providing health resources for these populations.

With a particular focus on refugees with disabilities, a group of people highly vulnerable to the "(un)reasonable public charge" designation, Monika Noble and co-authors Mathieu Simard, Lisa Eckenwiler, Ryoa Chung, Robyn Mellett, and Matthew Hunt offer an analysis akin to Wild et al.'s in mapping immigration processes for these new arrivals in Canada. In "Structural Health Vulnerabilities and Refugees with Disabilities in Canada," the authors identify obstacles to health justice within two critical domains: the legal domain and medical-social services. This essay explicitly deploys the notion of "structural health vulnerabilities" in its analysis: "an increased propensity to incur health risks directly related to social inequalities stemming from structural injustices that disproportionately affect an individual or social group" (Chung 2021, 201). Like Wild et al., the aim of their chapter is to identify opportunities for furthering health justice.

PART IV: RESPONSIBILITIES FOR HEALTH JUSTICE

With these vivid portrayals of the moral landscape, it becomes clear that responsibilities for justice are everywhere: with governments, government agencies, humanitarians and their organizations, health professionals, and ordinary people. What should they—what should we do to avoid worsening health injustice and, better yet, to advance health justice, for forced migrants?

In the first essay in this section, "Culpability, Liability, Responsibility, and Self-Interest: Analyzing the Reasons for Our Duties to Refugees and Migrants," Peter West-Oram sets out to present and examine three principal ways of answering the question of whether wealthy countries have obligations of global health justice to refugees and other migrants. For many people, after all, shared citizenship is an important parameter for responsibilities. At least, some say, we should prioritize our compatriots in conditions of scarcity, an unquestioned assumption in many debates that, according to some, warrants scrutiny (Schrecker 2008). Starting from the grounding assumption that the harms linked to forced migration and the needed remedies are structural, West-Oram outlines three prominent lines of thinking, along with their strengths and weaknesses, about responsibilities for the health needs of these migrants: an entitlement approach. That is, health is a human right, grounded in a wide array of ethical ideals and, furthermore, possibly realized for all people everywhere with existing global resources and with little burden to the privileged and overwhelming benefit to others; what some call a relational account of justice, that is, one grounded in connection and contribution to the conditions that lead to migration and that threaten health; and a self-interest account. West-Oram's goal is to offer an overview rather than defend a particular argument and to stimulate thought on how best to respond to the "structural nature of the injustices driving migration and the pursuit of refuge." Readers, especially those new to the debate, will benefit from West-Oram's clear presentation of major strands of argument in understanding contemporary debates and formulating or refining their own positions.

Shannon Fyfe's essay examines links between epistemic justice and health justice. Hers is another contribution centered on appalling conditions of migrant detention, specifically the horrifying—and mostly shielded from public view—health conditions in migrant detention facilities at the US-Mexico border in the late 2010s run by US Customs and Border Control, Immigration and Customs Enforcement, and the Department of Health and Human Services Administration for Children and Families. In these places people have been denied access to reproductive care, mental health services, preventive care for communicable diseases, and more, despite quite often being sick or injured from a journey and in many cases subjected to harmful conditions in custody. Fyfe's chapter, "Hidden Knowledge and Epistemic (in)Justice in US Migrant Detention," gives voice—at least obliquely—to migrants and people who work with them in detention settings and witness health injustice, highlighting the harms to health and also the injustice of their silencing and the necessity of accessing the knowledge they hold as migrants or "secondhand knowers" for health justice. We place her essay in this section because she suggests a possible path forward: reducing or even eliminating the incarceration of migrants and denouncing detention—especially in conditions of deprivation and threats to health—as a strategy and epistemic activism. That is, sharing their knowledge for the sake of justice. Fyfe concludes with a nuanced analysis of epistemic activism's complications, including "sourcing norms" and sorting out the risks and benefits of truth-telling under various conditions in the service of structural justice.

While Fyfe's analysis focuses on settings not intended for care, we should think here, too, about what can happen in places organized—at least ostensibly—around support for people forced from home, as Arawi and El Zouhbi as well as Makhoul and El Ashkar highlight. Their contributions call for more reflection on the responsibilities held by humanitarian actors and organizations. As Chung and Liu note, international humanitarian agencies have been conscripted into providing more services and filling more and more of the needs that once were met by nations. Theirs is an impossible and ever-expanding task. What *are* they responsible for? It seems easy to say at least "Do no harm," though this too seems hard to attain. At least three editors have spoken to this question either here in these pages or elsewhere. Chung and Liu call on the international community to find a way to fund health services for forcibly displaced people and, in a 2021 chapter, Eckenwiler and Wild call for humanitarian actors to be more intentional about accommodations for people ruptured from their roots and aim for what they call "ethical placemaking." Taking trauma more seriously in this effort is also in order (Eckenwiler 2024). There are many pressing questions around the nature and scope of humanitarians' obligations to support the health of afflicted populations, but perhaps the most urgent question is whether states will continue to make asylum elusive and treat displaced people and health justice as someone else's responsibility.

Amy Reed-Sandoval shines a light on the role of doctors in helping to facilitate migration for their patients, an issue that gets little attention or ethical analysis, in her essay, "Doctors as Immigration Agents: An Ethical Challenge." Reed-Sandoval points to the advice, the immigration paperwork, the logistical support, and more offered by doctors who assist—or refuse to assist—their patients crossing borders and argues that these doctors should be seen as immigration agents (to be distinguished from, for example, immigration officers). In this role, she argues, they are responsible for what she calls "structural competence" or understanding of the structural barriers that threaten their migrant patients' health in addition to being responsible for caring for them and advocating for their health. This echoes an earlier recommendation from Wolf and is significant for its call to physicians to look beyond the biomedical model and attend not just to social determinants of health but more specifically to structural injustice and its implications. Moreover, she maintains that doctors are responsible for working to uphold the principle of universal moral equality. Finally, Reed-Sandoval draws on the work of another author featured here, Ryan Essex, to argue that doctors have duties to engage in "healthcare resistance" and, in short, to stand up against policies and practices that are harmful or unjust.

Our last two essays, both from Australia, focus on actions available to, and perhaps obligatory for, health professionals in the context of detention. In his second chapter for the collection, "Resistance, Health, and Structural Injustice in the Context of Forced Displacement," Ryan Essex asks about the role of resistance and protest in challenging structural health injustice against migrants, again in the context of the Australian detention system. Essex is especially interested in what he calls disruptive resistance in health and healthcare. On his account, disruptive resistance, a practice that involves actions that challenge others to reevaluate what they believe, can serve as an effective response to "epistemic ignorance" around the treatment of detainees, its health implications, and structural injustice. Disruptive resistance also holds the potential to make "the structures that perpetuate injustice unsustainable." Like Fyfe, Essex sees epistemic justice as playing a vital role in advancing health justice.

The final chapter, "Dual Loyalties and Healthcare: The Weaponization of Suffering and the Ethics of Resistance," from co-editor Deborah Zion, examines four main forms of response taken by healthcare providers who provide care to asylum seekers in detention: complicity, subversion, withdrawal, and advocacy. While some of these may be indefensible, even the most justifiable leaves a "moral remainder." Zion concludes by arguing that the act of witnessing, or *temoinage*, is an ethical option.

As stated at the outset, the editors of this volume are committed to a relational conception of justice, most notably the one offered by Iris Marion Young in her paper "A Social Connection Model of Responsibility" (2006). If I may, in the closing paragraphs of this introduction, I want to take a bit of editorial license and point toward another line of thought, namely, imagining responsibilities for justice from an ontological perspective and, specifically, a relational ontology (a genre of which is embedded in Young's account, if inexplicitly). In other words, how might thinking about who/what we are—in ways that push beyond the ahistorical, myopic, and power-concealing confines of liberal individualist and nationalist accounts—help to inform our understanding of our responsibilities? For example, what might be the implications for our sense of responsibility for forced migrants if we embraced what Lorraine Code (2006) calls an "ecological" account and saw ourselves as interdependent with others, as "being made by and making relations in reciprocity with other subjects and diverse locations"? Or from a perspective like that of Martinique philosopher Edouard Glissant, who argues in *Poetics of Relation* (2005, 144) that "identity is a system of relation . . . produced in the chaotic network of Relation and not in the hidden violence of filiation; [this relational identity] does not devise any legitimacy as its guarantee of entitlement, but circulates, newly extended." What might we make of the work of Achille Mbembe (2019, 28) and if we conceived of ourselves as "a compound of other living beings and other species [who] belongs to all places together"? On his view, "we are all made up of diverse borrowings from foreign subjects and . . . have always been beings of the border" (30). And later, in his conclusion, "The Ethics of the Passerby," he writes, "Becoming human in the world is a question neither of birth nor of origin or race. It is a matter of journeying, of movement, of transfiguration" (187), of questioning how one is constituted and in relation to whom and how.

These authors and the others assembled in this collection compel us to consider how we are related to forced (indeed all) migrants and to the structural injustices that erode their health, and, in turn, ask what responsibilities we have. They also call on us, with much urgency, to "resist conceiv[ing] of the world as not simple and straightforward, with only one truth, mine" (Glissant, 2005, 154–155). More relational conceptions of who we are can surely propel us toward wanting to understand the knowledge and experiences of others for the sake of acting ethically and perhaps, too, toward accepting responsibility for health (and other) injustices. We may even come away with enriched understandings of ourselves.

REFERENCES

Acarturk, Ceren, Mustafa Cetinkaya, Ibrahim Senay, et al. 2018. "Prevalence and Predictors of Posttraumatic Stress and Depression Symptoms Among Syrian Refugees in a Refugee Camp." *Journal of Nervous and Mental Disease* 206 (1): 40–45.

Ahmad, Ayehsa, Outi Autii, Babitha George, et al. 2023. "Widening Understanding of Solastalgia Through Land-Based Violence: Why We Need to Create New Notions of Harm and Suffering Toward the Land to Understand Mental Distress Within and Beyond Land-Dependent and Indigenous Communities." *International and Comparative Journal of Human Rights* 6 (1): 141–161.

Ahmad, Ayesha, Ryoa Chung, Lisa Eckenwiler, et al. 2022. "What Does It Mean to Be Made Vulnerable in the Era of COVID 19?" *The Lancet* 395: 1481–1482.

Alpak, Gokay, A. Tamar Unal, Feridun Bulbul, et al. 2015. "Post-Traumatic Stress Disorder Among Syrian Refugees in Turkey: A Cross-Sectional Study." *International Journal of Psychiatry in Clinical Practice* 19 (1): 45–50.

Chung, Ryoa. 2021. "Structural Health Vulnerability: Health Inequalities, Structural and Epistemic Injustice." *Journal of Social Philosophy* 52 (2): 201–216.

Code, Lorraine. 2006. *Ecological Thinking: The Politics of Epistemic Location*. Oxford University Press.

Eckenwiler, Lisa. 2012. *Long-Term Care, Globalization, and Justice*. Johns Hopkins University Press.

Eckenwiler, Lisa. 2022. "An Eco-Structural Lens for Health Ethics." *Hastings Center Report*, December 2022, 3.

Eckenwiler, Lisa. 2024. "Ethical Place-Making, Trauma, and Health Justice in Humanitarian Settings." In *Trauma-Informed Placemaking*, edited by Cara Courage and Anita McKeown. Routledge.

Eckenwiler, Lisa, and Verina Wild. 2021. "Justice for Refugees Living Under Long-Term Displacement and Segregation: From Livelihoods to Place-Making." *Journal of Social Philosophy* 52 (2): 234–250.

Fiddian-Qasmiyeh, Elena, Gil Loescher, Katy Long, et al. 2014. *The Oxford Handbook of Refugee and Forced Migration Studies*. Oxford University Press.

Glissant, Edouard. 2005. *Poetics of Relation*. University of Michigan Press.

Lugones, María. 1987. "Playfulness, 'World'-Travelling, and Loving Perception." *Hypatia* 2 (2): 3–19.

Mbembe, Achille. 2019. *Necropolitics*. Duke University Press.

Nayeri, Dina. 2017. "The Ungrateful Refugee: We Have No Debt to Repay." *The Guardian*, April 4. https://www.theguardian.com/world/2017/apr/04/dina-nayeri-ungrateful-refugee.

Oliver, Kelly. 2017. *Carceral Humanitarianism: Logics of Refugee Detention*. University of Minnesota Press.

Parekh, Serena. 2016. *Refugees and the Ethics of Forced Displacement*. Routledge.
Powers, Madison, and Ruth Faden. 2008. *Social Justice: The Moral Foundations of Public Health and Health Policy*. Oxford University Press.
Schrecker, Ted. 2008. "Denaturalizing Scarcity: A Strategy of Enquiry for Public Health Ethics." *Bulletin of the World Health Organization* 86 (8): 600–605.
Tufan, Ali E., M. G. Alkin, and Sukriye Bosgelmez. 2013. "Post-Traumatic Stress Disorder Among Asylum-Seekers and Refugees in Istanbul May Be Predicted by Torture and Loss Due to Violence." *Nordic Journal of Psychiatry* 67 (3): 219–224.
UN Office for the Coordination of Humanitarian Affairs. 2019. *Global Humanitarian Review 2019*. https://www.unocha.org/sites/unocha/files/GHO2019.pdf.
Venkatapuram, Sridhar. 2011. *Health Justice: An Argument from the Capabilities Approach*. Cambridge University Press.
Wild, Verina. 2013. "Asylum-Seekers and Public Health Ethics." In *Ethics in Public Health and Health Policy: Concepts, Methods, Case Studies*, edited by Daniel Strech, Irene Hirschberg, and Georg Marckmann. Springer International.
Wild, Verina, Dilshad Jaff, Sarita Shah, and Mike Frick. 2017. "Tuberculosis, Human Rights and Ethics Considerations Along the Route of a Highly Vulnerable Migrant from Sub-Saharan Africa to Europe." *International Journal of Tuberculosis and Lung Disease* 21 (10): 1075–1085.
World Health Organization (WHO). 2022. "Refugee and Migrant Health, Fact Sheet." https://www.who.int/news-room/fact-sheets/detail/refugee-and-migrant-health.
Young, Iris Marion. 2006. "Responsibility and Global Justice: A Social Connection Model." *Social Philosophy and Policy* 23 (1): 102–130.
Young, Iris Marion. 2011. *Responsibility for Justice*. Oxford University Press.

A MAP OF THE WORLD

ANNA GOTLIB

I want to show you the map of the world
There, on the wall beside our window
It hangs, clearly outlined in red and blue and green
My precise arrows tell you precisely where to go
Where the land ends and mystery begins
Dark specters wander darker seas
And myths are weaved into star-blessed sand
Only to be washed away by morning and by time
An offering of life
No less than this.

I want to draw you the map of the world
To guide your unsteady hand
As it carves canyons
Moves from plain to town
And back again
I want to give you blue for water, bluer for the sky
And red for mountains of the desert
But save the black for those winter nights
When stillness moves the sacred and profane
In their eternal dance.

I want to give you the map of the world
To offer it to you whole and pure
To put it in your hands, fait accompli
Sheathed in the certainty of my steady hand.

But I refrain
Instead, I lay the paintbrush at your door

And leave a stack of parchment
Blank, untouched by me or any other
And slowly back away so as not to wake you
So when you tire of sleep
You will pick up the brushes and the parchment
And go where mapmakers go
Drawing that first unsteady line
Not meant for me
At last.

PART ONE

Forced to Flee

1

Tuberculosis, Human Rights, and Ethics Considerations Along the Route of a Highly Vulnerable Migrant from Sub-Saharan Africa to Europe

VERINA WILD, DILSHAD JAFF, N. SARITA SHAH, AND MIKE FRICK

1.1 INTRODUCTION

With more than 280 million people living outside their country of origin (United Nations 2020) migrant health is becoming a critical public health ethics issue (Wild and Dawson 2018).[1] A major barrier to migrants' access to healthcare is their legal status (Scholz 2016). Although a substantial number of migrants arriving from less to more industrialized countries migrate through official channels that involve pre-immigration health screening and/or post-arrival health services, many cross borders without documentation. For example, in 2023 a total of 155,754 undocumented migrants arrived in Italy (Info Migrants 2024).

As we will see in this chapter, this group of migrants is highly vulnerable in relation to their health and well-being (Dauvrin et al. 2012). Tuberculosis (TB) in migrants is a challenging issue due to the complexities in detection, diagnosis, and prolonged treatment during transit. Other challenges

1. This chapter has previously been published in the *International Journal of Tuberculosis and Lung Diseases*: Wild, Verina, Dilshad Jaff, N. Sarita Shah, and Mike Frick. 2017. "Tuberculosis, Human Rights and Ethics Considerations Along the Route of a Highly Vulnerable Migrant from Sub-Saharan Africa to Europe," *International Journal of Tuberculosis and Lung Diseases* 2: 1075–1085. It is reprinted here in a slightly updated version with friendly permission from International Union Against Tuberculosis and Lung Disease (The Union).

Verina Wild et al., *Tuberculosis, Human Rights, and Ethics Considerations Along the Route of a Highly Vulnerable Migrant from Sub-Saharan Africa to Europe*. In: *Forced Migration and Health Justice*. Edited by: Lisa A. Eckenwiler, Verina Wild, Anna Gotlib, Ryoa Chung, and Deborah Zion, Oxford University Press. © Oxford University Press (2026). DOI: 10.1093/oso/9780197795491.003.0001

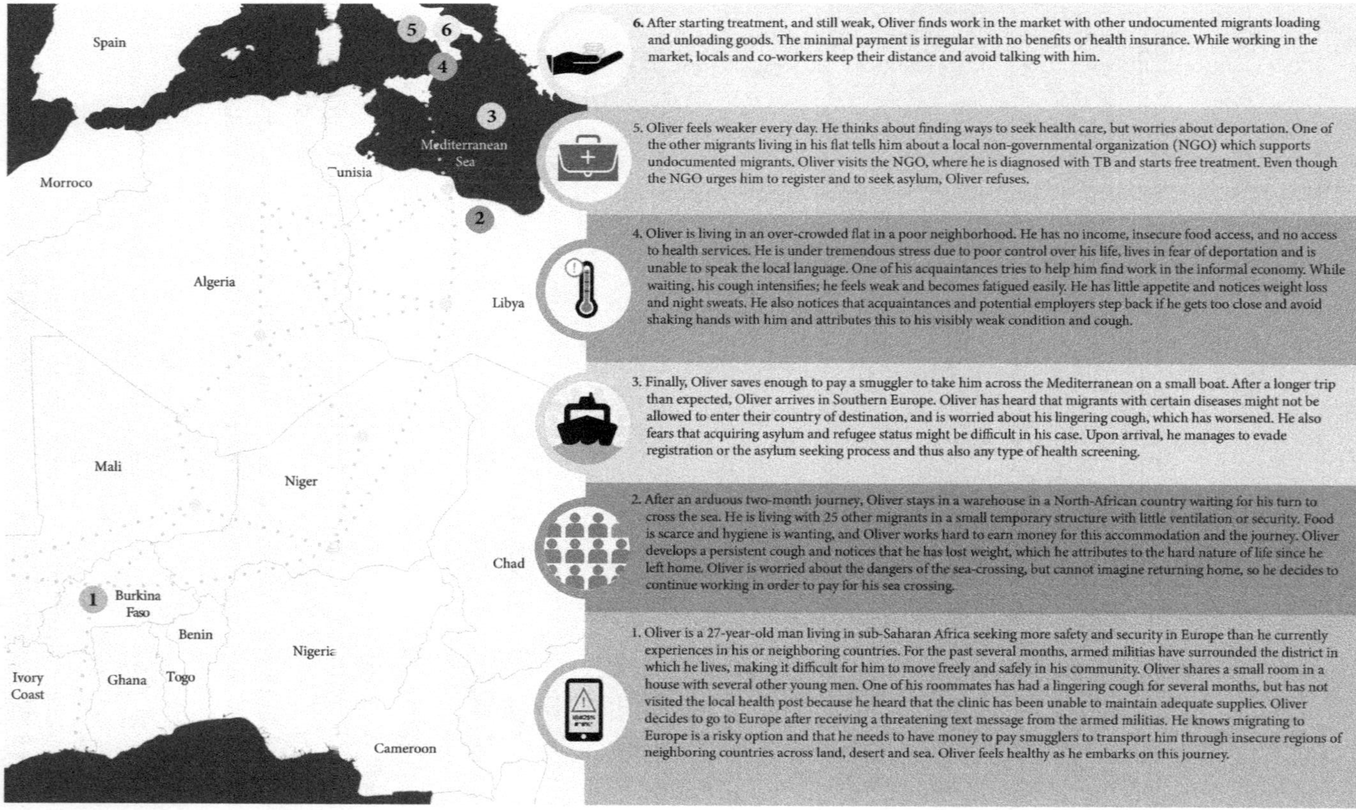

Figure 1.1: Oliver's hypothetical journey to Europe: tracing a common route of migration from sub-Saharan Africa to Europe. The map depicts a possible migrant route from sub-Saharan Africa to Europe and is loosely based on the migrant journeys reported in Patrick Kingsley's book, *The New Odyssey* (2016).

are related to a broad range of implications in terms of social and political determinants of health, and processes of stigmatization and discrimination occur frequently. Overall TB rates among native-born and foreign-born persons in low-incidence countries have declined since 2009 (Ködmön et al. 2016; Lönnroth et al. 2017). Most TB in migrants stems from post-arrival reactivation of remotely acquired latent tuberculous infection, although a portion may have TB due to primary progression of a recent tuberculous infection (Sandgren et al. 2014). Nevertheless, transmission within immigrant communities and workplaces post-arrival has been proven/detected (Sandgren et al. 2014; Lönnroth et al. 2017).

In the present chapter, we trace a commonly used route of a migrant from sub-Saharan Africa to Europe (see Figure 1.1 and Table 1.1) (Kingsley 2016). We have called the fictitious protagonist of our story Oliver, and the details of his story are loosely based on the migrant journeys reported in Patrick Kingsley's book, *The New Odyssey* (2016).

During each phase of the route, we identify situations in which human rights and ethical principles and values might be affected in relation to the provision of TB services. By illustrating the route, we aim to show how all steps are connected. We identify crucial points at which human rights principles and ethical values such as non discrimination, protection of health, well-being, and health justice are relevant for implementing public health policy and practice.

Throughout the chapter, we use the term "migrant" to refer to "any person who is moving or has moved across an international border or within a country away from their habitual place of residence, regardless of their legal status, whether their decision to move was voluntary or involuntary, the cause for the movement, and the length of stay" (International Organization for Migration [IOM] 2017). The United Nations Development Programme (2009) has noted that "the proliferation of migration categories obscures rather than illuminates the processes underlying the decision to move, with potentially harmful effects on policy-making."

We agree that a strict line between undocumented migrant and refugee can often not be drawn, as we will see in our case example. By adopting this approach to terminology, we aim to show how ethics and human rights can strengthen public health efforts to address TB among persons in migration, regardless of their reasons for movement or legal status.

At the same time, inclusive usage of the word "migrant" does not mean that we should lose sight of the legal protections established for specific groups, such as refugees and asylum seekers, and it does not preclude the possibility of applying human rights and ethics in the case of more specific categories, such as undocumented migrants or seasonal workers. Undocumented immigration takes on various forms, including, for example, undocumented entry, fraudulent documentation, or visa violation (Turner 2016). The case presented in this chapter and subsequent analyses focus on the first form of undocumented immigration.

We chose to develop Oliver's story in this way for several reasons:

1. Undocumented migrants are among the most vulnerable migrants. Those who care for these migrants in policy and practice have a special responsibility to identify and focus on vulnerabilities and discuss the issues at stake. Ethics and human rights approaches offer tools to discuss possible vulnerabilities in relation to health and to address health services for this subgroup. Oliver's case provides the opportunity to discuss these tools.
2. The route we chose is underrepresented in the literature on ethics and human rights of migrant health. While healthcare for undocumented migrants has been discussed, the larger focus taken here, on the entire migration route from sub-Saharan Africa to Europe, with its own particularities, has so far been neglected. Nevertheless, a substantial number of migrants are currently moving along this route, and understanding their health needs, especially in terms of TB, is of general urgency.
3. With our case selection, we aim to show that we are not dealing only with a nationally confined subpopulation with certain health issues that require a domestic response. A significant portion of the migration experience occurs before arrival in a host country, when a migrant is in preparation to depart and in transition (Dhavan et al. 2017). Ethics and human rights reflections should take these phases into account, in addition to considering the experience of being a newcomer to the country of destination. A geographically confined view tends to underestimate the biographical issues that come beforehand and which motivate a person to migrate, as well as those events that the migrant encounters during the journey. Issues encountered during all stages of the migration experience can affect the health and well-being of a person, and an examination thereof can show where the burdens and challenges lie.

1.2 HUMAN RIGHTS PERSPECTIVES ON THE CASE

A human rights–based approach to TB and migration opens several avenues for analysis and action. First, a rights-based analysis starts by examining the concordance between specific laws, policies, and practices related to TB, migration, and international and regional human rights law. Second,

Table 1.1. SUMMARY OF A COMMON CASE OF A MIGRANT TRAVELING FROM SUB-SAHARAN AFRICA TO EUROPE

Step	Migration Phase	General Situation	TB Status	Ethical and Human Rights Principles
1	In the country of origin/before departure.	Oliver (O.) lives in poverty in a high-TB burden country in sub-Saharan Africa. He and his family feel threatened by terror militia because of their faith. O. feels healthy and strong.	Latent TB infection.	Rights to life, food, education, and health not protected; no access to education for prevention of communicable diseases and other public health issues.*
2	During transit	O. lives in a cramped, overcrowded warehouse waiting for smugglers to take him to Europe. He experiences food scarcity and harsh working and living conditions. O. has a persistent cough and begins to lose weight.	Conversion to active TB; no diagnosis. Primary TB transmission possible.	No access to primary healthcare; weak or nonexistent health infrastructure; no access to education for diagnosis or treatment of TB disease; no access to safety and security; dire living conditions and food insecurity with detrimental mental and physical health effects.
3	At the border.	O. has heard that migrants with diseases will not be allowed to enter Europe. O. arrives on European soil and immediately goes underground to avoid registration, fearing expulsion for health reasons.	Active TB; no diagnosis. Primary TB transmission possible.	Failed efforts by region of destination to convey the message that (1) everyone has the right to seek asylum, and therefore the right to seek asylum is independent from health status, and that (2) everyone has a right to health, independent from residence status.

Continued

Table 1.1. CONTINUED

Step	Migration Phase	General Situation	TB Status	Ethical and Human Rights Principles
4	After arrival.	O. stays with acquaintances in an overcrowded flat while waiting for a work opportunity. O.'s cough persists, he starts to feel weaker, loses more weight, and starts looking ill. He notices that his potential employers are taking a step back when he approaches them.	Active TB; no diagnosis. Primary TB transmission possible.	Opportunity for country to reach out to newly arrived migrants and inform them about healthcare options. Because O. looks ill and coughs in addition to being an immigrant of lower social status, processes of stigmatization are exacerbated.
5	First half-year.	O. feels weaker and looks for healthcare. He hears of a local NGO that helps undocumented migrants. O. receives TB treatment but refuses to register officially at the immigration office.	TB diagnosis; TB treatment begins.	Healthcare system does not ensure universal right to health for everyone in the territory.
6	Long-term perspective.	O. works as an undocumented migrant. He feels better on treatment and is told that the risk of spreading TB to others is effectively gone, but he continues to feel reluctance from his co-workers and acquaintances to enter into contact with him, shake hands, share a meal, etc. Treatment continues through NGO.	TB is treated.	Process of stigmatization, stereotyping, exclusion based on limited understanding of TB transmission risk; failure to ensure transition from parallel NGO health program to routine primary healthcare.

* Not limited to potential migrants; the general population in the country also faces these issues. However, these conditions have a special impact on potential migrants, as they (1) can function as additional mobilizing factors and (2) contribute to systematic disadvantages for the migrants even during and after transit.

Source: migrant route adapted from Kingsley (2016).

a rights-based approach seeks to integrate human rights principles such as non-discrimination, participation, accountability, and transparency into migrant health programs. Third, such an approach draws on key elements of the right to health and interrelated rights to define standards for evaluating the success of these programs—standards that can be used in advocacy and litigation to hold governments accountable for meeting their obligations under international law. These obligations include the duties to respect, protect, and fulfill human rights. Briefly, the obligation to "respect" charges governments with not taking any actions that would interfere with or curtail human rights, including discriminatory policies (Forman 2015). "Protect" requires governments to prevent third parties from violating rights, while the duty to "fulfill" refers to creating an enabling environment in which individuals can fully exercise their rights.

1.2.1 Examining Laws and Policies

The human rights standards for the health and protection of migrants are not located in a single treaty, but instead find expression throughout numerous international and regional human rights instruments (Table 1.2) (International Organization for Migration [IOM] 2013). Central to understanding the individual in our fictive case study, Oliver (see Figure 1.1), is the right to health (e.g., Article 12 of the International Covenant on Economic, Social, and Cultural Rights [ICESCR]) (United Nations [UN] 1966). ICESCR Article 12 establishes the right of everyone to enjoy the highest attainable standard of physical and mental health and tasks states parties (i.e., governments that have ratified or acceded to the convention) with upholding the right by taking steps to prevent, treat, and control epidemic diseases and by "creating conditions which would ensure to all medical service and medical attention in the event of sickness." Importantly, in General Comment 14, the Committee on Economic, Social, Cultural Rights (CESCR) states that the right to health extends to the underlying determinants of health, including food, housing, and other socioeconomic factors; access to health-related information; and safe and healthy working conditions (UN 2000).

Throughout his journey, Oliver passed through territories in which governments were unable to fully protect and fulfill his right to health, as well as those in which governments failed to respect the health rights of migrants. In his home country, the rights to life, food, education, and health were not protected and there was no access to education for prevention of communicable diseases for the population at large (Haar and Rubenstein 2012). Oliver experienced severe deprivation while staying in

Table 1.2. INTERNATIONAL HUMAN RIGHTS INSTRUMENTS RELEVANT TO MIGRATION AND HEALTH

Universal Declaration of Human Rights
International Covenant on Economic, Social, and Cultural Rights
International Covenant on Civil and Political Rights
International Convention on the Protection of the Rights of All Migrant Workers and Members of their Families
Convention Against Torture
International Convention on the Elimination of All Forms of Racial Discrimination
Convention on the Elimination of All Forms of Discrimination Against Women
Convention on the Rights of the Child
Convention on the Rights of Persons with Disabilities

Note: These treaties enshrine the rights relevant to health and migration. In some cases, the treaty itself may not expressly focus on migrants, but the relevant human rights treaty bodies responsible for monitoring implementation of the rights therein have addressed the issue of migration in general comments clarifying the normative meaning and legal content of the treaty.
Source: adapted from International Organization for Migration (2013).

the warehouse in northern Africa, where his worsening condition went unaddressed. The lack of access to the underlying determinants of health, such as food, shelter, and safe working conditions, for migrants constituted a failure to both respect and protect the right to health (Haar and Rubenstein 2012). Once he reached southern Europe, Oliver feared that he would encounter a screening program oriented more toward securing the health of European nationals against "imported" diseases than toward promoting the health of undocumented migrant newcomers. Even if the country provided for screening, diagnosis, and treatment irrespective of residence status—as many European countries do for asylum seekers and sometimes also for undocumented migrants—Oliver mistrusted and feared the authorities based on, for example, information from fellow migrants. He had heard that persons found to have a communicable disease might face administrative penalties mimicking criminal penalties (e.g., deportation or detention) (UN 2010; Rubio-Marín 2014). Aware of his poor health, unsure about his chances of acquiring protection as a refugee, and worried about potential state-imposed penalties, Oliver chose to go underground, where he struggled to access medical care. This action was based partly on misinformation about his actual rights and opportunities—many places in Europe (municipalities and/or countries) provide TB services irrespective of residence status—and partly fueled by a general feeling of not being welcome (perhaps based on the observation that many countries seem to place the protection of the nation's citizens over the right to health for immigrants).

This resulted in his ultimately becoming an undocumented migrant with very little security and protection, although his chances of obtaining asylum and proper protection might even have been quite high. The phenomenon of immigrants delaying or avoiding treatment or preventive healthcare due to fear of penalties has already been described and discussed in the literature (Asch et al. 1998; Hampshire 2005; Toomey et al. 2014).

1.2.2 Integrating Human Rights Principles

In General Comment 14, the CESCR singles out the principle of non-discrimination as being central to the right to health, and notes that particular attention must be paid to ensuring that health facilities, goods, and services are made accessible to all "in law and in fact" (UN 2000). In several places, General Comment 14 refers specifically to migration, stating that governments must "refrain from denying or limiting equal access for all persons, including prisoners or detainees, minorities, asylum seekers, and illegal immigrants, to preventive, curative, and palliative health services." While ICESCR Article 2 provides for progressive realization—an acknowledgment that states are at various stages of development and may have resource constraints that preclude them from immediately providing for the full realization of rights—in General Comment 14, the CESCR notes that states parties have immediate obligations in relation to the right to health, including "a guarantee that the right will be exercised without discrimination of any kind." Moreover, progressive realization does not obviate the obligation of states to take concrete action toward realizing rights or to justify retrogressive measures. Retrogression could occur, for example, if states revise migration policies in ways that limit access to healthcare for migrants where it once existed or impose stricter penalties that amplify vulnerability or lead to worse health outcomes by dissuading migrants from seeking care.

In addition to non-discrimination, the participation of individuals in decision-making about programs and policies that affect their lives is a core tenet of the right to health; ideally, decisions should be made with the involvement of those who will bear their consequences (World Health Organization 1978; de Freitas 2017). Upholding the principle of participation may be particularly challenging when working with undocumented migrants due to the lack of trust and access, language barriers, and the lack of knowledge about their destination's healthcare system.

The process of incorporating human rights principles into policy and practice encourages health programs to consider the ways in which interventions are implemented, in addition to measuring their outcomes (Gruskin et al. 2007). Programs that adopt rights-based approaches will center on the welfare of persons in migration as an end in itself rather than treating migrant health only as a means of securing some other goal (e.g., public safety). In Oliver's case, it was not until his friend connected him to the migrant services nongovernmental organization (NGO) that Oliver had the impression of encountering a health service that was designed to meet the needs of migrants.

1.2.3 Defining Standards

Finally, a rights-based approach will draw on key elements of the right to health to define standards for judging the provision of TB services in the context of migration. The 3AQ (availability, accessibility, acceptability, and quality) framework outlined in General Comment 14 provides a starting point, specifying that the right to health must contain the following elements in all its forms and at all levels: the 3AQ of health goods and services (UN 2000). Each of these considerations forms a focal point around which to organize for change. The absence or partial fulfillment of these elements characterized Oliver's interaction with health services before his connection to the NGO.

1.2.4 Human Rights and International Humanitarian Law

In upholding obligations under the right to health in the context of TB and migration, governments need not act alone. The CESCR's interpretation of the right to health emphasizes cooperation among states in addressing cross-border health issues, and stresses that "the economically developed States Parties have a special responsibility . . . to assist" (UN 2000). This responsibility is closely related to the perspectives of global justice and global health ethics, discussed below. In addition, the duty of international assistance demonstrates that the drivers of TB and migration may be beyond the ability of any single state to address at its borders. Often these conditions stem from situations of conflict covered by international humanitarian law (IHL), which is designed to limit the violence of conflicts and protect the victims of those conflicts (International Committee of the Red Cross 2004). Oliver is a case in point, as he is affected by armed conflicts—directly, by the threatening messages received in his home country, and indirectly, by the lack of security and healthcare during his journey through countries in conflict. In all such situations, IHL is applicable. IHL is a set of rules designed to limit the violence of conflicts and protect the victims of those conflicts (International Committee of the Red Cross 2004). As a victim of armed conflict, Oliver is protected by rules stipulated in the Geneva Conventions and their Additional Protocols. For example, Article 3 and Article

14 of Protocol II provide for the protection of objects indispensable to survival, and Article 17 of Protocol II provides for the protection of civilian populations against forced displacement. The 1951 Convention concerns the rights of displaced persons within the host country with respect to legal status, employment, and housing (United Nations High Commission for Refugees 2011). The applicability of relevant human rights treaties, alongside IHL and the perspective of IHL in the case of migration and TB, is understudied and needs further investigation.

1.3 THREE HIGHLIGHTS FROM THE ETHICS AND JUSTICE LITERATURE

Traditionally, health ethics has mainly focused either on the domestic health of citizens, to seek better healthcare, or on obligations from high-income countries towards low- and middle-income countries. A specific ethics of migrant health and well-being that could be applied to Oliver's case is only in its early stages. The existing literature on migrant health ethics has so far focused mainly on the question of access to healthcare in receiving countries (Wild et al. 2015), but ethically relevant issues arise throughout the entire migration route. In line with the human rights perspective, and in an attempt to develop a more specific and comprehensive ethics of migrant health and well-being, we highlight three strands of discussions in the ethics and justice literature that can be derived from Oliver's case and that add weight to arguments for improving health along migration routes typified by Oliver's case.

1.3.1 Acknowledging a Global Justice and Global Health Ethics Perspective (Relevant for All Steps)

The link between global justice theories, global health ethics, and resulting obligations is not yet fully developed, but there is increasing interest among scholars of public health ethics and justice (Pinto and Upshur 2013; Benatar and Brock 2021). Traditionally, social justice theories have focused on the just distribution of goods and resources in the national context. In contrast, theories of global justice, particularly moral cosmopolitanism, emphasize the equal moral worth of every human being, independent of their place of birth (Heilinger 2020). These theories identify and trace the existing globalized social connections and resulting obligations between those countries that profit (e.g., from trade structures) and those that are less privileged, even if they are geographically far apart (Brock 2009; Pogge 2010; Young 2013).

This approach provides direct insights for global health ethics. It can show that a narrow focus on national healthcare is insufficient, given that global trade, communication, and travel have effectively created a global community. According to this approach, health and well-being should be understood as a global value to be ensured for everyone by a global effort. Nevertheless, even if one does not fully agree with such a cosmopolitan approach, there is a less controversial, minimalist demand: that a country's policies and practices must not harm other countries' population health (Daniels 2008; Hunter and Dawson 2011). This means that in all policies, even in migration policy, potentially harmful effects on the health outcomes for all those affected—not only domestically but also globally—should be taken into account (see also the firewall argument below). Beyond this limited demand to avoid harm, theories of global justice and global relational equality increasingly emphasize positive obligations to take action to improve the health of populations in or from low- and middle-income countries if a country is in a position to do so, and even more so if such a capable country benefits from an existing power imbalance (Farmer 2004; Hunter and Dawson 2011; Pinto and Upshur 2013). The approach to global health ethics includes the understanding that a single country should not focus only on those who are in its territory, but that the international community has a short- and long-term responsibility to secure health for all, in every country—in other words, to consider health to be a global project (Pinto and Upshur 2013; Benatar and Brock 2021). The response to COVID-19 shows the importance of such global obligations and that strengthening acute emergency responses to public health crises, as well as long-term strengthening of health systems, infrastructure, and social determinants of health in low-and middle-income countries, should be urgent priorities.

Regarding Oliver's case, we can see the short- and long-term importance for the international community to strengthen the health systems, infrastructure, and social determinants of health in his country of origin and in the countries he is passing through. This is based on the demands of global justice and the corresponding assignment of responsibilities (Caney 2006; Brock 2009), but such global responsibilities do not necessarily conflict with national interests. On the contrary, global health ethics suggests that the responsibility of one high-income country for its own citizen's health should also encompass efforts to improve the health systems in low- and middle-income countries to stabilize these regions, reduce migration pressure, and reduce the risk of communicable diseases for all.

The lens of global health ethics also reveals the simple, important fact that the same global obligations exist for migrants. Countries—and especially those that have the resources to do so—should consider it their responsibility to create a healthcare system that allows every person in a given territory to seek healthcare once they arrive at the country of destination, irrespective of his or her legal status. Details of the scope of health services offered would have to be determined in each country, based on the resources available and on what is included in the regular universal healthcare package, if one exists (Segall 2009; Brock 2015). There are various ethical arguments that call for equal access to healthcare for all, that is, the equal moral worth of every human being, which entails securing for every person the opportunity to live a flourishing life, health as a basic good for a flourishing life, reciprocity, and solidarity (Dwyer 2015; Illingworth and Parmet 2015; Wild 2015). Again, such responsibilities to provide universal healthcare for all people in a state's territory, regardless of their residence and citizenship status, do not necessarily conflict with pragmatic state interests, such as protection of public health, improved health, and thus a healthier workforce in the country, or even a reduction in costs for the national healthcare system (Bozorgmehr and Razum 2015; Dwyer 2015; Illingworth and Parmet 2015; Wild 2015).

1.3.2 Emphasizing the "Firewall Argument" (Especially Relevant to Steps 3–6)

Undocumented migrants are often effectively cut off from the protection of basic human rights or even from pursuing their basic human rights because they fear negative consequences of making the authorities aware of them. For example, if an undocumented migrant is a victim of violence, he or she might refrain from calling the police for fear of being deported (Carens 2015). As a remedy against undocumented migrants being effectively unable to claim their basic human rights, a so-called firewall has been proposed through an interpretation of the ethics of human rights. A thorough description and discussion of the argument can be found in the work of the philosopher Joseph Carens on the ethics of immigration. The important point is, as Carens (2015) writes, it does not make moral sense to formally provide a right under conditions that make it practically impossible to actually pursue this right. There is therefore an ethical obligation to develop mechanisms for the proper protection of basic human rights. Carens describes the firewall as follows: "Democratic states can and should build a firewall between the enforcement of immigration law, on the one hand, and the protection of general human rights, on the other. We ought to establish as a firm legal principle that no information gathered by those responsible for protecting general human rights can be used for immigration enforcement purposes" (133). Carens engages in a profound discussion of this argument and characterizes it as "idealistic in relation to the status quo" (296). On the basis of examples, he nevertheless describes in detail the feasibility of reasonably effective firewalls if there is the will to implement them.

As described in Oliver's case, studies show that fear of immigration law enforcement is in fact one of the main reasons why undocumented migrants refrain from seeking medical care, even if in principle legal ways to seek healthcare are available (Hacker et al. 2011). This has several negative consequences: Oliver does not receive the necessary—but in some European countries technically available—healthcare, which creates a risk both to himself and to the people around him. Even if there is contact with the medical system, healthcare workers might not be able to provide appropriate and effective care because Oliver might not disclose all his symptoms due to fear of deportation, resulting in a mistrust of the health system. A firewall would ensure that practitioners of each profession can fulfill their duties without worrying that their actions will interfere with immigration law enforcement.

The firewall argument has been taken up in more detail in the area of migrant health and is becoming inextricably tied to the acknowledgment and affirmation of human rights. It calls for a separation of immigration law and healthcare for migrants based on the importance of health, irrespective of the legal residence status of the person (Ashcroft 2005; *The Lancet* 2007). As there are fewer feasibility constraints in high-income countries, these countries have a special responsibility to care for everyone in their territory (Wild 2015).

This argument can increasingly be found in official international policy proposals. For example, the report of the UN Secretary General (2014) on the promotion and protection of human rights claims that "the absence of firewalls between public services and migration authorities is a vital force in the denial of basic rights" (7/18). With utmost clarity, the European Council emphasized the need for a firewall:

> It deals exclusively with the question of ensuring access by all persons . . . to those human rights which are guaranteed to them in international human rights instruments, in particular as concerns education, health care, housing, social security and assistance, labor protection and justice, while they are within the jurisdiction of a member State. To this end, this GPR [general policy recommendation] calls for the creation of effective measures (hereafter "firewalls") to prevent state and private sector actors from effectively denying human rights to irregularly present migrants by clearly prohibiting the sharing of the personal data of, or other information about, persons suspected of irregular presence or work, with the immigration authorities for purposes of immigration control and enforcement. (European Commission Against Racism and Intolerance 2016, 7)

The firewall argument can be used for different purposes. It can be used to highlight a harmful, nonexistent separation of immigration law enforcement and basic human rights. This is, for example, the case in the United Kingdom, the United States, and Australia, where asylum seekers are required to undergo pre-entry TB screening. This requirement denies the right to enter the country and claim asylum in the case of untreated, infectious TB (Aldridge et al. 2014; Wickramage and Mosca 2014; New South Wales Government 2015). Here the firewall argument helps to argue for a separation in principle. An empirical investigation as to whether it functions would be the second step.

The firewall argument can also be used in less controversial contexts. In continental Europe, where asylum seekers are allowed to enter the country without prior health screening, immigration authorities are interested in finding undocumented migrants and deporting them. In Germany, for example, a law requires public institutions—excluding physicians but including, for example, social workers, who are often involved in organizing access to healthcare—to denounce all undocumented migrants to the immigration authorities (Bundesministerium der Justiz 2004). The firewall argument can be used to discuss potential fundamental moral flaws of legal regulations.

Some European cities have used their autonomy to build firewalls around health provision for undocumented migrants and to provide secure, free, and confidential health care, irrespective of their residence status. Here, too, the demand of the firewall is to investigate whether these options are well communicated to the migrants and whether these firewalls function in practice (Platform for International Cooperation on Undocumented Migrants 2017).

1.3.3 Non-Stigmatization as Part of Health Justice Theories (Especially Relevant for Steps 4 and 6)

Various studies have shown that TB is stigmatized, which in itself constitutes a moral problem. Stigma can lead to harmful consequences, such as discrimination and negative socioeconomic outcomes, or can negatively impact healthcare-seeking behavior due to diagnostic delays and reduced treatment adherence (Courtwright and Turner 2010; Craig et al. 2017). Studies on stigma often distinguish three levels: individual stigma (e.g., in interactions between two people), institutional or structural stigma (e.g., through institutional practices, rules, and policies), and internalized self-stigmatization (Mahajan et al. 2008). Being a migrant can exacerbate stigma in relation to TB on all three levels, as being a migrant strongly correlates with experiencing stigma, prejudices, and implicit biases (Segrest Purkiss et al. 2006; Abarca et al. 2013; Green et al. 2016).

Stigma and the resulting discrimination also play an important role in theories of justice and of justice in health. A central concern of such theories is to reach equality in certain areas. In relation to stigma, theories demanding relational or democratic equality, participation, and respect for persons are particularly pertinent (Anderson 1999; Young 2010). These theories focus on the quality of interactions between persons and object to discrimination, exclusion, and domination. The central aim is to realize a society of equals in moral worth; stigmatization contradicts this aim.

An especially interesting health justice theory for Oliver's case is Madison Powers and Ruth Faden's theory of social justice in public health and health policy. At the core of their approach lies the assumption that social justice is the foundational moral justification of public health (Krieger and Birn 1998; Wolff and De-Shalit 2007; Venkatapuram and Marmot 2011; Green et al. 2016). Powers and Faden (2008) identify six fundamental dimensions of well-being that are essential for any human being at any time: health, personal security, reasoning, respect, attachment, and self-determination. Justice in their view requires sufficiency of every dimension. Each dimension of well-being can be influenced by one or multiple social determinants. In Oliver's case, we can detect insufficiency in most or all dimensions of well-being (Wild 2013). Here we want to focus on respect, which "requires an ability to see others as independent sources of moral worth" (Powers and Faden 2008, 22). Oliver might experience being "perceived as being of lesser value because of membership in a particular . . . group, about whom invidious judgments are made" (23). Lack of respect, stigmatization, and resulting discrimination constitute a serious assault on the person as a morally worthy agent.

According to Faden and Powers (2008) and Anderson (1999), those health inequalities matter most and thus require action most urgently when they travel with clusters of disadvantaging determinants that undermine multiple dimensions of well-being. As we have seen, stigma in relation to migrant status and TB is part of the clustering of disadvantage that Oliver experiences (Wild 2013). If the basic moral task to see others equally as independent sources of moral worth is taken seriously, individual and institutional stakeholders would be responsible in cases such as Oliver's for taking relevant actions to secure non-stigmatization and respect.

1.3.4 Other Ethical Issues in TB Care of Migrants

Other ethical issues are of significance in relation to TB and migration. For example, one could discuss the ethical legitimization of migrating or seeking asylum with the primary purpose of seeking TB care. Other questions are, for example, in relation to the case where the patient does not speak the language of the healthcare providers or does not want to follow through with isolation or other TB care procedures because he or she is on the move. Another question is whether compulsory screening at the border is ethically defensible when there is weak evidence that it helps to reduce transmission or improve individuals' health outcomes (Wickramage and Mosca 2014).

All these issues are highly relevant, but not in Oliver's case, as he stays undiagnosed and untreated for most of the journey. This chapter puts special emphasis on this type of problem, as Oliver's story might be representative of many other migrants with TB or other communicable diseases. A different migrant story, of a migrant who is diagnosed and treated during the journey, will help to identify and address more fields. This shows the importance of continuing to analyze different case studies of migrants affected by TB for their significance as regards ethics and human rights. Ethics discussions in relation to human rights discourses, and vice versa, should focus on these questions much more systematically than is currently done to provide a sound and appropriate ground for argumentation and adequate responses in policy and practice.

1.4 PUTTING HUMAN RIGHTS AND ETHICS INTO PRACTICE

Implementing ethical values and human rights, as outlined here, in TB and migrant health services poses a considerable challenge. Countries receiving undocumented migrants should respond to the surge in human mobility through public health policies based on evidence, ethics, and human rights to ensure that migrant health issues are addressed.

The turn toward nationalist dynamics in some Western nations can make the task of affirming ethics and rights in migrant health even more challenging. Policies based on fear, discrimination, and exclusion may affect not only the health of migrants but also that of the host communities where migrants live and work or of others in their countries of transit. In this context, it is critical that the TB community stay with the task of upholding ethics and affirming rights. Incremental victories protecting the health and rights of migrants with TB may occur first in individual programs or for individual cases, before building into bigger policies. TB programs and practitioners should build active solidarity and alliances with migrant rights movements and other groups that are defending human rights and working toward global health justice; they also should collaborate with more general anti-discrimination, ethics education, and right-to-health initiatives. Aligned with others, TB programs can become spaces where alternatives to stigmatizing, dehumanizing, and rights-denying approaches to migrant health are tried and shown to succeed. Ultimately it is the responsibility of states to uphold their obligations under international human rights law and enact policies that reflect the ethical and moral underpinnings of public health. However, single states acting alone cannot solve a problem as complex in its genesis as migration-associated TB. Cross-border projects are necessary to make progress against the global drivers of TB. Such projects should acknowledge the obligations of international human rights and humanitarian law throughout the migration route and reaffirm the insight of global health ethics—that health for all is a shared project, and that responsibility increases with the privilege, wealth, and advantages that a country holds. In working with peers from other nations, health professionals will be creating the foundation on which approaches to TB and migration based on evidence, ethics, and human rights can be strengthened.

REFERENCES

Abarca, Tomás Bruno, Christopher Pell, Aurora Bueno Cavanillas, José Guillén Solvas, Robert Pool, and María Roura. 2013. "Tuberculosis in Migrant populations. A Systematic Review of the Qualitative Literature." *PLoS One* 8: e82440.

Aldridge, Robert W., Tom A. Yates, Dominik Zenner, Peter J. White, Ibrahim Abubakar, and Andrew C. Hayward. 2014. "Pre-Entry Screening Programmes for Tuberculosis in Migrants to Low-Incidence Countries: A Systematic Review and Meta-Analysis." *Lancet Infectious Disease* 14: 1240–1249.

Anderson, Elizabeth S. 1999. "What Is the Point of Equality?" *Ethics* 109: 287–337.

Asch, Steven, Barbara Leake, Ronald Anderson, and Lillian Gelberg. 1998. "Why Do Symptomatic Patients Delay Obtaining Care for Tuberculosis?" *American Journal of Respiratory and Critical Care Medicine* 157: 1244–1248.

Ashcroft, Richard E. 2005. "Standing Up for the Medical Rights of Asylum Seekers." *Journal of Medical Ethics* 31: 125–126.

Benatar, Solomon, and Gillian Brock, eds. 2021. *Global Health: Ethical Challenges*. Cambridge University Press.

Bozorgmehr, Kayvan, and Oliver Razum. 2015. "Effect of Restricting Access to Healthcare on Health Expenditures Among Asylum-Seekers and Refugees: A Quasi-Experimental Study in Germany, 1994–2013." *PLoS One* 10: e0131483.

Brock, Gillian. 2009. *Global Justice: A Cosmopolitan Account*. Oxford University Press.

Brock, Gillian. 2015. "Global Justice, Cosmopolitan Duties and Duties to Compatriots: The Case of Healthcare." *Public Health Ethics* 8: 110–120.

Bundesministerium der Justiz. 2004. "Gesetz über den Aufenthalt, die Erwerbstätigkeit und die Integration von Ausländern im Bundesgebiet, § 87 Übermittlungen an Ausländerbehörden." Accessed May 2024. https://www.gesetze-im-internet.de/aufenthg_2004/index.html#BJNR195010004BJNE009406116.

Caney, Simon. 2006. *Justice Beyond Borders: A Global Political Theory*. Oxford University Press.

Carens, Joseph H. 2015. *The Ethics of Immigration*. Oxford University Press.

Courtwright, Andrew, and Abigail Norris Turner. 2010. "Tuberculosis and Stigmatization: Pathways and Interventions." *Public Health Reports* 125 (4): 34–42.

Craig, Gillian M., A. Daftary, N. Engel, S. O'Driscoll, and A. Ioannaki. 2017. "Tuberculosis Stigma as a Social Determinant of Health: A Systematic Mapping Review of Research in Low-Incidence Countries." *International Journal of Infectious Diseases* 56: 90–100.

Daniels, Norman. 2008. *Just Health: Meeting Health Needs Fairly*. Cambridge University Press.

Dauvrin, Marie, Vincent Lorant, Sima Sandhu, et al. 2012. "Healthcare for Irregular Migrants: Pragmatism Across Europe. A Qualitative Study." *BMC Research Notes* 5 (99).

de Freitas, Cláudia. 2017. "Public and Patient Participation in Health Policy, Care and Research." *Porto Biomedical Journal* 2: 31–32.

Dhavan, Purnima, H. M. Dias, J. Creswell, and D. Weil. 2017. "An Overview of Tuberculosis and Migration." *International Journal of Tuberculosis and Lung Disease* 21: 610–623.

Dwyer, James. 2015. "On Taking Responsibility for Undocumented Migrants." *Public Health Ethics* 8: 139–147.

European Commission Against Racism and Intolerance. 2016. "On Safeguarding Irregularly Present Migrants from Discrimination: ECRI General Policy Recommendation No 16." https://www.coe.int/en/web/european-commission-against-racism-and-intolerance/recommendation-no.16.

Farmer, Paul. 2004. *Pathologies of Power: Health, Human Rights, and the New War on the Poor*. University of California Press.

Forman, Lisa. 2015. "Decoding the Right to Health: What Could It Offer to Global Health?" *Bioethics Forum* 8: 91–97.

Green, Eva G. T., Oriane Sarrasin, Robert Baur, and Nicole Fasel. 2016. "From Stigmatized Immigrants to Radical Right Voting: A Multilevel Study on the Role of Threat and Contact." *Political Psychology* 37: 465–480.

Gruskin, Sofia, E. J. Mills, and Daniel Tarantola. 2007. "History, Principles, and Practice of Health and Human Rights." *The Lancet* 370: 449–455.

Haar, Rohini Jonnalagadda, and Leonard S. Rubenstein. 2012. "Health in Post Conflict and Fragile States." https://www.usip.org/sites/default/files/SR_301.pdf.

Hacker, Karen, Joycelyn Chu, Carloyn Leung, et al. 2011. "The Impact of Immigration and Customs Enforcement on Immigrant Health: Perceptions of Immigrants in Everett, Massachusetts, USA." *Social Science & Medicine* 73: 586–594.

Hampshire, James. 2005. "The Politics of Immigration and Public Health." *Political Quarterly* 76: 190–198.

Heilinger, Jan-Christoph. 2020. *Cosmopolitan Responsibility: Global Injustice, Relational Equality, and Individual Agency*. De Gruyter.

Hunter, David, and Angus J. Dawson. 2011. "Is There a Need for Global Health Ethics? For and Against." In *Global Health Ethics*, edited by S. Benatar and G. Brock. Cambridge University Press.

Illingworth, Patricia, and Wendy E. Parmet. 2015. "The Right to Health: Why It Should Apply to Immigrants." *Public Health Ethics* 8: 148–161.

Info Migrants. 2024. "Italy Reports 50% Increase in Migrant Landings in 2023." https://www.infomigrants.net/en/post/54260/italy-reports-50-increase-in-migrant-landings-in-2023.

International Committee of the Red Cross. 2004. "What Is International Humanitarian Law?" Accessed May 2024. https://www.icrc.org/en/document/what-international-humanitarian-law.

International Organization for Migration. 2013. "International Migration, Health, and Human Rights." https://publications.iom.int/books/international-migration-health-and-human-rights.

International Organization for Migration. 2017. "Who Is a Migrant?" https://www.iom.int/who-is-a-migrant.

Kingsley, Patrick. 2016. *The New Odyssey: The Story of Europe's Refugee Crisis*. Guardian Books.

Ködmön, Csaba, Phillip Zucs, and Marieke J. van der Werf. 2016. "Migration-Related Tuberculosis: Epidemiology and Characteristics of Tuberculosis Cases Originating Outside the European Union and European Economic Area, 2007 to 2013." *Eurosurveillance* 21 (12): 30164.

Krieger, Nancy, and Anne-Emanuelle Birn. 1998. "A Vision of Social Justice as the Foundation of Public Health: Commemorating 150 Years of the Spirit of 1848." *American Journal of Public Health* 88: 1603–1606.

The Lancet. 2007. "Access to Healthcare for Undocumented Migrants in Europe." 370: 2070. https://www.thelancet.com/journals/lancet/article/PIIS0140-6736(07)61872-8/fulltext.

Lönnroth, Knut, Zohar Mor, Connie Erkens, et al. 2017. "Tuberculosis in Migrants in Low-Incidence Countries: Epidemiology and Intervention Entry Points." *International Journal of Tuberculosis and Lung Disease* 21: 624–637.

Mahajan, Anish P., Jennifer N. Sayles, Vishal A. Patel, et al. 2008. "Stigma in the HIV/AIDS Epidemic: A Review of the Literature and Recommendations for the Way Forward." *AIDS* 22 (2): S67–S79.

New South Wales Government. 2015. "Refugee Screening and Follow Up." https://www.health.nsw.gov.au/Infectious/tuberculosis/Pages/refugee-screening.aspx.

Pinto, Andrew D., and Ross Upshur. 2013. *An Introduction to Global Health Ethics*. Routledge.

Platform for International Cooperation on Undocumented Migrants. 2017. "Cities of Rights: Ensuring Healthcare for Undocumented Residents." https://picum.org/wp-content/uploads/2023/08/CityOfRights_Health_EN.pdf.

Pogge, Thomas W. 2010. *World Poverty and Human Rights: Cosmopolitan Responsibilities and Reforms*. 2nd ed. Polity Press.

Powers, Madison, and Ruth R. Faden. 2008. *Social Justice: The Moral Foundations of Public Health and Health Policy*. Oxford University Press.

Rubio-Marín, Ruth, ed. 2014. *Human Rights and Immigration*. Oxford University Press.

Sandgren, Andreas, Monica Sañe Schepisi, Giovanni Sotgiu, et al. 2014. "Tuberculosis Transmission Between Foreign- and Native-Born Populations in the EU/EEA: A Systematic Review." *European Respiratory Journal* 43: 1159–1171.

Scholz, Nicole. 2016. "The Public Health Dimension of the European Migrant Crisis." European Parliament. http://www.europarl.europa.eu/RegData/etudes/BRIE/2016/573908/EPRS_BRI(2016)573908_EN.pdf.

Segall, Shlomi. 2009. *Health, Luck, and Justice*. Princeton University Press.

Segrest Purkiss, Sharon L., Pamela L. Perrewé, Treena L. Gillespie, Bronston T. Mayes, and Gerald R. Ferris. 2006. "Implicit Sources of Bias in Employment Interview Judgments and Decisions." *Organizational Behavior and Human Decision Processes* 101: 152–167.

Toomey, Russell B., Adriana J. Umaña-Taylor, David R. Williams, Elizabeth Harvey-Mendoza, Laudan B. Jahromi, and Kimberly A. Updegraff. 2014. "Impact of Arizona's SB 1070 Immigration Law on Utilization of Healthcare and Public Assistance Among Mexican-Origin Adolescent Mothers and Their Mother Figures." *American Journal of Public Health* 104 (1): S28–S34.

Turner, Neil. 2016. "Undocumented Migration: A Global Problem." *Perspectives in Anthropology*. https://perspectivesinanthropology.wordpress.com/2016/06/01/illegal-immigration-a-global-problem/.

United Nations. 1966. "International Covenant on Economic, Social and Cultural Rights, International Covenant on Civil and Political Rights. A/RES/21/2200." https://www.ohchr.org/en/resources/educators/human-rights-education-training/2-international-covenant-economic-social-and-cultural-rights-1966.

United Nations. 2010. "Report of the Special Rapporteur on the Human Rights of Migrants—Impact of the Criminalization of Migration on the Protection and Enjoyment of Human Rights. A/65/222." https://www.ohchr.org/en/special-procedures/sr-migrants/annual-reports.

United Nations Committee on Economic, Social and Cultural Rights. 2000. "General Comment No 14: The Right to the Highest Attainable Standard of Health (Art 12)." http://www.refworld.org/pdfid/4538838d0.pdf.

United Nations, Department of Economic and Social Affairs. 2020. "International Migration 2020." https://www.un.org/development/desa/pd/sites/www.un.org.development.desa.pd/files/undesa_pd_2020_international_migration_highlights.pdf.

United Nations Development Programme. 2009. "Human Development Report, 2009. Overcoming Barriers: Human Mobility and Development." http://hdr.undp.org/en/content/human-development-report-2009.

United Nations High Commission for Refugees. 2011. "The 1951 Convention Relating to the Status of Refugees and Its 1967 Protocol." https://www.unhcr.org/sites/default/files/legacy-pdf/4ec262df9.pdf.

United Nations Secretary General. 2014. "Promotion and Protection of Human Rights, Including Ways and Means to Promote the Human Rights of Migrants: Report of the Secretary-General. A/69/277." https://digitallibrary.un.org/record/778942?v=pdf.

Venkatapuram, Sridhar, and Michael G. Marmot. 2011. *Health Justice: An Argument from the Capabilities Approach*. Polity.

Wickramage, Kolitha, and Davide Mosca. 2014. "Can Migration Health Assessments Become a Mechanism for Global Public Health Good?" *International Journal of Environmental Research and Public Health* 11: 9954–9963.

Wild, Verina. 2013. "Asylum-Seekers and Public Health Ethics." In *Ethics in Public Health and Health Policy: Concepts, Methods, Case Studies*, edited by Daniel Strech, Irene Marckmann, and Georg Marckmann. Springer.

Wild, Verina. 2015. "Universal Access to Healthcare for Migrants: Applying Cosmopolitanism to the Domestic Realm." *Public Health Ethics* 8: 162–172.

Wild, Verina, and Angus J. Dawson. 2018. "Migration: A Core Public Health Ethics Issue." *Public Health* 158: 66–70.

Wild, Verina, Deborah Zion, and Richard Ashcroft. 2015. "Health of Migrants: Approaches from a Public Health Ethics Perspective." *Public Health Ethics* 8: 107–109.

Wolff, Jonathan, and Avner De-Shalit. 2007. *Disadvantage*. Oxford University Press.

World Health Organization. 1978. "Primary Healthcare." http://apps.who.int/iris/bitstream/10665/39228/1/9241800011.pdf.

Young, Iris M. 2010. *Inclusion and Democracy*. Oxford University Press.

Young, Iris M. 2013. *Responsibility for Justice*. Oxford University Press.

2

Environmental Migrants, Structural Injustice, and Moral Responsibility

JAMES DWYER

2.1 INTRODUCTION

The English word "refugee" comes from the Latin *refugere*, which means "to run away" or "flee."[1] In common understanding, refugees are people who have fled wars, oppression, or persecution. In international law, refugees are people who are outside their country and are unwilling to return because they have a "well-founded fear of being persecuted for reasons of race, religion, nationality, membership of a particular social group or political opinion" (United Nations 1951). Even in this narrow legal sense, there are about 43.7 million refugees in the world today. Another 73.5 million people are internally displaced (United Nations High Commissioner for Refugees 2024). They fled within their own country in order to escape wars, oppression, or persecution.

Images, stories, and accounts of refugees and internally displaced people prompt us to recognize and raise deep ethical issues. What responsibilities do we have to address the root causes of displacement? What is the moral violation when people are deprived of a sense of home? What responsibilities do we have to care about and for people who cannot return home safely? What claims do these people have to protection and healthcare? What differences should receiving communities accommodate when providing healthcare? Bioethics, broadly conceived, has taken up these issues (Wild et al. 2015; Klingler et al. 2018).

In this chapter, I want to focus ethical attention on people who move or are forced to move because of environmental problems. I will refer to

1. This chapter has previously been published as: James Dwyer, 2020. "Environmental migrants, structural injustice, and moral responsibility," Bioethics 34: 562–569. It is reprinted here with friendly permission from John Wiley and Sons / Wiley Company.

James Dwyer, *Environmental Migrants, Structural Injustice, and Moral Responsibility*. In: *Forced Migration and Health Justice*. Edited by: Lisa A. Eckenwiler, Verina Wild, Anna Gotlib, Ryoa Chung, and Deborah Zion, Oxford University Press. DOI: 10.1093/oso/9780197795491.003.0002 these people as "environmental migrants." This broad term includes people who are fleeing environmental disasters to save their lives and people who have lost their homes and a sense of belonging in a place. But the term also includes people whose lives have been affected by environmental problems in different ways and to different degrees.

My first aim in this chapter is to describe environmental migration in a way that recognizes its diversity and complexity. I do not want to focus on a small subset of environmental migrants, for example, those people who will become stateless when their small island nations become uninhabitable (Risse 2009; Wyman 2013). I want to say something about the ethical issues raised by the broader, more complex phenomenon. And I want to recognize how often multiple factors overlap and combine to result in migration.

My second aim is to show how environmental migration raises issues of structural justice. Although I will form and explain some particular judgments of justice as I go along, I will not try to derive these judgments from an abstract theory of justice. In this context, I believe that the particular judgments are more warranted than the abstract theories. Because I believe that the unfairness of the situation is relatively clear and compelling, at least upon reflection, I focus more attention on issues of responsibility and responsiveness.

My third aim is to articulate an account of responsibility that fits the phenomenon of environmental migration that I describe and the judgments of justice that I make. I do not aim to show that this account of responsibility is the best general account of duties and obligations. Rather, I suggest that this account complements other conceptions of responsibility because it makes sense of some important features of environmental migration, addresses judgments of justice, and points to ways to respond. My aims are *theoretically* modest: to describe environmental migration in a certain way, show how issues of justice arise, and articulate a complementary view of responsibility.

2.2 ENVIRONMENTAL PROBLEMS AND MIGRATION

To live, people have to cope with environmental problems. Some people have to cope with rising sea levels, storms, and flooding. Others have to cope with droughts and shortages of fresh water. Some have to cope with melting glaciers that result in flooding in the short term and lack of water in the long term. Others have to cope with soil degradation, salinization, and desertification. Some have to cope with deforestation and forest fires. Many have to cope with air pollution, water pollution, and food insecurity.

Some people have responded and will respond to environmental problems by migrating. Since environmental migration is as old as human migration, we should expect that some humans will migrate when faced with contemporary environmental problems. In describing environmental migration in this section, I want to recognize its complexity: many factors coexist, interact, and vary by degree. To describe this complexity, I will use a stylistic device: I pose six questions that assume a dichotomy and show why the dichotomy poses a false choice. I believe this stylistic device will help to show the complexity of the phenomenon that I want to address.

First, are the causes of environmental problems slow-onset changes or sudden-onset events? The causes of environmental problems often involve both slow-onset changes in the background conditions and sudden-onset events that precipitate the acute problem. While changes in sea levels are slow-onset, and storms are sudden-onset, the problems that people face from storm surges are a combination of these and other factors. Furthermore, some of the sudden-onset events, such as flooding, now seem to be cycles within the background of a changed climate. In fact, many environmental problems involve factors that range over a continuum from slow-onset to sudden-onset, and the risks that people face include factors in the natural, built, and social environments. I will return to this point in the section on justice.

Second, are the causes of environmental problems local or global? In many cases, local, regional, and global factors combine and contribute to environmental problems. For example, the people who live in the Pearl River Delta in China are at increased risk of flooding. Global climate change exacerbates the risks. Industrialization and regional economic development also play a large part. Urban development and local destruction of wetlands contribute to the risks. In practice, it may be difficult to separate out causes and assign probabilities in a precise way. We need to recognize this complexity and develop ethical accounts that fit the complexity. As a first step, we might think about how assigning or taking responsibility at one level does not necessarily exclude assigning or taking responsibility at another level.

Third, are people who move in response to various environmental problems really environmental migrants, or are they economic migrants? They may be both. Sometimes environmental problems may lead to economic problems. Consider one example. Because climate change will probably make droughts in the Sahel more frequent and intense, small farmers in this region will find it harder to grow food and support their families. When their incomes and resources fall too low, they or someone in their family may decide to migrate. In this case, people who are responding to underlying environmental problems may look like—and be dismissed as—economic migrants.

In most cases of migration, environmental factors or conditions combine with economic, social, and political factors (McAdam 2012). We need to acknowledge this complexity and overcome the simplistic and sharp division between environmental refugees and economic migrants. In practice, it may not be possible to separate different factors and to assign them an exact weight. I deal with this complexity by focusing ethical attention on unjust structures and background conditions. I simply refer to people as environmental migrants when I think the environmental factors are the dominant and underlying factors or when I want to focus ethical attention on certain problems and responses.

Fourth, should we not make a sharp distinction between people who move to avoid war and conflict and people who move to avoid environmental problems? No, this sharp distinction does not hold up causally or ethically. Environmental problems like desertification, water shortages, and population growth may lead to or exacerbate armed conflict. The conflict and genocide in Rwanda and the civil war in Syria occurred in a context of serious environmental problems (Munien 2010; Kelley et al. 2015). Of course, an environmental problem is rarely the only factor behind an armed conflict, but climate change has increased and may continue to increase the probability of conflicts in some regions. Furthermore, a sharp distinction between armed conflicts and environmental problems reflects international legal practices more than ethical differences. People who move to escape environmental problems as well as people who move to escape armed conflict have often been treated unjustly, have been deprived of rights, and have moral claims on others.

Fifth, are people forced to flee, or do they voluntarily choose to move in search of a better life? This formulation is misleading because, on the one side, it diminishes the role of agency, and, on the other side, it leaves out the dire and unjust circumstances from which people are migrating. Furthermore, it suggests that force is the only or most salient moral feature. Even when storms, floods, and fires endanger people's lives and threaten their homes, they are not passive victims. Often they are active agents who make choices and respond to difficult situations in ways that promise a better life. In other cases, gradual changes affect ecosystems, and people who depend most directly on these systems find it harder and harder to maintain their livelihood. So they may decide to move. Here again people respond to difficult situations in ways that promise a better life. In most cases, terrible circumstances and difficult situations do not exclude choice and agency, but people's responses hardly seem like a voluntary choice and decision. Perhaps, as Alexander Betts (2013) suggests, "survival migrants" is a better term for many people who are not legally recognized as refugees.

Furthermore, the element of force may not be the most salient ethical feature in some contexts. Later I shall articulate an account of the ethical issues that focuses less attention on force and more attention on the fairness of the background conditions.

Sixth, in thinking about environmental migrants, should we focus attention on people who move across international borders or on people who move within their own country? As I noted earlier, international law makes a big distinction between international refugees and internally displaced people. However, this distinction does not merit so much ethical weight in the case of environmental problems. Where people migrate to often depends on the nature of the problem, their starting location, their economic resources, and their social networks. I worry that the legal distinction between externally and internally displaced people will be used to avoid taking ethical responsibility for unjust structures and conditions that induce people to move within their own country.

Many of the environmental problems that induce people to migrate will be exacerbated by climate change (Intergovernmental Panel on Climate Change [IPCC] 2014). Because of human activity, greenhouse gases are increasing in the atmosphere. The increase in these gases is changing temperatures, altering precipitation patterns, increasing the intensity of storms, raising sea levels, acidifying the oceans, and more (IPCC 2014). These changes contribute to a range of environmental problems: floods, droughts, salinization, soil degradation, crop failures, shortages of fresh water, heatwaves, and more (IPCC 2014). All these problems impact human health and welfare.

In the short term, the impact of climate change on livelihoods, food production, and fresh water may affect the most people (IPCC 2014). Environmental problems may induce more people to migrate in the 21st century than wars, oppression, and persecution did in the 20th century. Estimates vary widely because researchers use different concepts and resolve uncertainties in different ways. There is uncertainty about who to count as environmental refugees or environmental migrants. There is also uncertainty about how much societies will reduce greenhouse gas emissions. And there is uncertainty about how adaptive and resilient societies will become. It is not clear whether low-income countries will have the resources to fund insurance schemes, manage floods, protect fresh water, adapt agriculture, strengthen public health systems, and so on. And it is not clear whether some high-income countries will have the political will and foresight to do the same.

The International Organization for Migration ([IOM] 2017) defines environmental migrants as "persons or groups of persons who, for compelling reasons of sudden or progressive changes in the environment that adversely affect their lives or living conditions, are obliged to leave their habitual homes, or choose to do so, either temporarily or permanently, and who move either within their country or abroad." This definition avoids many of the dichotomies that I discussed. By referring to compelling reasons, it recognizes the role of agency. It includes both sudden- and slow-onset changes, and it recognizes the effect that these changes have on livelihoods and living conditions. It does not place too much weight on whether the migrants cross borders and whether they can or intend to return home. With this definition and some moderate assumptions, the IOM (2017) estimates that climate change will induce 200 million people to migrate by the year 2050.

With a sense of the magnitude and urgency of the problem of environmental migration, I now turn to the ethical issues. I shall focus attention on issues of justice and then on issues of responsibility.

2.3 ISSUES OF JUSTICE

We are all at risk of becoming environmental migrants, but we are not equally at risk. Our particular risk depends on many factors, some obvious, some less so. In order to show how the risks are distributed, I will consider four broad categories of risks: temporal position, geographic location, kind of society, and position in society.

The first category is people's temporal position, the generation to which they belong. Greenhouse gases are accumulating in the atmosphere faster than the natural world can recycle them. In preindustrial times, the level of carbon dioxide was probably about 280 parts per million (ppm); in 1959, it was 316 ppm; in 2013, it surpassed 400 ppm for the first time (National Oceanic and Atmospheric Administration, Earth Systems Research Laboratory 2013). Because of the accumulation of greenhouse gases, the climate is changing rapidly. Without better preventive and adaptive actions, younger people will face higher risks over their lifetime than older people will, and future generations will face higher risks than the current generation will.

The second category is geographic location. The physical features of the places people live affect their risk. For example, people who live in coastal areas are at increased risk of inundation from rising sea levels and storm surges. This includes people who live on small island states, coastal plains, and river deltas. A sea level rise of two meters would displace about 35 million people in the deltas of the Nile, Mekong, and Ganges rivers (Warner et al. 2009). Other people will be affected by droughts and shortages of fresh water. The livelihoods of millions of small farmers depend on regular patterns of rainfall. When it becomes more and more difficult for them to earn a living, many will be induced to migrate. And billions of people in Asia depend for fresh water on the regular accumulation and melting of the Himalayan glaciers. In the short term, these glaciers will melt faster; in the long term, less fresh water will be available. The geographic factors can be exacerbated or attenuated by the social factors that I consider next.

The third category is the kind of society in which people live. In general, high-income countries will be better able to respond and adapt to changes in the climate. They have the resources to change infrastructure, strengthen public health systems, develop insurance schemes, and so on. But it is not just a question of money. Those high-income countries that are governed with fairness, foresight, and consultation will protect more of their citizens. But it is not just a question of good governance. Civil society makes a difference. Those societies that cultivate civic engagement, social solidarity, and neighborly care are better constituted to deal with the risks that arise. Historical practices and knowledge may make a difference. The Netherlands has a tradition of maintaining dikes; Pakistan has a tradition of responding to floods; and Bangladesh has developed warning systems for cyclones. However, even good traditions and systems may break down at some point.

The fourth category is people's position within their society. For example, wealthy people who live on the coast of Florida are at risk because of their geographic location, but they are somewhat protected by their wealth and social position. They have economic resources to call upon, insurance schemes to back them up, and powerful networks upon which they may rely. Moreover, their livelihoods do not depend so directly on fragile ecosystems. Many other people in society are less protected and at greater risk. In general, the following factors will affect people's risk and ability to respond: power, wealth, income, type of livelihood, education, housing, race, and gender. These factors parallel the social determinants of health (Commission on Social Determinants of Health 2008). Here I want to note an obvious point: people are simply born into a certain generation, in a certain place, in a certain kind of society, and into some social position. All these factors profoundly affect their risk of becoming environmental migrants. By noting how these factors bear on risk, I do not mean to deny that people may exercise some control over some factors. After all, I view migration as an attempt to exercise control. Although the distribution of the risk is very important, it is only part of the story that bears on justice. Contributions to the problems are also relevant.

In the world at large, many people have contributed relatively little to the environmental problems that may induce them to migrate. This is most apparent with respect to greenhouse gas emissions. Many of the people who are at risk because of climate change are people with a low carbon footprint in a low-income country. Per capita emissions in the United States are twice as high as in Japan, another high-income country; they are five times as high as in Chile, a moderate-income country; and they are 60 times as high as in Bangladesh, a low-income country (Boden et al. 2007). Although national averages are important, they obscure the differences within countries. In every country, some people emit much more than average. The wealthiest 11% of the people in the world are responsible for 50% of the carbon emissions (Chakravarty et al. 2009). Yet because of their power, wealth, and social position, they face fewer risks. The differences between people's emissions and their risks raise deep issues of justice.

Justice is not only about how the risks of and the contributions to environmental problems are distributed. It is also about respect, dignity, and meaningful participation (Rawls 1971). Indeed, ideals of social democracy emphasize the need to foster the participation of people who are affected by social practices, policies, and values (Dewey 1954). There are good reasons behind these ideals. Fostering participation works to show respect for all people, gather insights from those with different perspectives, and increase the effectiveness of the resulting policies. To make livelihoods and communities more resilient to environmental changes will probably require the meaningful participation of many people. For example, to increase resilience, societies might try to develop schemes that provide crop failure insurance for small farmers. But to develop a scheme without consulting and engaging small farmers in deliberation shows a lack of respect for their experience and needs and is more likely to result in schemes that favor large farmers or provide wrong incentives.

To sum up, it seems unfair that people who have contributed very little to environmental problems face high risks from those problems, while people who have contributed to and benefited much more from high emissions face lower risks. Furthermore, it seems unfair that many people have not been allowed or encouraged to participate more meaningfully in forming policies that so profoundly affect their lives. I am not going to try to derive these judgments of justice from more general and abstract theories of justice. Among people who have studied and reflected on the environmental problems, there seems to be more agreement about these judgments than about abstract theories. In spite of differences in theoretical approaches, most (but not all) philosophical thinkers tend to converge on some basic judgments of justice: that it is unfair that societies and people with high emissions, and wealth generated by past emissions, are not doing more to prevent further climate change and to help others adapt to the changes that have occurred and will occur (Gardiner et al. 2010). So now I am going to explore issues of responsibility. This exploration presupposes some rough and overlapping judgments of justice, but it does not require agreement on a general and abstract theory of justice.

2.4 CONCEPTIONS OF RESPONSIBILITY

I will sketch three conceptions of responsibility in order to consider how well they fit the problem of environmental migration. My purpose is not to show that the third conception provides a better general account of responsibility or that it rests on a better foundation. My purpose is to show that it takes into account many of the features that I noted in the previous sections and that it outlines why and how we should respond.

The first conception develops the idea that we have responsibilities to aid other people simply because we are human beings. The idea is that some of our responsibilities are not based on promises we make, actions we take, or roles that we assume. These responsibilities are based on our nature as human beings. This idea may take different forms and be explicated in different ways. A contemporary form is the discourse about human rights and responsibilities. People may have some rights in virtue of their status and dignity as human beings, and we may have responsibilities to uphold and protect those rights. Another form of this idea draws on Kant's philosophy. Kant grounds some positive duties to aid in our status as rational and autonomous beings. According to Kant (1981), not to acknowledge positive duties to aid others leads to a contradiction in will. In accounts based on Kantian philosophy as well as accounts based on human rights, our personal, societal, and international relations need to include positive duties to aid other people. (Of course, other philosophies and accounts may also explain a duty to aid others.) Simply because we are human beings with the ability to help, we may have some responsibilities to prevent environmental problems, help people to adapt, and aid those who have compelling reasons to migrate. I accept the idea that we have some responsibilities that cannot be traced back to explicit consent, particular actions, or specific roles. I also accept that these responsibilities bear on the problem of environmental migration. However, this conception of responsibility does not directly address the injustices that I tried to articulate in the previous section. It does not get at how human conduct contributes to the environmental problems, social structures, and background conditions that induce some people to migrate.

The second conception of responsibility is akin to the idea of legal liability. Accounts of legal liability try to set out the conditions under which it would be right to punish people for acts or to hold them liable for harms (Hart 2008). Although these accounts sometimes include the idea of deterrence, they tend to be backward-looking: they focus on a particular harm in the past. Then they hold an individual person liable if a clear causal chain connects that person's actions to the harm and if that person acted intentionally, recklessly, or negligently. (In a few rare contexts, legal accounts include a notion of strict liability, but I will set that aside.) A conception of responsibility based on causal links and wrongdoing can be developed and used to address some environmental harms and problems, and as scientific understanding and public awareness increase, it could be extended to more environmental harms and problems. However, this conception does not really fit the features and concerns that I tried to describe in the previous two sections. The links between climate change and extreme weather events, for example, are rarely clear causal chains. Rather, emissions of greenhouse gases change the probability that extreme weather events will occur (Huber and Gulledge 2011). Furthermore, the global, regional, and local contributions to environmental problems are often difficult or impossible to tease out. And migration is often multifactorial: environmental, economic, social, political, and personal factors bear upon people's decisions to migrate (McAdam 2012; Wyman 2013). Nor is the element of wrongdoing so clear. Many people contributed to environmental problems before they knew, even before they should have known, about the risks to others. And many contributions to environmental problems are individually very small but cumulatively very important.

The second conception of responsibility insists that the connections between the harm and the people held responsible be clear causal chains that link the harm to a form of wrongdoing. The first conception of responsibility ignores all connections; it focuses on people's ability to provide aid to those in need. Both views offer incomplete accounts with respect to environmental migration. A complementary account of responsibility would examine conduct that accords with accepted norms, as well as actions that violate norms because they are intentionally harmful, reckless, or negligent. It would shift the focus from discrete acts and omissions to social structures and background conditions because these structures and conditions shape the situations in which people make decisions about migration and because these structures and conditions unfairly disadvantage some people. It would take into account the probabilities of future risks brought about by cumulative actions, and thereby shift the focus from a few individual actors to include millions of people, many corporations, and many governments. A complementary account of responsibility might even change the tone of the discussion from liability to responsiveness—to why and how we should respond in a more caring way.

The third conception of responsibility uses the idea of a responsibility to address structural injustice. Before her untimely death, Iris Marion Young (2011) developed an account of responsibility for structural injustice. I want to use this account to consider responsibilities to prevent environmental problems, to help people to adapt to environmental changes, and to aid those who have compelling reasons to migrate. I shall sketch this account as I use it to address four key questions, but I shall not try to justify it except in a theoretically modest way: by showing how it illuminates aspects of the ethical problem and helps to address important questions.

2.4.1 For What Should I (and People Who Are Situated Like Me) Take Responsibility?

No sensible conception of responsibility will focus on natural events that are beyond human control, for example, on eclipses or tsunamis. Although it does not make sense to assign or take responsibility for a tsunami, it makes good sense to develop warning systems, build sea walls, locate power plants safely, strengthen emergency responses, foster neighborliness, and so on. Acts of preparation are within human control and subject to ethical evaluation. The same can be said of social structures, background conditions, economic systems, political processes, and accepted practices (Young 2011). These human constructs influence whether some environmental problems occur, how serious they become, what groups are placed at risk, and what responses are ready at hand. For example, these constructs influence the combustion of fossil fuels, which increase carbon emissions, which increase temperatures, which increase sea levels, which lead to greater storm surges, which tend to displace more people. In particular cases, these links may not amount to clear causal chains. The influence of human constructs may be a matter of frameworks in which things happen or a matter of probabilities that certain things will occur. This is what I and other people need to take responsibility for: those social structures that unfairly increase the probabilities that people will be induced to migrate for environmental reasons.

2.4.2 Why Should I (and People Who Are Situated Like Me) Take Responsibility?

Some responsibilities arise from the ways that I am related to or situated with respect to environmental problems. As I go about my life, I participate in and reinforce structures, processes, conditions, and norms that unfairly increase the risk that certain groups will need to migrate for environmental reasons. My involvement grounds my responsibility. Young writes:

> The ground of my responsibility lies in the fact that I participate in the structural processes that have unjust outcomes. These processes are ongoing and ought to be transformed so they are less unjust. Thus I share with others the responsibility to transform these processes to reduce and eliminate the injustice that they cause. My responsibility is essentially shared with others because the harms are produced by many of us acting together within accepted institutions and practices, and because it is not possible for any of us to identify just what in our own actions results in which aspects of the injustice that particular individuals suffer. (2011, 110)

This responsibility is not grounded in or explicated by a clear causal chain that links my particular action to a particular harm. That is the way of legal liability. Nor is it grounded in or explicated by a common humanity. That is the way of natural duty. This responsibility is grounded in my relationship to the problem. Because of how I am related to the structures that influence the risks and problems, I have a shared responsibility to change those structures that unfairly disadvantage people, including people in distant places and future generations.

2.4.3 How Should I (and People Who Are Situated Like Me) Take Responsibility?

Unjust structures influence environmental problems and social conditions that will induce millions of people to migrate. Because I and many other people are implicated in these structures, we share some responsibility to change them. Appropriate changes might include forms of environmental protection, limitations on political lobbying, carbon taxes, caps on emissions, corrections of externalities, insurance schemes for people at risk, changes in agriculture, changes in infrastructure, new forms of economic life, more responsive public health systems, more responsive networks of neighbors, and so on. Changes like these require political action, in the best and broadest sense of that term. Young views political action as "public communicative engagement with others for the sake of organizing our relationships and coordinating our actions most justly" (2011, 112). This form of engagement relies on communication in some public space and community. It aims to organize relationships and coordinate actions so that they are less unjust. Although this form of action is collective, and the responsibility is political or civic, the responsibility itself is individual. This form of responsibility arises when individual people are structurally situated, have the capacity to communicate, and live in social contexts where political actions have some realistic chance of bringing about social change. In this sense, political action includes not only action that tries to influence governmental policies but also actions that citizens take in civil society. Young notes that those "who share responsibility for structural injustice may also find ways of making social changes through collective action in civil society independent of or as a supplement to state policies and programs" (2011, 112). Action in civil society is promising because state policies are often influenced and protected by vested interests like the fossil fuel industry. Action in civil society is also promising because it can form coalitions that span international borders, just as environmental problems do. But the task is enormous: to generate political will to create new structures or adapt old structures to address injustices. This daunting task leads to the next question.

2.4.4 How Much Responsibility Should I (and People Who Are Situated Like Me) Take?

Although I cannot give an exact answer to this question, I will point out three factors that seem salient. How much responsibility I should take depends on how serious the problem is. The more serious the problem, the more responsibility I should take. For the people at high risk, environmental problems often threaten their lives, health, and livelihoods. The number of people who may be affected is staggering. As I noted before, a moderate estimate is that 200 million people will be induced to migrate by the year 2050. How much responsibility I should take also depends on my relationship to the problem. The more I am privileged by the unjust structures that shape the problem, the more responsibility I should take. Many wealthy countries and people have profited from and depend on high levels of consumption and emissions. Even ordinary people in high-income countries are somewhat privileged by these patterns. When I examine my own situation, I see that I am relatively privileged by the structures of the carbon-intensive society in which I live. Like many people in this society, I heat my home, use a computer, ride in cars, fly in airplanes, and do many other things that depend on fossil fuels. These and other activities have unsustainable footprints that disadvantage others. The amount of responsibility that I should take may also depend on the nature of the unjust structures. Structures that privilege race or gender seem, other things being equal, even worse than structures that privilege geographic location or neighborliness. In the United States, with its history of slavery and unequal rights, African American communities face more risk from a number of environmental problems: the presence of toxic dumps, exposure to air pollution, and permanent displacement from hurricanes (Bullard and Wright 2012). Of course, it is not easy to separate the effects of race from the effects of wealth, but the distribution of wealth is conditioned by past practices of discrimination and exclusion. The general point seems sound: the moral nature of the privilege is relevant to how much responsibility I should take.

2.5 CONCLUSION

To begin, I described the phenomenon of environmental migration in a way that recognizes its complexity and diversity. Then I noted some of the injustices behind this form of migration. Since these judgments of justice seem warranted to me, I focused more attention on issues of responsibility. I articulated and used an account of responsibility for unjust social structures and background conditions. This form of responsibility is grounded in our relationship to these structures and conditions. Many of us participate in and benefit from structures and conditions that unfairly disadvantage others. Taking responsibility often requires political action to change these structures and conditions. Although I believe that the third conception of responsibility helps to focus attention on important features and aspects of environmental migration, I did not try to justify this conception in a theoretical way or show that it is generally better than other conceptions of responsibility. Indeed, I believe that the three conceptions I considered are complementary in the sense that social responses to environmental migration will need to include all of them. The first conception of responsibility emphasizes human responsibility and the duty to aid. The second conception emphasizes juridical responsibility and the assignment of liabilities and costs. The third conception emphasizes political responsibility and the need to change structures and conditions. I emphasized the third conception because I believe it focuses ethical attention on ways needed to respond to the current situation.

ACKNOWLEDGMENTS

I would like to thank Ruth Macklin and William Ruddick for their probing questions and heartfelt encouragement. I would also like to thank the two anonymous reviewers for their very helpful comments.

REFERENCES

Betts, Alexander. 2013. *Survival Migration: Failed Governance and the Crisis of Displacement*. Cornell University Press.

Boden, T., G. Marland, and B. Andres. 2007. "Ranking of the World's Countries by 2007 Per Capita Fossil-Fuel CO_2 Emission Rates." Carbon Dioxide Information Analysis Center. https://www.eea.europa.eu/data-and-maps/data-providers-and-partners/carbon-dioxide-information-and-analysis.

Chakravarty, Shoilbal, Ananth Chikkatur, Heleen de Coninck, Stephen Pacala, Robert Socolow, and Massimo Tavoni. 2009. "Sharing Global CO_2 Emissions Reductions

Among One Billion High Emitters." *Proceedings of the National Academy of Sciences* 106 (29): 11884–11888.
Commission on Social Determinants of Health. 2008. "Closing the Gap in a Generation: Health Equity Through Action on the Social Determinants of Health." http://apps.who.int/iris/bitstream/handle/10665/43943/9789241563703_eng.pdf;jsessionid=F2CC4EE133E2D4932241A31A929F904D?sequence=1.
Dewey, John. 1954. *The Public and Its Problems*. Swallow Press.
Gardiner, Stephen, Simon Caney, Dale Jamieson, and Henry Shue. 2010. *Climate Ethics: Essential Readings*. Oxford University Press.
Hart, H. L. A. 2008. *Punishment and Responsibility: Essays in the Philosophy of Law*. 2nd ed. Oxford University Press.
Huber, D., and J. Gulledge. 2011. "Extreme Weather and Climate Change: Understanding the Link and Managing the Risk." C2ES. http://www.c2es.org/publications/extreme-weather-and-climate-change.
Intergovernmental Panel on Climate Change. 2014. *Climate Change 2014: Impacts, Adaptation, and Vulnerability*. World Meteorological Organization.
International Organization for Migration. 2017. "Migration and Climate Change." https://environmentalmigration.iom.int/iom-and-migration-environment-and-climate-change-mecc.
Kant, Immanuel. 1981. *Grounding for the Metaphysics of Morals*. Hackett.
Kelley, Colin P., Shahrzad Mohtadi, Mark A. Cane, Richard Seager, and Yochanan Kushnir 2015. "Climate Change and the Recent Syrian Drought." *Proceedings of the National Academy of Sciences* 112 (11): 3241–3246.
Klingler, Corina, Dennis Odudoya, and Katja Kuehlmeyer. 2018. "Migration, Health, and Ethics." *Bioethics* 32: 330–333.
McAdam, Jane. 2012. *Climate Change, Forced Migration, and International Law*. Oxford University Press.
Moodley, Vadi, Alphonse Gahima, and Suveshnee Munien. 2010. "Environmental Causes and Impacts of the Genocide in Rwanda: Case Studies of the Towns of Butare and Cyangugu." *Accord*, October 26. https://www.accord.org.za/ajcr-issues/environmental-causes-and-impacts-of-the-genocide-in-rwanda/.
National Oceanic and Atmospheric Administration, Earth Systems Research Laboratory. 2013. "Trends in Atmospheric Carbon Dioxide." Global Monitoring Laboratory. https://gml.noaa.gov/ccgg/trends/.
Rawls, John. 1971. *A Theory of Justice*. Harvard University Press.
Risse, Matthias. 2009. "The Right to Relocation: Disappearing Island Nations and the Common Ownership of the Earth." *Ethics & International Affairs* 23 (3): 281–299.
Robert D. Bulllard, and Beverly Wright. 2012. *The Wrong Complexion for Protection: How the Government Response to Disaster Endangers African American Communities*. NYU Press.
United Nations. 1951. "Convention and Protocol Relating to the Status of Refugees." https://cms.emergency.unhcr.org/documents/11982/55726/Convention+relat.
United Nations High Commissioner for Refugees. 2024. "UNHCR Statistics—The World in Numbers." https://data.unhcr.org/en/dataviz/6.
Moodley, V., A. Gahima, & S. Munien. 2010. "Environmental causes and impacts of the genocide in Rwanda: Case studies of the towns of Butare and Cyangugu." *African Journal on Conflict Resolution*, 10 (2).
Warner, Koko, Charles Ehrhart, Alex de Sherbinin, Susana B. Adamo, and Tricia Chai-Onn. 2009. "In Search of Shelter: Mapping the Effects of Climate Change on

Human Migration and Displacement." Columbia University. nfccc.int/resource/docs/2009/smsn/igo/056.pdf.
Wild, Verina, Deborah Zion, and Richard Ashcroft. 2015. "Health of Migrants: Approaches from a Public Health Ethics Perspective." *Public Health Ethics* 8: 107–109.
Wyman, Katrina. 2013. "Are We Morally Obligated to Assist Climate Change Migrants?" *Law & Ethics of Human Rights* 7 (2): 185–212.
Young, Iris M. 2011. *Responsibility for Justice*. Oxford University Press.

3

Health Challenges and the "Forced" Migration of the Cameroonian Middle Class

THIERRY NGOSSO

3.1 INTRODUCTION: DISRUPTING THE "FORCED" VERSUS "VOLUNTARY" DISTINCTION

Migration issues remain among the most important at the heart of the national and international political agendas. According to some polls, immigration was considered voters' primary concern in future American presidential elections (Saad 2024). Consider the ongoing legal and political battle over the agreement between the UK and Rwanda to send people who have made asylum claims to the UK government to Rwanda (Sen et al. 2022). Let us also think about the European pact on migration and asylum that the European Parliament recently validated, and which aims to harmonize the rules and conditions for welcoming migrants on European soil (De Bruycker 2022). Finally, let's consider questions related to climate migration and the fact that climate change represents the primary source of contemporary migration (Ghosh and Orchiston 2022). While it remains a crucial political issue, the migration phenomenon raises deep ethical concerns, including the moral relevance of borders and the conceptual status of "illegal" aliens. Beyond such considerations, what is even of greater relevance from an ethical standpoint regarding migration is how Western scholars have dominantly framed the discourse on migration and migration policies and how two debatable distinctions within Western politics have shaped our perception and handling of the migration phenomenon.

A subtle distinction is frequently made between refugees (political migrants) and economic migrants, assuming that refugees or political migrants are "forced" to leave their countries, while economic migrants have

Thierry Ngosso, *Health Challenges and the "Forced" Migration of the Cameroonian Middle Class*. In: *Forced Migration and Health Justice*. Edited by: Lisa A. Eckenwiler, Verina Wild, Anna Gotlib, Ryoa Chung, and Deborah Zion, Oxford University Press. © Oxford University Press (2026). DOI: 10.1093/oso/9780197795491.003.0003 "chosen" to do so (Ngosso and Oberprantacher 2018). This distinction has led to public immigration policies based on what has been called "selected migration" or "chosen immigration." The implications here are twofold: on the one hand, this distinction provides grounds for the claim that it is legitimate for a sovereign state to choose its immigrants. On the other hand, it suggests that the strength of the legitimacy of a sovereign state in choosing its immigrants is proportional to the lack of choice of the migrants. The more migration is considered "forced," the less select migration or chosen immigration policies are considered legitimate. When migrants are genuinely forced to leave their country of origin, the state's choice of immigrants becomes more problematic.

In attempting to counter such a distinction and its implications, one might argue that imminent threats to people's lives can be both political as well as economic, and hence that the very notion of "forced migration" itself as a scholarly concept raises some relevant ethical questions (Gibney 2018, 48–59). Being forced to do something or coerced to leave one's country does not necessarily eliminate the possibility of choosing. As Marylin Frye (1983) points out when discussing the role of coercion in the oppression and exploitation of women from a lesbian feminist perspective, coercion is less about the absence or lack of choice than about creating the conditions that make it impossible to choose "freely." For instance, if I am coerced or forced by an armed robber to choose between my life and handing over my car or my wallet, I am still "afforded" the possibility of choosing among several options (Card 1986, 153). However, the request of the armed robber is seriously tampering with my options or leaving me with options that are humanly very costly. With that understanding of coercion in mind, framing the notion of "forced migration" in the context of the political/economic migration distinction can be ethically problematic. In this respect, there are no genuine reasons to think that those who take the perilous path of the Mediterranean Sea, which each year swallows up thousands of Africans on the route toward the European "El Dorado," are less forced to leave their country than those whose government persecutes them for their political ideas or sexual orientation.

Another distinction concerning "economic migrants" is between middle-class and poor or lower-class immigrants. It is assumed that migrating to wealthier countries is a matter of coercion only for poor or lower-class people and, therefore, that the degrees of freedom and therefore of choice are greater for middle-class people. This may be true to some extent, but it should also be put into perspective, all things considered. Given the tortuous path of the Western Mediterranean route, which for sub-Saharans includes the thorny crossing of the Sahara before taking the boats and makeshift pirogues leading to Lampedusa, one might find it evident that few citizens of the African middle class would undertake such a dangerous and deadly adventure. According to the United Nations Refugee Agency, no fewer than 3,231 people were reported dead or missing at sea in the Mediterranean and the northwest Atlantic in 2021, compared to 1,881 in 2020, 1,510 in 2019, and more than 2,277 in 2018 (United Nations High Commissioner for Refugees 2022). The number of migrants who lost their lives on the road across the Sahara Desert and in remote border areas is believed to be even higher. The number of people dead or missing is still increasing, despite the relative decline in the total number of migrants.

The macabre and tragic toll of the route to the Western Mediterranean could explain why those who are part of the African middle class would be less constrained than poor migrants to resort to it if they wish to migrate to the West. Moreover, unlike poor migrants, migrants from the middle class have less dangerous and more comfortable options. For instance, in countries like Canada that practice selective immigration based on quotas, there are immigration programs and policies that are intended essentially to attract members of the middle classes from underdeveloped or emerging countries. Even if these programs are not explicitly presented as such, the requirements for submitting applications and the often very long and onerous nature of consular and other procedures de facto exclude poor people and those from the lowest social classes. Because they have the means to undertake such procedures without undue constraint, people from the middle class can weigh the pros and cons of their emigration and choose what best serves their interests. It is, therefore, not a question of life or death, as might be the case for people of modest social class. This reinforces the position that the immigration of economic migrants from the African middle class is more voluntary than that of poor economic migrants.

This conclusion must, however, be put into perspective. On the one hand, contrary to what many may think and as dangerous as the Western Mediterranean route may be, this journey is not just the preserve of poor immigrants. The Western Mediterranean route is not only dangerous but also very onerous. The road to the European El Dorado has become a lucrative business for many smugglers; it is estimated that some economic migrants must pay smugglers several thousand dollars. Therefore, even if the journey involving crossing the Mediterranean Sea is not absolutely inaccessible for poor immigrants, it is not easily accessible to many poor people. On the other hand, while one might think that African middle-class people can provide most of their essential needs for themselves and their families and may not need to leave their country of origin, there are circumstances and specific local challenges, such as the structurally poor conditions of the educational or healthcare systems, that can "force" them to migrate.

3.2 HEALTH INJUSTICE IN CAMEROON

The structurally poor conditions of the healthcare system in many sub-Saharan African countries, such as Cameroon, play a crucial role in the decision of many from the African middle class to migrate, and it provides an interesting case of how the issue of "forced migration" could play out in developing countries. Of course, this is not specific to Cameroon, but using Cameroon as a case study here provides some insights into the ethical dynamics that health issues and concerns play in the decision-making of the Cameroonian middle class to migrate.

Despite being the largest economy in Central Africa, with a GDP estimated in 2018 at $38.445 billion, Cameroon is a developing country ranked 98th in terms of its GDP and 152nd in terms of its gross income per capita, established at $1,544 in 2018. Even if Cameroon has a high literacy rate, 75%, and has one of the most educated populations in sub-Saharan Africa, the average duration of schooling remains five years, and life expectancy at birth was only 58.51 years in 2017. These data mean that the Human Development Index has been evaluated at 0.563, which puts Cameroon 150th out of 187 countries.

In terms of health, Cameroon is one of the countries ranked low by the World Health Organization (WHO), in particular because of the lack of a functional health insurance system, which makes access to basic healthcare extremely difficult for a good part of the population. This is true despite recent progress and even the launch in March 2024 of the pilot phase of the universal health coverage (UHC) program. Less than 10% of the population has health insurance, leaving households to contribute almost 83% of the cost of healthcare. Most people, therefore, rely mainly on their family and sometimes social networks to cover even their most basic healthcare needs. This context also favors using other therapeutic sources, such as churches or traditional medicine. Infectious and parasitic diseases and an increasing prevalence of cardiovascular disease, diabetes, and cancer dominate Cameroon's epidemiological profile. Infant mortality was around 9.5% in 2012, some of the leading causes of which were neonatal complications such as severe infections, asphyxia, prematurity, malaria, pneumonia, and diarrhea. In the larger population, the leading causes of death remain HIV/AIDS, respiratory infections, malaria, and diarrhea. These communicable diseases must be added to nutrition problems and perinatal conditions, which are the significant causes of morbidity and mortality. Note that the prevalence of HIV is 4.5%, and that of tuberculosis is about 23%. In addition, many other conditions have considerable prevalence, such as diabetes and high blood pressure, which represent significant costs in health expenditure. In addition, Cameroon is going through a human resources crisis, with a ratio of 1.1 doctors and 7.8 nurses and midwives per 10,000 inhabitants (WHO et al. 2010), partly due to the brain drain of healthcare personnel.

Despite some improvement, the Cameroonian healthcare system is still hindered by several significant challenges, including an underfunded and stressed health system with outdated or poorly maintained/managed infrastructure. Health expenditures continue to represent a very low percentage of GDP, despite the country's commitment under the Abuja Declaration, when many African Union member states met in Abuja, Nigeria, in April 2001 to allocate 15% of each country's GDP of the Union's budget to health. Other challenges include the lack of a robust healthcare workforce and the lack of equity in access to healthcare due to inadequate and unequal distribution of equipment, worsened by corruption and loose regulations that increase the system's inefficiency, to name a few. To address most of these challenges, in 2015 the Cameroonian government set up the "Health Sector Strategy 2016–2027" (Cameroon Ministry of Public Health 2015), which details public health policies with a dual perspective: contributing to accelerating the development of human capital for growth and sustainable development and aligning with the UN's Sustainable Development Goals by accelerating the implementation of universal health coverage.

3.2.1 Developmental Disabilities in the Cameroonian Healthcare System and Society

If there is little progress on improving healthcare in Cameroon, especially in ensuring a universal health coverage program, mental disorders of development and other intellectual handicaps or mental disabilities, especially among children, remain a blind spot within the structurally poor conditions of the Cameroonian health system (Djifack Tetinou et al. 2020). "Developmental disorders" generally refer to impairments in children's cognitive, behavioral, or language development (Hemming and Bouras 2016). Intellectual disabilities and comorbidities associated with diseases such as epilepsy, autism, and other conditions related to mental development are the poor cousins of public health policies in Cameroon (Toguem et al. 2022).

This is not, of course, a problem specific to Cameroon. Equity regarding developmental disorders, intellectual/mental disabilities, and mental health more broadly is a global structural injustice problem. There is a trend of neglecting developmental disabilities in many healthcare systems across the globe, irrespective of a country's economic status, which results in structural discrimination of people with mental illness or intellectual disabilities

(Gren Voldby et al. 2022). There is, therefore, a double structural injustice suffered by people with intellectual or mental disabilities.

On the one hand, their health needs are very rarely considered in either legislation or health systems in most countries, increasing health disparities with the rest of the population. They have less access to healthcare, affecting their health outcomes and making them more vulnerable to other social determinants. In the context of autism or language disorders, it is possible to remedy the disability or at least limit its pervasive effects if it is detected early and if potentially ill people receive appropriate care in time. But the fact that some health systems cannot even allow this type of diagnosis upstream worsens the already precarious situation of people living with or likely to develop a pathology linked to developmental disorders.

On the other hand, these people are stigmatized socially and discriminated against in the labor market, which profoundly affects their social status and self-esteem. According to a report by the WHO and UNICEF (2023), children and young people suffer most of the social exclusion and prejudice that come with a mental or intellectual disability diagnosis. According to that report, around 317 million children and young people had some health conditions that contributed to developmental disabilities in 2019.

This problem of structural injustice suffered by children and young people with developmental disorders or intellectual disabilities or those likely to become mentally disabled is made worse by the already critical situation of a health system as deficient as that of Cameroon. The lack of infrastructure, the lack of specialized medical personnel, geographical and financial inaccessibility, the poor care of diseases related to intellectual and mental disabilities in medical as well as in other social environments (schools, universities, churches, etc.) are made even worse in the Cameroonian context, where these intellectual or mental deficiencies are often associated with witchcraft.

Only two public medical structures suitable for people with intellectual and mental disabilities exist in the entire country. According to a 2019 report by the Organisation Suisse d'Aide aux Réfugiés (OSAR), access to specialized care, such as neurology or speech therapy, that significantly affects developmental disabilities in children and young people is seriously compromised in Cameroon. Not only is specialized care expensive and services often under-equipped, but the lack of specialist medical personnel is even more telling. For instance, in 2019 there were only 15 neurologists in the entire country, one neuro-pediatrician, and around five speech therapists, all of them in the private sector and all based in Douala, the economic capital of Cameroon (OSAR 2019). Such personnel scarcity makes it nearly impossible for children and young people who need mental care to access it. Nearby facilities are lacking, and traveling to Douala is impossible for most; even if one could travel, there are long waits to access services, averaging two months before obtaining a consultation. Consultation and other therapy costs are beyond many people's financial reach: a speech therapy assessment costs between 30,000 and 250,000 CFA francs, or between US$50 and US$415; the price of a consultation with assessment is 30,000 CFA francs, or US$50; and a simple consultation costs 10,000 CFA francs, or US$17 (OSAR 2019).

Besides the struggles of the Cameroonian healthcare system to accommodate the needs of children and young people with developmental disabilities, there is a very limited number of specialized schools that can take care of children with neuromotor disorders. The only specialized, but under-equipped, public school in the entire country that can accommodate these children is the Center for the Rehabilitation of the Disabled in Yaoundé. A very limited number of private specialized schools do exist, in Yaoundé and Douala, but they do not generally specialize in the care of children with neuromotor disorders and their fees are very high: between 400,000 and 3 million CFA francs, or between US$665 and US$5,000 for one year of support (ASAR 2019). Furthermore, there is no university training program in the field of speech therapy in Cameroon, and even though the Cameroon Academy of Neurology, created in 2018 and which has 15 members, offers a certain number of postgraduate training courses, it cannot compensate for the lack of more traditional training in public universities.[1]

The medical, educational, or social structural problems posed or revealed by the lack of adequate care for intellectually disabled people or children affected by some kind of developmental disorder are due to the lack of an adequate legislative framework in Cameroon to guide public mental health policy (medical, educational, security, etc.) and to protect the fundamental rights of people with mental or intellectual disabilities. There is incremental progress and recognition by the Cameroonian government of the importance of addressing the needs of people living with intellectual and mental disabilities, which recently led to "the introduction of a mental health curriculum in the national harmonized program for medical schools" (Ngasa et al. 2022, 693) and with the development of some pieces of mental health–related policies, laws, or decisions, such as those included in the National Health Development Plan for 2016–2020 (Minsanté 2016). Nevertheless, given the need for a multisectoral and multifaceted approach to mental health, only mental health legislation would be able to account for "the perspectives of the private sector, the finance system, the justice system, the education system, religious healers, traditional healers, traditional

1. See Cameroon Academy of Neurology (cameroon-academy-of-neurology.org).

leaders, and people living with mental illness and their families" (Ngasa et al. 2022, 693) and holistically address the issues following the ratification of the United Nations Convention of the Rights of Persons with Disabilities by the Cameroonian government in 2021.

This is the broader context that many in the Cameroonian middle class face and that puts them in a position where they may be "forced" to migrate to other countries, most often countries where there is not only adequate care for children living with disabilities but also a legislative framework and public policies that allow for the support of the mentally disabled children beyond the medical care they need, their better integration into society, and relief for families for whom this care can be both financially and emotionally costly. The issue for most Cameroonian middle-class families whose children are affected by these pathologies is not that they are unable to cover all the medical costs of treating the mental development-related illnesses, such as epilepsy, respiratory injuries, or choking. Often those who belong to the Cameroonian middle class have the financial means to make a single trip to another country to receive treatment for specific pathologies (a delicate surgical operation, the treatment of a specific pathology for which there is no specialist in Cameroon, etc.). This is a common practice even in wealthy countries.

Nevertheless, the nature of the pathologies linked to intellectual disabilities and what they require in terms of extra-medical measures raise very different issues for the families concerned, such as long-term support for children outside medical care, particularly when they are affected by an incurable mental disability or even when they require both medical care and supra-medical structures for optimal and permanent monitoring of their handicap. For many Cameroonian middle-class families with children suffering from mental disorders, intellectual handicaps, and mental developmental pathologies, what really matters is the permanent and long-term effective management of these pathologies.

Achieving such long-term management of mental and developmental illnesses goes beyond what may be required financially, either for the Cameroonian government or for the families themselves. If it were only about the affordability of medical care, perhaps many of those families would not be "forced" to migrate. But the long-term management of mental and developmental pathologies requires a complete reorganization of society: building specialized schools, developing new designs for roads and public buildings, adding provisions in labor market policies, setting up national campaigns against the stigmatization of people living with intellectual disabilities, and more. Such a complete reorganization of Cameroonian society seems to be a very long shot timewise for many of those families who need to address now the pressing need of their intellectually disabled child and who are therefore "forced" to migrate to give their children a chance to live a meaningful life despite their handicaps.

3.3 HEALTH AND OTHER INJUSTICES FACING CAREGIVERS

Cameroonian middle-class families are "forced" to migrate not just to find adequate medical and social support for their children suffering from mental disabilities. An equally important factor that would "force" them to migrate is the stress and anxiety that take hold of parents and other members of the extended family who must accompany their children through the ups and downs of their handicap, which can, in turn, affect the mental health of these family members. In this case, it is essential to point out that mothers are the ones who often bear the more significant part of the emotional, physical, and mental burdens of accompanying children with mental disabilities and who are, therefore, disproportionately affected (Wamba et al. 2021).

Seeing the health of one's mentally disabled child not being addressed optimally due to the structural deficiencies of the Cameroonian health system, along with the risk of sinking into depression or suffering mental health issues oneself due to the heavy burden of supporting one's child in such a precarious environment is often enough to "force" those who have the capacity and the "luck" to emigrate to do so. The notion of "luck" is worth mentioning here because, at the other end of the migration process, potential host countries such as Canada will limit migration that is too costly to their national healthcare system in the name of "reasonable public charge." Nevertheless, "health" migrants from Cameroon may be "lucky" enough to get admitted if the intellectual handicap of their child is not profoundly severe and therefore not too costly for the receiving country and if the expertise they themselves bring to that country overrides the costs associated with caring for their child. Moreover, once they are "forced" to migrate, these Cameroonian middle-class families may look for other countries that provide the same overall care and multifaceted support for their intellectually disabled child, but with fewer health restrictions or conditions of entry.

Overall, this case study allows us to put the notion of "forced migration" into perspective. It is no longer the prerogative of people persecuted for various reasons nor of people whose economic opportunities are seriously compromised in their country of origin. It could and should be legitimately extended and applied to people with more than enough or high income in many African developing countries such as Cameroon, whose governments are unable or unwilling to set up or develop a comprehensive healthcare and social system that can holistically address the conditions of people affected by mental and developmental illness, especially children and young people, and the conditions of their families who can be vulnerable to potential mental health issues themselves.

3.4 PERPETUATING INEQUITIES AND UNDERMINING SOLIDARITY AND SOCIAL CHANGE

Beyond the health-grounded recalibration of the notion of "forced migration," it is essential to note that the forced migration of the Cameroonian middle class is not the only morally problematic consequence of a structurally weak health system when it comes to intellectual disabilities and other mental and developmental illnesses. The other morally problematic consequences are the reinforcement of inequalities of opportunity and even of outcomes between middle-class families and poor families having to support children with mental disabilities (Ngui et al. 2010) and the neutralization of any catalyst for the convergence of social and political struggles, which could lead to substantial improvements in the health system and post-medical support for the mentally disabled.

On the one hand, when Cameroonian middle-class and poor families face the same situation in supporting a mentally disabled child or young person, the poor families cannot even choose to emigrate due to their very limited resources. This does not mean that Cameroonian middle-class families are not forced to migrate because they can choose to do so. Recall Frye's interpretation of "coercion." Being forced to do something does not nullify the possibility of choosing. Coercion tampers with the options or choices we are given. It only means, ironically, that poor families are not even afforded the choice of being "forced" to migrate. Such lack of equality of opportunities, especially for children with mental disabilities, is morally wrong and can be addressed only by a reformed health and social system in Cameroon that will allow all Cameroonian families to locally support their mentally disabled members equally.

On the other hand, the fact that Cameroonian middle-class families are "forced" to migrate prevents the emergence of solidarity among the various economic classes, which would force leaders and policymakers to take these health problems and their social consequences seriously. In fact, most Cameroonian families do not have one or more mentally disabled children or young people who require rigorous medical and post-medical monitoring. Therefore, this health and social issue is not at the heart of the most vocal social demands. Only families who share the burden of supporting mentally disabled people, especially children and young people, know the obstacle course that this represents in a health and social context such as that of Cameroon and can coalesce their civic efforts to put these issues at the heart of public discussion. But the fact that some families are forced to emigrate and have the financial means to do so short-circuits any potential solidarity between these families, reinforces an unhealthy individualism between members of the same national community, and contributes to the status quo of a system that does not take the care of mentally disabled people seriously.

People can be "forced" to leave their country because they are poor or threatened. But a structurally broken health and social system that cannot provide adequate care and extra-medical support for families whose children suffer from intellectual handicaps or mental disabilities, as is the case in Cameroon, can also force middle-class families from developing countries to emigrate to wealthier countries that offer better care, even if it means giving up an advantageous social status in their home country. Such a move does not only increase and worsen health inequalities and the gap between middle-class and poor families in contexts like Cameroon, where the government is either unable or unwilling to build a healthcare system that can provide basic healthcare and extra-medical support for mentally disabled people, especially children. Such a move also prevents social forces that may help address this enormous health challenge from coalescing in the long run.

REFERENCES

Cameroon Ministry of Public Health. 2015. "Health Sector Strategy 2016–2027." https://www.minsante.cm/site/?q=en/content/health-sector-strategy-2016-2027-0.

Card, Claudia. 1986. "Oppression and Resistance: Frye's Politics of Reality." *Hypatia* 1, no. 1: 149–166.

De Bruycker, Philippe. 2022. "The New Pact on Migration and Asylum: What It Is Not and What It Could Have Been." In *Reforming the Common European Asylum System: Opportunities, Pitfalls, and Downsides of the Commission Proposals for a New Pact on Migration and Asylum*, edited by Daniel Thym and Odysseus Academic Network. Baden-Baden.

Djifack Tetinou, Franklin, Seraphin Nguefack, Félécité Ndongmo Nguefack, et al. 2020. "Comorbidities Associated with Pediatric Epilepsy at a Cameroonian Tertiary Teaching Hospital: A Cross-Sectional Study." *PAMJ Clinical Medicine* 3 (127). https://www.clinical-medicine.panafrican-med-journal.com//content/article/3/127/full.

Frye, Marilyn. 1983. *Politics of Reality: Essays in Feminist Theory*. Crossing Press.

Ghosh, Rajan Chandra, and Caroline Orchiston. 2022. "A Systematic Review of Climate Migration Research: Gaps in Existing Literature." *SN Social Sciences* 2: 47. https://doi.org/10.1007/s43545-022-00341-8.

Gibney, Matthew J. 2018. "Political Theory, Ethics and Forced Migration." In *The Oxford Handbook of Refugee and Forced Migration Studies*, edited by Elena Fiddian-Qasmiyeh and Gil Loescher. Oxford University Press.

Gren Voldby, Katrine, Lone Christina Hellström, Marie Eva Berg, and Lena Eplov. 2022. "Structural Discrimination Against People with Mental Illness: A Scoping Review." *SSM Mental Health* 2: 100117. https://doi.org/10.1016/j.ssmmh.2022.100117.

Hemmings, Colin, and Nick Bouras, eds. 2016. *Psychiatric and Behavioural Disorders in Intellectual and Developmental Disabilities*. Cambridge University Press.

Minsanté. 2016. "National Health Development Plan 2016–2020." https://www.minsante.cm/site/?q=en/content/national-health-development-plan-nhdp-2016-2020.

Ngasa, Stewart, Didier Demassosso, Neh Chang, and Etienne Assonganyi. 2022. "Mental Health Legislation: A Defect in Cameroon's Health System." *The Lancet Psychiatry* 9 (9): 693–694.

Ngosso, Thierry, and Andreas Oberprantacher. 2018. "Réfugiés ou Migrants? Réflexion Critique sur une Populaire, mais Problématique Distinction." *Ethica* 2 (2): 63–90.

Ngui, Emmanuel, Lincoln Khasakhala, David Ndetei, and Laura Weiss Roberts. 2010. "Mental Disorders, Health Inequalities, and Ethics: A Global Perspective." *International Review of Psychiatry* 22 (3): 235–244.

Organisation Suisse d'aide aux Réfugiés. 2019. "Cameroon: Accès à des Soins de Santé et à une Education Spécialisée: Recherche rapide de l'analyse-pays de l'OSAR." Berne, February 15. https://www.refugeecouncil.ch/fileadmin/user_upload/Publikationen/Herkunftslaenderberichte/Afrika/Kamerun/190215-kam-acces-soins-medicaux-f.pdf.

Piyal, Sen, Grace Crowley, Paul Arnell, et al. 2022. "The UK's Exportation of Asylum Obligations to Rwanda: A Challenge to Mental Health, Ethics and the Law." *Medicine, Science and the Law* 62 (3): 165–167.

Saad, Lydia. 2024. "Inflation, Immigration Rank Among Top U.S. Issue Concerns." Gallup. https://news.gallup.com/poll/642887/inflation-immigration-rank-among-top-issue-concerns.aspx.

Toguem, Michael Guy, Manasi Kumar, David Ndetei, François Erero Njiengwe, and Frederick Owiti. 2022. "A Situational Analysis of the Mental Health System of the West Region of Cameroon Using the World Health Organization's Assessment Instrument for Mental Health Systems (WHO-AIM3)." *International Journal of Mental Health Systems* 16 (18). https://doi.org/10.1186/s13033-022-00528-9.

United Nations High Commissioner for Refugees. 2022. "Les statistiques du HCR sur les traversées de la Méditerranée révèlent un nombre croissant de morts et de tragédies en mer." https://www.unhcr.org/fr/actualites/briefing-notes/les-statistiques-du-hcr-sur-les-traversees-de-la-mediterranee-revelent-un.

Wamba, Nguimabou Valdés, and Jacques-Philippe Tsala Tsala. 2021. "Intellectual Disability in Children and Family Resilience: Clinical Case of Cameroonian Families." *Acta Scientific Medical Sciences* 5 (4): 48–61.

World Health Organization and UNICEF. 2023. "Global Report on Children with Development Disabilities." September 15. https://www.unicef.org/documents/global-report-children-developmental-disabilities.

World Health Organization. 2010. AHWO Cameroon Fact Sheet.

4

"You Venezuelans Are Shameless!"

Connecting Reproductive and Immigration (In)Justice

ALLISON B. WOLF

4.1 INTRODUCTION

When the 22-year-old Afro-Venezuelan woman Rosmary Acacio discovered she was pregnant, she did not know what to do. Having only recently arrived in Colombia, she knew neither her rights nor the services available to her as a Venezuelan migrant. Luckily for Acacio, one of her neighbors helped her, and she sought care in her third trimester at Erasmo Meoz University Hospital in Cúcuta, where she was informed that receiving prenatal care at their facility was required for her to give birth there. She did seek such services for a month before going into labor, despite enduring mistreatment and indignities during her prenatal visits by the head nurse, who treated her with disgust. Acacio explained through tears, "I think she was racist. She looked at me with disdain and I felt humiliated. She always tried to avoid attending to me. If I came in second, she would see me last; sometimes she wouldn't even give me the bracelet to enter the clinic and get in line. When it was time for a vaginal exam or some other type of check, she would avoid doing it at all costs; she would always have students do it" (Telléz 2022).

Despite these experiences, Acacio hoped the birth would proceed without incident, and at first, it did. Things changed, however, when her baby started crowning. After the physician on call prepared Acacio for delivery and started wheeling her into a newly renovated delivery room, they were stopped by a nurse and told they could not enter the delivery room because one of the hospital's administrators had arrived to see the new facility. Acacio recounted, "When the nurse did that, the doctor reprimanded her and told her to stop because she was risking mine and my son's lives. . . . At the

Allison B. Wolf, *"You Venezuelans Are Shameless!"*. In: *Forced Migration and Health Justice*. Edited by: Lisa A. Eckenwiler, Verina Wild, Anna Gotlib, Ryoa Chung, and Deborah Zion, Oxford University Press. © Oxford University Press (2026). DOI: 10.1093/oso/9780197795491.003.0004 same time, two doctors were physically pulling me in different directions by my hands and feet to force me onto a special stretcher. In the midst of all of that, they then told me I had too much urine in my bladder, which was a risk to the baby" (Telléz 2022).

In response to the situation and still fighting with hospital staff, the physician adjusted the baby's position and inserted a catheter to remove the urine. When the procedure was completed, they removed the catheter with such force that the baby was born with a hole in his jaw. And then, during the delivery itself, the physician performed an episiotomy without Acacio's knowledge or consent.

Acacio's mistreatment did not end with the birth of her son. The hospital staff did not let her see her son for several hours and provided no explanation for the delay or information about his health. When staff brought Acacio her son around six o'clock in the evening, he was bloody and dark; it appeared that nobody had cleaned him. When they finally bathed her son the next morning, Acacio noticed that he had a four-centimeter-long cut on his face, for which, again, she received no explanation (Téllez 2022).

Acacio is one of many pregnant Venezuelan migrants who are increasingly enduring obstetric violence and other injustices when they seek reproductive care in Colombia. Scholars have documented immigration injustices related to gender, race, class, and sexual orientation; however, they rarely explore the connections between reproductive injustice (including obstetric violence) and immigration injustice, leading them to miss key aspects of both. And remedying this gap in our understanding requires connecting the dots between obstetric (and other reproductive) care and immigration status, country of origin, and the treatment of migrants and asylum seekers in the host nation.

This essay aspires to do just that by utilizing a feminist framework of immigration justice. To accomplish this, I will begin by offering a brief overview of recent Venezuelan migration to Colombia and the core push factors driving pregnant Venezuelans specifically to migrate. Then I present some fundamental challenges pregnant Venezuelans like Acacio face in relation to reproductive healthcare in Colombia. Finally, I suggest some inherent connections between reproductive healthcare injustices, principally obstetric violence, and immigration injustice.

4.2 MIGRATION OF PREGNANT VENEZUELANS TO COLOMBIA: A BRIEF OVERVIEW

Pregnant Venezuelans are just one group of the millions of Venezuelans who have fled their country in recent years. The phenomenon began when Hugo

Chávez assumed power and wealthy, highly educated Venezuelans left for the United States, Spain, and Colombia (LaRosa and Mejía 2017). They were followed by middle-class Venezuelan professionals (Economía y Negocios 2019). But starting around 2015, Venezuelans began to flee *en masse* amid a complex humanitarian crisis with an economy in free fall, runaway inflation, a collapsed healthcare system, pervasive political instability and unrest that left many without food or access to medical treatment (Inter-American Commission on Human Rights 2019). As of late 2019, over 4.5 million Venezuelans had left their country (United Nations High Commissioner for Refugees [UNHCR] 2019, 2020), over 13% of its total population (Organization of American States 2019). By March 2020, the number had reached 5 million, or 16% of Venezuela's total population (International Organization for Migration 2025). As of October 2021, there were nearly 6 million displaced Venezuelans throughout the world (R4V 2021). And according to the UN Refugee Agency, as of early 2024 roughly 7.7 million Venezuelan nationals had left, almost 3 million of whom reside in Colombia (UNHCR 2024).

Colombia has done more to welcome Venezuelans than any other nation. For example, Colombia kept its borders open to Venezuelans (except during the COVID-19 pandemic) and extended citizenship to children born to Venezuelan parents on Colombian soil (Bartsfield 2019; Kurmanaev and González 2019). In 2017, it created a permit exclusively for Venezuelan nationals called *Permiso Especial de Permanencia*, allowing its holder to work and access healthcare and education for two years. Most recently, in February 2021, the Colombian government announced that it would regularize recently arrived Venezuelans by offering them Temporary Protective Status for up to 10 years (Ministerio de Relaciones Exteriores, Colombia 2021).

With respect to healthcare, all migrants in Colombia are entitled to emergency and public health services, regardless of their status (Ministerio de Salud y Protección Social, Colombia 2018). Since 2017, pregnant migrants have also had the legal right to prenatal, obstetric, and postpartum care (Quintero et al. 2023). Access to these and other healthcare services have expanded even further since 2021 as part of Temporary Status Protection that allows Venezuelans, "to affiliate with an insurance program through their places of employment or be covered by the social assistance program for lower income or vulnerable populations" (Giraldo et al. 2021, 2).

Beyond formal access to healthcare, the availability and quality of reproductive health services in Colombia stands in stark contrast with the reality in Venezuela. Whereas Colombia has a strong healthcare system that offers high-quality services, Venezuela's healthcare system collapsed long ago, and there are severe shortages of medicines (Martinez 2019). Maternal mortality is skyrocketing, extreme maternal morbidity has increased fourfold, cases of low-birthweight infants and perinatal deaths have more than doubled, and cases of gestational syphilis have dramatically increased (Solano et al. 2024). Under these circumstances, pregnant Venezuelans are afraid to give birth in their home nation. And even when they would prefer doing so, it is often economically impossible since the pregnant person must buy and bring their own supplies to the birth (which costs roughly $14.50 at a time when the monthly minimum wage in Venezuela is less than $1) (Martinez 2019). So pregnant Venezuelans feel compelled (if not forced) to seek reproductive care in Colombia, where, despite the legal framework, extensive healthcare infrastructure, and well-trained healthcare providers, they face various barriers to acquiring care and all too often are victims of both immigration injustice and obstetric violence when they do.

4.3 REPRODUCTIVE INJUSTICES MIGRANTS FACE IN COLOMBIA

Generally speaking, pregnant Venezuelans in Colombia face barriers to accessing reproductive care that include, but are not limited to, a lack of information or outright disinformation about their rights to access healthcare services, denial of healthcare services, cost, xenophobia, and violence (Jaramillo et al. 2021). Among undocumented pregnant Venezuelan migrants who arrived in Colombia before the first trimester of pregnancy, 42.4% received no prenatal care (Giraldo et al. 2021). As for those who became pregnant in Colombia, only 22.1% received prenatal care during the first trimester (compared to 97.5% of Colombian women) (Fernández-Niño et al. 2019). The Ministry of External Affairs reports that 76.8% of the 8,209 undocumented pregnant Venezuelan migrants registered in 2018 received no form of prenatal care at all. Rather than focusing on these broader issues, though, I will center the ways in which some migrants, like Acacio, experience obstetric violence in the process of receiving reproductive care (Ministerio de Relaciones Exteriores, Colombia. 2018).

"Obstetric violence" refers to violence committed by medical practitioners while delivering healthcare related to pregnancy and childbirth. Most commonly, "obstetric violence" references abuses and assaults that occur in the course of labor and delivery—forced cesarean sections, procedures (such as episiotomies, vaginal exams, and rupturing membranes) performed without the laboring person's knowledge or consent, physically trying to prevent birth while waiting for a doctor to arrive, and physically restraining the laboring person—but it may also refer to abuses, indignities, and assaults incurred during prenatal or postpartum care via the denial of treatment, verbal humiliations, invasive practices, a disregard for pain, lack of privacy during vaginal exams, unnecessary use of medication, and sexual assault (Seals Allers 2020). Anna Annborn and Hafrún Rafnar Finnbogadóttir (2022) divide these experiences into four categories: (1) lack of information and consent, (2) insufficient pain relief, (3) lack of trust and security, and (4) the experience of abuse, including threats of violence from healthcare providers and birth experiences compared to rape. Farah Diaz-Tello (2016) adds threats of calling law enforcement or child protective services against pregnant persons who refuse recommended procedures. I have argued that obstetric violence also includes any action during prenatal care, labor and delivery, and postpartum care that perpetrates "metaphysical violence," or "violence that affects who or what one is" (Wolf 2013, 104).

Consistent with these definitions, we can identify various ways in which pregnant Venezuelan migrants, like Acacio, experience this type of violence in Colombia (Wolf 2022). First, they face verbal abuse and xenophobia when seeking or receiving obstetric care; pregnant migrants are constantly being told that they should go back to their country, are chastised for "coming to Colombia to have babies," and are being told that they somehow deserve their mistreatment. More specifically, migrants report being told the following:

- "I don't care if you die, and I don't care about your mental health issues. I am only here to attend to your wounds." (Téllez 2022)
- "You Venezuelans are shameless coming to Colombia to have babies!" (Téllez 2022)
- "Child, you better pack your things and go back to your country where they can attend to you because here, we are already doing too much to help the Venezuelans who come." (Arenas 2019)
- "[Losing your baby] is your fault for getting pregnant. . . . [Y]ou Venezuelans need to take better care of yourselves." (Téllez 2022)
- "It's fun to make babies, but not to have them." (Vallana-Sala 2019, 1)
- "Here we are doing you a favor." (Arenas 2019)

In addition to verbal abuse and xenophobia, pregnant Venezuelans endure physical and emotional violence, including (but not limited to) healthcare providers performing procedures and examinations without the patient's knowledge, not letting new mothers see their babies, physical restraint during birth, and verbal and racist abuse (Téllez 2022). In fact, we saw most of these in Acacio's case. For example, she was physically restrained by two healthcare providers, who then performed an episiotomy without her knowledge or consent, and she was unable to see her son. And pregnant migrants face these issues regardless of their legal status and formal efforts by the Colombian government granting them access to such services, which suggests that the injustices result more from oppression than, for example, a lack of rights or formal legal status. Since the core guiding analytic concept of feminist ethics and philosophy is identifying and resisting oppression, a feminist approach can provide understanding in addressing these issues, which is what I will do in the remainder of this analysis.

4.4 CONNECTING REPRODUCTIVE AND IMMIGRATION (IN)JUSTICES: A FEMINIST APPROACH

Showing the connections between reproductive and immigration injustices requires briefly defining "immigration (in)justice." While some define immigration justice as being about protecting immigrants' human rights or a nation's border and admissions policies (such that immigration justice is achieved with more open or closed borders), I employ a feminist approach to immigration justice based on Iris Marion Young's (1990) account of social justice elaborated in *Justice and the Politics of Difference*. According to that conception, justice is neither synonymous with nor reducible to distributive justice; justice is, instead, concerned with social justice, the degree to which a society contains and supports the institutional conditions necessary for the realization of values needed to live a good life.

According to Young (1990, 37), such values can be encompassed by the ability to (1) develop and exercise one's capacities and express one's experience and (2) participate in determining one's actions and the conditions of one's action. And, Young suggests, since the institutional and social conditions required for the development of these capacities is the absence of structural domination and oppression, we can extrapolate that two social conditions define injustice: "oppression, the institutional constraint on self-development, and domination, the institutional constraint on self-determination" (37). In other words, justice is the absence of oppression and domination.

I have extended Young's ideas about justice to the context of migration. More specifically, I have argued elsewhere that immigration justice is fundamentally about identifying and resisting the oppression of immigrants, asylum seekers, refugees, and displaced persons in policies, practices, and norms related to migration and their effects such that if a policy or practice related to migration creates, perpetrates, and/or reflects oppression, it is unjust (Wolf 2020). Understanding what this entails, though, requires explaining more on the nature of oppression.

As Marilyn Frye (1983) explains in her landmark essay, oppression is like a bird cage that traps social groups and their members simply because they are members of those groups. Oppression catches these groups and their members "between or among forces and barriers which are so related to each other that jointly they restrain, restrict, or prevent the thing's motion or mobility" (2) in ways that are neither random, accidental, occasional, avoidable, nor the result of bad luck or the actions of a few bad apples. Under oppression, structures "work *together* to reduce, immobilize, and mold the oppressed" and placing them in a double bind, or a situation where their "options are reduced to a very few and all of them expose one to penalty, censure, or deprivation" (Frye 1983, 3).

People belong to multiple social groups, however, which means that (1) individuals may both experience and perpetuate oppression depending on the context, and (2) oppression is perpetuated and experienced in various manifestations (or, as Young refers to them, faces). According to Young, there are at least five faces of oppression: exploitation, marginalization, powerlessness, cultural imperialism, and systemic violence. I have argued elsewhere that the migration context includes at least two more: xenophobia and derivatization (Wolf 2019, 2020, 2021). The larger point, though, is that any time immigration policies, practices, and/or norms manifest one (or more) of these faces, they are oppressive, and thus, by definition, unjust.

This feminist conception of immigration justice makes evident that evaluating policies and practices toward migrants, asylum seekers, refugees, and displaced persons requires probing whether such policies, including those related to healthcare, create, perpetuate, or reflect oppression. And when this is our task, not only the ways that reproductive healthcare for pregnant migrants is oppressive become visible but also the fact that obstetric violence is not incidentally or randomly being perpetrated on migrant bodies. To the contrary, such treatment forms part of the larger cage of oppression that traps pregnant migrants in double binds just because of their gender and nationality. In particular, obstetric violence is a manifestation of oppression against migrants, a way of furthering oppression against migrants, and a consequence of oppression against pregnant migrants (Wolf 2022). In other words, it is one way immigration injustice is concretely experienced by pregnant migrants, it is a mechanism for treating such migrants unjustly, and it is the result of other types of immigration injustices.

Returning to Acacio's experience illuminates how obstetric violence and immigration injustice are connected in the ways that I just described. While it is true that Colombian women experience obstetric violence, the reasons, and ways Acacio experienced it is inseparable from her being a pregnant Afro-Venezuelan migrant in Colombia. More specifically, the obstetric violence she faced was a manifestation of anti-Venezuelan xenophobia specifically, was a tool to carry out immigration injustice against Acacio and was a result of immigration injustice against Venezuelans in Colombia.

First, obstetric violence forms part of the cage that traps pregnant migrants in double binds because of their immigration status and nationality. As such, it is a way that oppression manifests itself in the lives of specific migrants. As we saw in Acacio's case, for example, if a migrant does not seek prenatal care, then she is told she cannot access obstetric care. But when she sought prenatal care, she faced discrimination, violence, xenophobic comments, and other indignities. In this way, as Juliana Mateus Téllez (2022) puts it, "obstetric violence in Colombia against Venezuelan women mixes with xenophobia, discrimination and even racism." In other words, it is one way immigration injustice manifests in the lives of pregnant migrants.

Second, obstetric violence is a tool to carry out immigration injustice; it is both an implicit and an explicit tool for sending the message "You are not welcome." That is, obstetric violence is a way to communicate the message to migrants that if they get "out of their place" (e.g., by demanding rights, care, and sanctioned inclusion in the host nation), then they will face the consequences (e.g., abuse, violence, and discrimination). Let me be clear: I am not saying that this is (or at least is not necessarily) intentional. To the contrary, like many expressions of oppression, it is likely not. Nevertheless, the connection between oppression and immigration injustice is clearly evident, for example, in comments made to Acacio (as well as other pregnant Venezuelans) recounted earlier, insinuating or explicitly stating that Venezuelans should stop having babies in Colombia, should go home, or, most clearly, that they deserve the mistreatment they receive for having gotten pregnant and that Colombians are doing them a favor by providing any care to them at all. In these cases, obstetric violence is an especially pernicious form of both structural health injustice and immigration injustice since it both reflects inherent sexism in obstetric care and, simultaneously, serves to uphold colonialist, racist, classist, and sexist norms that inform immigration policy.

Finally, obstetric violence results from (indeed, is made possible by) existing immigration injustices such that existing anti-immigrant oppression (as opposed to legal status) makes this kind of treatment possible in the first place. I think Amy Reed-Sandoval's (2020b) conception of being socially (rather than legally) undocumented is useful here. According to Reed-Sandoval, being socially undocumented refers to the fact that, despite having documents or other permissions to reside in the US, many Latinx migrants are perceived as being in irregular status or as being in the country illegitimately. While I do not have the space to rehearse Reed-Sandoval's account and its implications in depth here, I do think that her account of being socially undocumented indicates how many of the reasons that undocumented immigrants do or do not face oppression is often not because of legal status but rather "because of how [they are] perceived" (2020b, 4).

In Acacio's case, the fact that she is perceived as an undocumented migrant without rights or claims to health services creates the conditions under which it is seen as acceptable to mistreat her in the ways described. For example, if she were not perceived as an undocumented migrant, healthcare providers would not say things like "You Venezuelans are shameless" or "Pack your things and go back to your country" or "We are doing you a favor." And I certainly think it is plausible that a nurse thought it acceptable to block the entrance into a delivery room or not bathe a newborn baby precisely because they did not fear repercussions that they would certainly have been vulnerable to had upper-class Colombians received such treatment. In this way, again, obstetric violence and other abuses related to reproductive healthcare are a consequence of immigration injustice.

4.5 CONCLUDING THOUGHTS

Given my insistence that identifying and addressing the inherent connections between reproductive injustice and immigration injustice requires using a feminist framework of immigration justice that centers oppression, before concluding I want to offer a few general suggestions of what doing so might accomplish. Of course, I do not have the space to offer in-depth solutions, but here are some initial ideas:

1. Colombia and the international community must create policies that go beyond mere formal access to reproductive healthcare services to also provide resources for programs to combat xenophobia in the healthcare setting.
2. Healthcare providers and staff must be held accountable for treating pregnant migrants in oppressive ways. This could include, for example, consequences for hiring and promotion for nurses, like those who Acacio dealt with, who mistreat pregnant migrants.
3. The Colombian government should do more outreach to inform migrants of how and where to receive reproductive healthcare. This could include working with hospitals and other healthcare facilities as well as creating public service campaigns.
4. Healthcare providers need to be educated on the circumstances surrounding immigration—both the circumstances in Venezuela and what migrants face on the journey (sexual violence, the conditions of the paths, etc.) so that they learn what care/services they will require. While it may be naive, I think this will also humanize Venezuelan migrants, including those who are pregnant, to combat xenophobia and the injustices discussed here.

5. The Colombian government and other actors (both domestic and international) need to take steps to respond to oppression and other barriers migrants face and generate specific reproductive healthcare needs. For example, they must do more to prevent sexual assault and rape, which results in unwanted pregnancy and increased need for reproductive health services and mental health services.
6. Bioethicists, immigration scholars, and activists need to join forces to fight these problems.

I am a philosopher, not a policymaker, and these are only some initial ideas that require further development. Still, this analysis shows that addressing the injustices that Acacio and so many other pregnant Venezuelans face requires seeing reproductive justice and immigration injustice as inherently connected via overlapping and intersecting oppressions. What happened to Rosmary Acacio happened because she was a pregnant, poor, Afro-Venezuelan immigrant. Improving the healthcare system for her, and everyone else, requires resisting all the oppressions she endured. I hope that what I have said here advances our efforts in doing just that.

REFERENCES

Annborn, Anna and Hafrún Rafnar Finnbogadóttir. 2022. "Obstetric Violence: A Qualitive Interview Study." *Midwifery* 105: 3–6.

Arenas, Natalia. 2019. "Para las Venezolanas el Embarazo es una Encrucijada." *070*, July 12. https://cerosetenta.uniandes.edu.co/para-las-venezolanas-el-embarazo-es-una-encrucijada/.

Bartsfield, Jenny. 2019. "Colombia Gives Venezuela Newborns a Start in Life." United Nations Refugee Agency. https://www.unhcr.org/en-us/news/stories/2019/10/5da42be64/colombia-gives-venezuela-newborns-start-life.html.

Calderón Jaramillo, Mariana, Rocío Murad, Natalia Acevado Guerrero, Luz Janeth Forero, and Juan Carlos Rivillas. 2021. "Sexual and Reproductive Health Needs: Perspectives of Venezuelan Migrant Population at Four Border Cities." *La Manzana de la Discordia* 16 (1): 3–23.

Diaz-Tello, Farah. 2016. "Invisible wounds: obstetric violence in the United States." *Reproductive Health Matters* 24 (47): 56–64, DOI: 10.1016/j.rhm.2016.04.004.

Economía y Negocios. 2019. "Cuánto ganan, dónde, y qué tipo de empleo tienen los venezolanos." *El Tiempo*, September 19. https://www.eltiempo.com/economia/sectores/salario-de-venezolanos-en-colombia-donde-trabajan-y-en-que-empleos-segun-dane-413732.

Fernández-Niño, Julián Alfredo, Maylen Liseth Rojas-Botero, Ietza Bojorquez-Chapela, et al. 2019. "Situación de Salud de Gestantes Migrantes Venezolanas en el Caribe Colombiano: Primer Reporte para una Respuesta Rápida en Salud Pública." *Revista Universidad Industrial Santander Salud* 51 (3): 208–219.

Frye, Marilyn. 1983. *The Politics of Reality*. Crossing Press.

Giraldo, Vanesa, Rita Sobxzyk, Julian Alfredo, Maylen Fernández-Niño, Liseth Rojas-Botero, and Ietza Bojorquez. 2021. "Prenatal Care of Venezuelans in

Colombia: Migrants Navigating the Healthcare System." *Revista de Saúde Pública* 55 (2): 49.

International Organization for Migration. 2025. "Venezuelan Refugee and Migrant Crisis." https://www.iom.int/venezuela-refugee-and-migrant-crisis.

Kurmanaev, Anatoly, and Jenny Carolina González. 2019. "Colombia Offers Citizenship to 24,000 Children of Venezuelan Refugees." *New York Times*, August 5. https://www.nytimes.com/2019/08/05/world/americas/colombia-citizenship-venezuelans.html.

LaRosa, Michael J. and Germán R. Mejía. 2017. *Colombia: A Concise Contemporary History*. Rowman & Littlefield.

Martinez, Marta. 2019. "Inside the Colombian 'War Hospital' Treating Venezuela's Pregnancy Crisis." *New Humanitarian*, November 27. https://www.thenewhumanitarian.org/news-feature/2019/11/27/Venezuela-Colombia-pregnant-women-birth-reproductive-rights-migration-Cucuta-maternal-care-migrants-refugees.

Ministerio de Relaciones Exteriores, Colombia. 2018. "RAMV Informe Final: Registro Administrativo de Migrantes Venezolanos en Colombia."

Ministerio de Relaciones Exteriores, Colombia. 2021. "Decreto 216 de 2021." https://www.funcionpublica.gov.co/eva/gestornormativo/norma.php?i=159606.

Ministerio de Salud y Protección Social, Colombia. 2018. "*Plan de Respuesta del Sector Salud al Fenómeno Migratorio*." Bogotá.

Organization of American States. 2019. "Report to Address the Regional Crisis Caused by Venezuela's Migrant and Refugee Flows." https://www.oas.org/documents/eng/press/OAS-Report-to-Address-the-regional-crisis-caused-by-Venezuelas-migrant.pdf.

Quintero, Lus Dary, Osorio Osorio, Yetza Habid, Laura Isaza Bojorquez-Chapel, Jorge Acosta-Reyes, and Kristina Fernández-Niño. 2023. "Interrupción Voluntaria del Embarazo y Salud Sexual y Reproductiva en Mujeres Migrantes en Barranquilla." *Revista Panamericana de Salud Pública/Pan American Journal of Public Health* 47 (49): 1–9. https://doi.org/10.26633/RPSP.2023.49.

Reed-Sandoval, Amy. 2020a. "Maternity and Migration." *Philosophy Compass* 15: 1–11.

Reed-Sandoval, Amy. 2020b. *Socially Undocumented: Identity and Immigration Justice*. Oxford University Press.

R4V. 2021. "Venezuelan Refugees and Migrants in the Region." https://www.r4v.info/en/refugeeandmigrants.

Seals Allers, Kimberly. 2020. "Obstetric Violence is a Real Problem. Evelyn Yang's Experience is Just One Example." *The Washington Post*, February 6. https://www.washingtonpost.com/lifestyle/2020/02/06/obstetric-violence-is-real-problem-evelyn-yangs-experience-is-just-one-example/.

Solano, Armando, Kristina Gemzell-Daniellsen, and Jorge Rubio. 2024. "FIGO Statement on Health of Refugees and Migrants in Colombia." International Federation of Gynecology and Obstetrics. https://www.figo.org/figo-statement-health-refugees-and-migrants-colombia.

Telléz, Juliana Mateus. 2022. "Migrar y Parir: Dar a Luz Lejos de Casa." Poder Parir. https://manifiesta.org/migrar-y-parir-dar-a-luz-lejos-de-casa/.

United Nations High Commissioner for Refugees. 2019. "Refugees and Migrants from Venezuela Top 4 Million." June 7. https://www.unhcr.org/en-us/news/press/2019/6/5cfa2a4a4/refugees-migrants-venezuela-top-4-million-unhcr-iom.html.

United Nations High Commissioner for Refugees. 2020. "Venezuela Situation." https://www.unhcr.org/venezuela-emergency.html.

United Nations High Commissioner for Refugees. 2024. "Venezuela Situation." https://www.unhcr.org/sites/default/files/2025-06/Venezuela%20GR2024%20Situation%20Summary%20FINAL%20v3.pdf.

Vallana-Sala, Viviana Valeria. 2019. "'Es Rico Hacerlos, Pero No Tenerlos': Análisis de la Violencia Obstétrica durante la Atención del Parto en Colombia." Special issue, *Revista Ciencias de la Salud* 17: 128–144. https://cerosetenta.uniandes.edu.co/tenemos-que-hablar-de-violencia-obstetrica/.

Wolf, Allison B. 2019. "Dying in Detention as an Example of Oppression." *Hispanic/Latino Issues in Philosophy Newsletter of the American Philosophical Association* 19 (1).

Wolf, Allison B. 2020. *Just Immigration in the Americas: A Feminist Account*. Rowman and Littlefield.

Wolf, Allison B. 2021. "Immigration Injustice in Colombia: Beyond the Question of Borders." *Border Criminologies Blog*. https://blogs.law.ox.ac.uk/research-subject-groups/centre-criminology/centreborder-criminologies/blog/2021/04/immigration.

Wolf, Allison B. 2022. "Obstetric Violence as Immigration Injustice: A View from the United States and Colombia." *Developing World Bioethics* 23 (2): 176–184.

Young, Iris Marion. 1990. *Justice and the Politics of Difference.* Princeton University Press.

Crossing the Volta

ALISON PHIPPS

The water spirits
take no prisoners.
On the islands
the snakes writhe.
You can land
and walk there
but contrary
to common speech
the island
does not belong
to the hotel.

The river spits forth plastic.
The boats sing
with the beat of the ghetto.
The continent stirs,
sluggish
and sleepy despite Her being up since dawn.
Irritated by the tin music,
She prefers the birdsong and the palm-leaf shaker,
the stroke of the lobster paddle.

She has seen us before on this river.
White skinned and black skinned,
making and spending our coins,
throwing out our bridges like ropes of progress
heaping up gold-earthen dams like sand-papered termite hills.

"Listen"
She whispers in a terrible tone
from deep inside the ripples.
"The birds are loyal to me, returning from afar with every season.
They swoop away from your grasping hands. They circle and soar.
Sentinels."

"Watch" she murmurs.
"Your children
all lathered in key soap
know my secrets as they

dive

through the shallows
and into
my flow."

The river is not for coins.

PART TWO

Detention and Encampment

5

Immigration Detention and Health in Australia

A Structural Perspective

RYAN ESSEX

5.1 INTRODUCTION

In this chapter I will discuss Australia's approach to immigration detention, how this can be understood as an issue of structural injustice, and the impact of this for refugees' and asylum seekers' health. I will outline what a structural approach means for those concerned about refugee health in Australia and how this moves us beyond simply meeting more immediate health needs, instead calling for the abolition of detention while challenging the background conditions that enable and sustain these policies.

First, I will provide an outline of Australia's approach to immigration detention and its impact on those detained. Second, I will argue that struggles for health cannot be separated from struggles for the abolition of detention. In making this claim I will show not only that immigration detention has a significant and negative impact on health but also that we should be skeptical that incremental change, such as calls for greater transparency or oversight, will lead to any substantive improvement. Instead, if we are concerned about the health of detainees in Australia, we should aim for the abolition of detention. Third, I will outline how we could begin to think about Australian immigration detention in light of discussions about structural injustice. I reason that while there is still a clear case to hold the Australian government responsible for the more direct harms of immigration detention, the lens of structural injustice is particularly useful in helping us contemplate the background conditions which have enabled and perpetuated these policies. Finally, I will draw this together and discuss

Ryan Essex, *Immigration Detention and Health in Australia*. In: *Forced Migration and Health Justice*. Edited by: Lisa A. Eckenwiler, Verina Wild, Anna Gotlib, Ryoa Chung, and Deborah Zion, Oxford University Press.
 DOI: 10.1093/oso/9780197795491.003.0005

how structural injustice can help us reflect on the abolition of detention and health in Australian immigration detention.

5.2 REFUGEES, ASYLUM, AND IMMIGRATION DETENTION IN AUSTRALIA

Australia has historically had an inconsistent and incongruous approach to migration. On the one hand Australia has welcomed over 900,000 refugees and millions of migrants since the end of World War II (Refugee Council of Australia 2023). A founding member of the UN, today Australia remains signatory to every major human rights instrument and resettles between 10,000 and 20,000 refugees a year through its humanitarian program (Essex 2020). This can be contrasted with Australia's approach to asylum seekers who arrive by boat. While Australian immigration detention is mandatory and indefinite, meaning anyone without a valid visa can be detained, it has been asylum seekers who have been singled out for uniquely harsh treatment. Since its introduction in 1992 hundreds of thousands of people have been detained in Australian immigration detention centers, the vast majority of whom have been asylum seekers.

At different times, Australia has maintained detention centers on the mainland, in every state, in designated centers, community settings, and, more recently, hotels. Australia also presently has a policy of offshore processing. Originally introduced in 2001, repealed and then re-introduced in 2012, this policy has forcibly removed asylum seeker boat arrivals to detention centers on Nauru and Manus Island (Papua New Guinea). Since 2013 the Australian government has maintained that nobody detained offshore will be resettled in the country. While many people have been moved to Australia and many have now been resettled in third countries, this policy has resulted in the detention of thousands of people, hundreds remaining offshore to this day with little hope for safety or security.

In understanding Australia's approach to immigration detention, it is not just the length or location of detention that matters. Underpinning the human costs and the various criticisms leveled at these policies is the fact that Australian immigration detention is primarily geared to deter. That is, successive Australian governments have deliberately implemented increasingly harsh policies in an attempt to stop further arrivals; this point is also particularly crucial for discussions about structural injustice later in this chapter.

Immigration detention may be described as a last resort among a range of actions the government has taken to stop asylum boats arriving in Australia, which has included turning boats back at sea (Phipps 2015). These policies have been openly promoted by successive Australian governments, with some even capitalizing on this during elections. For example, on the day of the most recent federal election, the Liberal government (soon to be defeated) released news that two boats carrying asylum seekers had been intercepted, with then Defense Minister Peter Dutton (the current opposition leader at the time of writing) claiming that people smugglers "have obviously decided who is going to win the election and the boats have already started" (quoted in Galloway 2022).

Deterrence has not only been leveraged politically; it has also had far-reaching consequences for those who have been detained, providing insight into why Australia has persevered with these policies despite the human toll within centers. Asylum seekers, particularly those offshore—in addition to being detained for years—have had to contend with "squalid" conditions (Amnesty International 2016), along with physical and sexual abuse, violence, and riots (Australian Parliamentary Select Committee 2015). This has occurred, at times quite blatantly, with the Australian government taking no action to address these issues or hold perpetrators to account (Amnesty International 2017).

Deterrence has also meant the Australian government has been particularly hostile to critics of these policies and unwilling to entertain alternatives. Center staff have been removed from their positions and publicly attacked (Farrell 2015), while advocates have been investigated by the Australian Federal Police (Farrell 2016). Public figures have also been attacked; most notably, then Australian Human Rights Commissioner Gillian Triggs was singled out and attacked throughout late 2015 after the release of the "Forgotten Children Report" (Australian Human Rights Commission [AHRC] 2014).

Perhaps unsurprisingly, these policies have had a devastating impact on health and transformed the delivery of healthcare within detention centers. I will discuss this further below, with a specific focus on structural injustice, namely, how a consideration of structural injustice could inform advocacy and activism in relation to health and healthcare for asylum seekers in Australia. First, I will examine the link between the abolition of detention and health, arguing that reform will do little to address the long-standing issues related to health and healthcare and that abolition of detention should be the overarching goal for anyone concerned about Australia's treatment of asylum seekers. I will then discuss how we should approach these issues, utilizing the literature on structural injustice.

Approaching this issue as one of structural injustice may at first seem an awkward fit; after all, the Australian government clearly has the capacity to do something about these issues, but it has made decisions that have resulted in the suffering of tens of thousands of vulnerable people. I will argue, however, that structural injustice helps us identify and respond to the underlying factors and background conditions that have led to and perpetuated the use of immigration detention in Australia, which factors have enabled the Australian government to maintain this punitive approach. I want to move beyond simple calls for abolition of detention or reform to begin to sketch out what would need to change to move toward abolition. I will then discuss the implications of this approach for the health and well-being of refugees and asylum seekers in Australia.

5.3 HEALTH, IMMIGRATION DETENTION, AND ABOLITION OF DETENTION

There is near consensus among those who have researched, worked, or been detained in Australian immigration detention centers that any reasonable standard of health is unobtainable within current detention arrangements. It is both tacitly and explicitly acknowledged throughout the literature that "a focus on maintaining and incrementally improving the system is vexed and the aspiration must be the abolition of the detention system" (Briskman and Zion 2014, 284). Below I want to briefly expand on this point, sketching how health and the abolition of detention are related. I will argue that it is simply not possible to meet the health needs of those who remain detained under current arrangements or through reform and that any attempt to do so is largely futile. For anyone who is concerned about refugee health in Australia (and elsewhere), we must demand abolition of detention; we cannot disentangle this from health (or a range of other factors, such as justice, for that matter).

In making my point, it is first necessary to introduce the empirical evidence in this area. One of the earliest studies to emerge about the health and well-being of detainees came from within an immigration detention center, carried out by a detained asylum seeker in collaboration with a psychologist who worked in an onshore center. Among the 33 participants surveyed, almost all (85%) displayed depressive symptoms, and well over half (65%) expressed suicidal ideation. The authors note that symptoms often got worse with length of time detained (Sultan and O'Sullivan 2001). Subsequent studies have painted a similar picture, detailing substantially more mental health symptoms and distress, increasing over time detained (Green and Eagar 2010; Bull et al. 2013).

While there are fewer studies, available evidence also suggests that physical health is impacted substantially, again deteriorating with length of time detained (Bull et al. 2013). These impacts have also been seen among children and families (Mares and Jureidini 2004; Steel et al. 2004). The AHRC's (2014) "Forgotten Children Report" examined children's health and well-being and the impact of onshore and offshore immigration detention. It found that immigration detention was having "profound negative impacts on the mental and emotional health of children" (29). In relation to offshore detention on Nauru, the report found that "[c]hildren detained indefinitely on Nauru are suffering from extreme levels of physical, emotional, psychological and developmental distress" (13).

In addition to this evidence, it is worth noting that refugees who are detained fare worse than those who are not. Globally, studies suggest poorer health among detained refugees (von Werthern et al. 2018), and a growing body of work speaks to this point in relation to Australian immigration detention. In Australia asylum seekers in detention have far worse health outcomes than asylum seekers and refugees in the Australian community, including higher rates of self-harm (Hedrick et al. 2019). We can also find evidence that those who are detained offshore compared to those onshore require far greater support from healthcare services (Essex, Kalocsányiová, Scott, et al. 2022) and have poorer mental health outcomes (Essex, Kalocsányiová, Young, et al. 2022).

In presenting this literature, I am hoping to make two points: that Australian immigration detention has a devastating impact on health, and that it is a clear and particularly potent factor when it comes to poor health; that is, it has a substantial impact regardless of the vulnerability of the populations detained and the range of other factors which may otherwise explain their relatively poor health outcomes.

In furthering the case for the abolition of detention, it is worth considering if these harms can be mediated, for example, through improved delivery of healthcare or increased oversight. On this point, we find a general consensus in the literature that while any small improvements should be welcomed, we should be skeptical that any such changes would make any substantive difference. In regard to the delivery of healthcare, I have argued elsewhere that health will not be addressed by improving healthcare delivery because it is "limited and transformed by design" and that this will remain the case as long as "Australian immigration detention is geared to promote suffering as a means of deterrence" (Essex 2016, 979). Similar sentiments can be found elsewhere. Peter Young, former medical director of International Health and Medical Services (IHMS; the private provider that has held the majority of contracts to deliver healthcare in detention), described the provision of care as "inherently futile" because the system itself is designed as a deterrent to cause suffering (Marr and Laughland 2014).

During hearings of the Australian Parliamentary Joint Select Committee on Australia's Immigration Detention Network (2012, 82–83) Professor Louise Newman was quoted as saying, "The irony of the current situation—even though IHMS might be attempting to improve service provision, which

I think is a very positive thing—is that, within the system of prolonged restrictive detention, people's mental health is unlikely to improve significantly. Even if we threw in there another 1000 mental health workers, be they psychologists or psychiatrists, we would still have a crisis which is a broad, systemic crisis."

It should be clear that immigration detention has a significant and negative impact on health, and we should be skeptical that this can be addressed with anything short of the abolition of detention. In this respect the struggles for health and the abolition of detention are linked. Beyond health there are several other obvious and pressing reasons to push for abolition of detention, on human rights and other grounds and the fact that it is morally repugnant to hold people in detention indefinitely as a deterrent to others.

5.4 ABOLITION OF DETENTION AND STRUCTURAL INJUSTICE

I have argued that the abolition of immigration detention would be an important step in improving the health of asylum seekers in Australia. Importantly, when it comes to Australian immigration detention, abolition is not a new idea; it has long been demanded by advocacy groups. What I want to do, however, is consider how scholarship on structural injustice could help inform those seeking abolition of detention and in turn impact the health of asylum seekers in Australia. I will first outline what I mean by structural injustice and then consider how it can inform efforts related to the abolition of Australian immigration detention.

Structural injustice exists as the end result of a number of large-scale social processes that often interact with and reinforce one another. These processes advantage some while disadvantaging others by constraining or limiting their opportunities. The end result is that these groups stand in different and most often unfair social positions (Young 2011b, 52–64).

While the broader social processes that create and perpetuate structural injustice are driven by individual actions, these actions are not necessarily malicious and can even be well-meaning. The sources of the unjust situation are "multiple, large-scale and relatively long term. Many policies both public and private and the actions of thousands of individuals according to normal rules and accepted practices contribute to producing these circumstances" (Young 2011b, 48). Consider the contribution that millions of individuals in wealthy countries make to climate change. While many of us may be taking steps to minimize our carbon footprint, we all contribute to climate change; if we use electricity or shop at any major supermarket we are likely to be responsible for carbon emissions, at least in some small way, for example. We are also likely to make a larger contribution than those in low- and middle-income countries. This list could of course go on; structural injustice has been applied to a range of other issues, such as gender inequality, racism, and homelessness. Structural injustice creates a distinct moral problem in that the actions of individuals often with good intent result in collective harm to certain other individuals or groups. That is, structural injustice is maintained even in the absence of malicious actors and those engaging in deliberate wrongdoing.

A number of theorists have more recently expanded on Young's work, identifying different forms of structural injustice. For example, Nuti (2019, 66) argues that there are at least two forms of structural injustice, historical structural injustice and structural injustices that do not stem from history. Historical structural injustice includes groups like women and others who have been socially or politically excluded in some ways. Groups that could be categorized as being disadvantaged by present-day structural injustices include the homeless.

Similarly, McKeown argues that there are three different types of structural injustice: (1) pure structural injustice refers to the type of injustice that Young was interested in, where "there is no identifiable perpetrator, and the injustice is the sum of multiple agents"; (2) avoidable structural injustice refers to situations where powerful agents could change unjust structures but fail or refuse to do so; and (3) deliberate structural injustice refers to circumstances "where agents are deliberately perpetuating unjust background conditions for their own gain, and they have the power to change them" (2021, 5; 2024).

Beyond these examples, structural injustice has also been applied to better understand our responsibilities toward refugees globally. Parekh (2020) argues that, traditionally, a focus on resettlement and asylum has obscured the broader responsibilities we have when it comes to refugees and asylum seekers. Similar to McKeown, first drawing a distinction between direct and structural injustice, Parekh argues that there are at least two distinct harms that deserve focus: the circumstances that drive asylum seekers from their home and the conditions created by the international community that leave the vast majority in limbo while seeking asylum. While this is a relatively cursory summary of this literature, one question that may seem obvious is what constitutes direct and structural injustice, which is particularly important for the discussion below.

At first glance, turning to theories of structural injustice may seem an awkward fit with current discussions in relation to Australian immigration detention; after all, the Australian government, which clearly has the capacity to help, has instead implemented policies that harm tens of thousands of vulnerable people. In fact, the Australian government has benefited politically from these policies, capitalizing on them in an attempt to win elections (and often being successful).

Australian immigration detention is what Hillier-Smith (2022, 8) labels a direct injustice, as opposed to structural injustice, namely because "it becomes clear that the containment of refugees and their prevention from accessing refuge is not an unintended, unfortunate, by-product of structural processes, but instead the direct harmful and unjust outcome of explicit and intentional policies." Hillier-Smith goes on to argue that we cannot consider immigration detention a structural injustice, as Australia is "among the most affluent and stable states on the globe, and thus ha[s] the capacity and resources to respond to refugees in ways that do not cause such harms, but instead protect refugees' wellbeing and human rights." (11) In many respects I agree. Successive Australian governments could and should have helped and should be held responsible for their actions. At worst, Hillier-Smith argues that focusing on structural injustice at the expense of direct injustice may even fail refugees who would be protected if we more directly challenged such harms.

While I believe this is a potential risk, I do not believe we necessarily lose sight of more direct injustice when focusing on structural injustice. If anything, in the case of Australian immigration detention a structural focus could complement existing efforts that seek to address these more direct injustices. I will outline this below, along with how structural injustice could help in advancing efforts not only in relation to abolition of detention but in addressing the health of asylum seekers in Australia.

5.5 HOW COULD AN UNDERSTANDING OF STRUCTURAL INJUSTICE CONTRIBUTE TO REFUGEE HEALTH IN AUSTRALIA?

I have argued that efforts to improve the health of immigration detainees in Australia cannot be separated from efforts aimed at abolition of detention. I have explored how an understanding of structural injustice could be applied to Australian immigration detention. Now I will outline what I perceive to be some of the advantages of turning to structural injustice, particularly as this relates to efforts aimed at abolition of detention and improving the health of asylum seekers in Australia.

First, there is a clear case to address forced displacement in the first instance. Turning to structural injustice helps us see the overarching and complex factors that drive forced displacement and how many of us in higher-income countries contribute. (See my brief example as it relates to climate change, above.) Addressing forced displacement at its source by addressing wealth inequalities, violence, and the drivers of corruption would ensure there was no need for people to flee their homes, let alone for states to turn to immigration detention. This of course is no small task; when we begin to think about forced displacement, its causes, and how it could be addressed, we can begin to imagine the change that would need to occur, arguably a complete social, political, and economic reordering of the world, something which is well beyond the scope of this chapter. This, however, raises a second point, namely that structural injustice helps us think through the background conditions that drive forced displacement, what maintains these conditions, and the responsibility we all have in working toward justice, three points I will deal with below.

Second, and on the point of responsibility, turning to structural injustice helps shift our focus from states as solely responsible. Australia is one state among many that have almost completely failed in relation to providing asylum. Despite this, the majority of the literature regarding asylum seekers focuses on state-based solutions. This of course would be ideal, as states and particularly wealthy states certainly have the power to do more and therefore have substantial responsibilities when it comes to asylum seekers (Wild 2015). Rather than isolating states and others involved in deliberate wrongdoing as solely responsible, a structural approach recognizes that multiple agents are almost always implicated, including those who might be ignorant and who have no malicious motives. Put another way, and as Lu (2011, 262) notes, focusing on individual and state wrongdoing misses the bigger picture; we need to also scrutinize the "social structural processes that enable and even encourage individual or state wrongdoing, and produce and reproduce unjust outcomes."

Similar sentiments are expressed by Hoover (2012, 234), who argues that "emerging understandings of responsibility in world politics have been too focused on the actions of individuals, leading to the neglect of structural causes of mass violence and more indirect lines of responsibility revealed by attending to the wider social context. Related to this limited focus on individual actors, academic accounts of moral agency have tended to downplay the political aspects of this focus on the individual's failure to uphold their obligations, which obscures the power inequalities and particular interests that are served by focusing on individual actors over enabling conditions and social structures."

Put another way, structural injustice shows us how we are all responsible in small ways for creating and sustaining the political and social conditions that drive asylum seekers to find safety and in enabling wealthy countries to exclude asylum seekers.

Third, structural injustice helps us to identify the background conditions that enable the use of immigration detention. While there remains a case to challenge deliberate wrongdoing and while present efforts should continue, structural injustice directs us away from being purely reactionary, pointing toward questions such as what underpins these policies and what it would take for it to no longer be acceptable that a government utilize immigration detention. In the case of Australia we could look at how the government has leveraged "unjust background conditions for their own gain" (McKeown 2021, 5).

On this point, there is a small body of research, most notably the work developed by Nethery (2010), which explores why Australia acts this way when it comes to immigration detention. Nethery offers three broad explanations. The first locates Australian immigration detention within the history of administrative detention, charting a lineage of similar forms of detention, identifying similarities and continuities with other forms of administrative detention which have been used since European settlement in Australia, such as Aboriginal reserves, quarantine stations, and enemy alien internment camps.

Nethery (2010) contends that immigration detention is "a response to a latent fear of invasion in the Australian psyche," (47) which can be attributed to two aspects of Australia's history: "our colonial history, based on the legal fiction of *terra nullius*, means that territory in Australia has always been contested [and] Australia's geographical location, as a white 'outpost' on the 'edge' of Asia, has resulted in a sense of vulnerability." (60) Nethery traces these anxieties to the present day, showing that immigration detention serves several social and political functions but that it is primarily "deployed to respond to actual and perceived political anxieties about Australian identity, the impact of globalization, and economic security for its citizens."(2)

One of the most crucial contributions of Nethery's thesis is to illustrate Australian immigration detention in its social, political, and historical context. It shows that we should be skeptical of simplistic, singular explanations for detention, such as racism. Perhaps most important, Nethery's thesis takes steps toward explaining Australia's actions. Within this broader picture, while not off the hook in regard to its responsibility to refugees in Australia, we can see how the government often operates under certain constraints. We also see how many contemporary and historical factors have enabled these policies. We cannot divorce Australia's colonialist and racist history from how asylum seekers are treated today.

Moreover, it is clear that the Australian government has not only failed to support asylum seekers but has acted to perpetuate unjust background conditions, like racism and xenophobia (which are also entangled with Australia's settler-colonial history), which allow the government to continue to turn to immigration detention and even use detainees for political ends. Perhaps most fundamentally, a structural approach helps us trace the origins of these issues. In other words, it helps to explain why Australia has turned to and maintained detention as its primary response to immigration, despite its drastic impact on health. This question is fundamental if we are to achieve the abolition of detention, yet it is often overlooked.

Fourth, it naturally follows that there is a case to spread awareness on several fronts, such as how people contribute to and enable structural injustice, which is maintained via "the normal processes of everyday life" (Young 2011a, 41). Raising awareness is key to showing how we all may contribute to broader injustices, but also how we may enable governments and others to treat refugees poorly.

Beyond this we need to consider more fundamental issues: why is it generally accepted that borders are inevitable and that refugees are undeserving of certain rights? A structural lens moves us beyond making demands or imagining simple solutions to what might be needed to establish better health for refugees in Australia to dealing with the messy realities of how this may be achieved: by challenging racism, by reckoning with our own history, and by realizing how we may contribute to and sustain systems or cultures which enable the use of detention. Perhaps most fundamentally, however, and returning to the core question of this chapter, if health can be addressed only through the reform or abolition of immigration detention, it is a fight that will need to occur on multiple fronts and must reckon with Australia's racist and colonial history and its contemporary social and political order.

REFERENCES

Amnesty International. 2016. "Island of Despair: Australia's 'Processing' of Refugees on Nauru." https://www.amnesty.org/en/documents/asa12/4934/2016/en/.

Amnesty International. 2017. "Australia/Papua New Guinea: Immigration Dept.'s Claims About Shooting on Manus Island Refuted." https://www.amnesty.org/en/latest/press-release/2017/05/australia-papua-new-guinea-immigration-depts-claims-about-shooting-on-manus-island-refuted/.

Australian Human Rights Commission. 2014. "The Forgotten Children: National Inquiry into Children in Immigration Detention." https://humanrights.gov.au/our-work/asylum-seekers-and-refugees/national-inquiry-children-immigration-detention-2014.

Australian Parliamentary Joint Select Committee on Australia's Immigration Detention Network. 2012. "Final Report." https://www.aph.gov.au/Parliamentary_Business/Committees/Joint/Former_Committees/immigrationdetention/index.

Australian Parliamentary Select Committee. 2015. "Taking Responsibility: Conditions and Circumstances at Australia's Regional Processing Centre in Nauru." https://www.aph.gov.au/parliamentary_business/committees/senate/regional_processing_nauru/regional_processing_nauru/final_report.

Briskman, Linda, and Deborah Zion. 2014. “Dual Loyalties and Impossible Dilemmas: Health Care in Immigration Detention.” *Public Health Ethics* 7 (3): 277–286.

Bull, Melissa, Emily Schindeler, David Berkman, and Janet Ransley. 2013. “Sickness in the System of Long-Term Immigration Detention.” *Journal of Refugee Studies* 26 (1): 47–68.

Essex, Ryan. 2016. “A Community Standard: Equivalency of Healthcare in Australian Immigration Detention.” *Journal of Immigrant and Minority Health* 19: 974–981.

Essex, Ryan. 2020. *The Healthcare Community and Australian Immigration Detention: The Case for Non-Violent Resistance*. Palgrave Macmillan.

Essex, Ryan, Erika Kalocsányiová, James G. Scott, and Rosana Pacella. 2022. “Health of Children in Australian Immigration Detention Centres: An Analysis of the Quarterly Health Reports from 2014 to 2017.” *Journal of Paediatrics and Child Health* 58 (6): 985–990.

Essex, Ryan, Erika Kalocsányiová, Peter Young, and Paul McCrone. 2022. “Psychological Distress in Australian Onshore and Offshore Immigration Detention Centres from 2014–2018.” *Journal of Immigrant and Minority Health* 24: 868–874

Farrell, P. 2015. “Police Carry Out More Raids on Save the Children Staff at Nauru Detention Centre.” *The Guardian*, October 22. http://www.theguardian.com/world/2015/oct/22/police-carry-out-more-raids-on-save-the-children-staff-at-nauru-detention-centre.

Farrell, P. 2016. “Australian Police Accessed Phone Records of Asylum Whistleblower.” *The Guardian*, May 23. https://www.theguardian.com/australia-news/2016/may/24/australian-police-accessed-phone-records-of-asylum-whistleblower.

Galloway, A. 2022. “Asylum Seeker Boat Stopped off Christmas Island as Morrison Trumpets Border Security on Election Day.” *Sydney Morning Herald*, May 21. https://www.smh.com.au/politics/federal/asylum-seeker-boat-stopped-off-christmas-island-as-morrison-trumpets-border-security-on-election-day-20220521-p5anb1.html.

Green, Janette P., and Kathy Eagar. 2010. “The Health of People in Australian Immigration Detention Centres.” *Medical Journal of Australia* 192: 65–70.

Hedrick, Kyli, Gregory Armstrong, Guy Coffey, and Rohan Borschmann. 2019. “Self-Harm in the Australian Asylum Seeker Population: A National Records-Based Study.” *SSM-Population Health* 8: 100452.

Hillier-Smith, Bradley. 2022. “Direct and Structural Injustice Against Refugees.” *Journal of Social Philosophy* 54 (2): 262–284.

Hoover, Joseph. 2012. “Reconstructing Responsibility and Moral Agency in World Politics.” *IT* 4 (2): 233–268.

Lu, Catherine. 2011. “Colonialism as Structural Injustice: Historical Responsibility and Contemporary Redress.” *Journal of Political Philosophy* 19 (3): 261–281.

Mares, Sarah, and J. Jureidini. 2004. “Psychiatric Assessment of Children and Families in Immigration Detention: Clinical, Administrative and Ethical issues.” *Australian & New Zealand Journal of Public Health* 28 (6): 520–526.

Marr, D., and O. Laughland. 2014. “Australia’s Detention Regime Sets Out to Make Asylum Seekers Suffer, Says Chief Immigration Psychiatrist.” *The Guardian*, August 4. https://www.theguardian.com/world/2014/aug/05/-sp-australias-detention-regime-sets-out-to-make-asylum-seekers-suffer-says-chief-immigration-psychiatrist.

McKeown, Maeve. 2021. “Structural Injustice.” *Philosophy Compass* 16 (7): e12757.

McKeown, Maeve. 2024. *With Power Comes Responsibility: The Politics of Structural Injustice*. Bloomsbury Academic.

Nethery, Amy. 2010. "Immigration Detention in Australia." PhD diss., Deakin University.

Nuti, Alasia. 2019. *Injustice and the Reproduction of History: Structural Inequalities, Gender and Redress*. Cambridge University Press.

Parekh, Serena. 2020. *No Refuge: Ethics and the Global Refugee Crisis*. Oxford University Press.

Phipps, Claire. 2015. "Did Australia Pay People-Smugglers to Turn Back Asylum-Seekers?" *The Guardian*, June 17. https://www.theguardian.com/world/2015/jun/17/did-australia-pay-people-smugglers-to-turn-back-boats.

Refugee Council of Australia. 2023. "How Many Refugees Have Come to Australia?" https://www.refugeecouncil.org.au/how-many-refugees-have-come/.

Steel, Zachary, Shakeh Momartin, Catherine Bateman, et al. 2004. "Psychiatric Status of Asylum-Seeker Families Held for a Protracted Period in a Remote Detention Centre in Australia." *Australian and New Zealand Journal of Public Health* 28 (6): 527–536.

Sultan, A. and K. O'Sullivan. 2001. "Psychological Disturbances in Asylum-Seekers Held in Long-Term Detention." *Medical Journal of Australia* 175 (11–12): 593–596.

von Werthern, Martha, Katy Robjant, Z. Chui, et al. 2018. "The Impact of Immigration Detention on Mental Health: A Systematic Review." *BMC Psychiatry* 18 (1): 1–19.

Wild, Verina. 2015. "Universal Access to Health Care for Migrants: Applying Cosmopolitanism to the Domestic Realm." *Public Health Ethics* 8 (2): 162–172.

Young, Iris Marion. 2011a. *Justice and the Politics of Difference*. Princeton University Press.

Young, Iris Marion. 2011b. *Responsibility for Justice*. Oxford University Press.

Place?

SYLVIA AGBIH

Tents, containers, site trailers, sport halls, out-of-use old army barracks, provisional shelters. Camp beds and bunk beds. No privacy. Basic food packages. Provisional mass showers and toilets. No place to take care of your needs. No place to go to – away from the closed, segregated space with guarded entrance and exit. Constant presence of strangers and of precarity. A liminal place. Not here, not there. Passing through. Passing by? Non-permanent. Not belonging to this place. Not part of this community. How long will one be allowed to stay? How long will we have to stay? Where next? Is there a place for us somewhere?

6

The Health Impacts of Immigration Detention

Examining Moral Injury

SURESH SUNDRAM, DEBBIE C. HOCKING, AND SANDRA PASSARDI

The use of immigration detention for asylum seekers by host countries has attracted considerable interest as a potential mechanism of deterrence for unauthorized transnational movement of people (Australian Human Rights Commission 2004). Although attracting considerable criticism from human rights and health perspectives, the practice has been extended to include processing of asylum claims in third countries (Australian Human Rights Commission 2013). At the forefront of these practices has been Australia, which introduced third-country regional processing of asylum seekers in 2001. Concerns about the physical and mental health impacts of this immigration detention have been repeatedly raised; however, detailed evidence is sparse. This chapter outlines the evolution of the policy and its health impacts, focusing on the psychological consequences of immigration detention.

6.1 AUSTRALIAN IMMIGRATION POLICY REGARDING ASYLUM SEEKERS: IMMIGRATION DETENTION AND OFFSHORE PROCESSING

Australia has a long-standing policy of deterrence against those seeking asylum; the first legislation passed immediately after national federation as the Immigration Restriction Act of 1901, otherwise known as the White Australia Policy (Meaney 1995). More recently, those who arrive on Australian

Suresh Sundram, Debbie C. Hocking, and Sandra Passardi, *The Health Impacts of Immigration Detention*. In: *Forced Migration and Health Justice*. Edited by: Lisa A. Eckenwiler, Verina Wild, Anna Gotlib, Ryoa Chung, and Deborah Zion, Oxford University Press.
DOI: 10.1093/oso/9780197795491.003.0006

territories without valid entry documents, such as unauthorized maritime arrivals, are subject to mandatory detention in immigration detention centers. Although they are able to lodge an asylum claim, they remain in detention at the minister for immigration's discretion for the duration of their refugee status determination process, which may last for years (Refugee Council of Australia 2020).

This policy of mandatory detention for unauthorized arrivals was introduced in 1992 with bipartisan political support and has continued unabated, with its primary intent to be a deterrent for those who may want to seek asylum in Australia but who arrive without authorization. The legality of the policy, despite key challenges to its constitutional basis, was initially upheld by the High Court of Australia, when it determined that immigration detention can be indefinite (Refugee Council of Australia 2020). However, in 2023, the Court revised this to exclude those detainees who have no prospect of return.[1] In response, in late 2024, the Australian parliament passed further amendments to the Migration Act, allowing the government to transfer non-citizens, to third countries (in this case Nauru) under "third country reception arrangements". The places of detention have often been isolated, remote, and difficult to access, such as Christmas Island, northwest Western Australia, and outback South Australia. In 2001, the mandatory detention policy was expanded to non-Australian offshore regional processing centers on the Pacific Island nation of Nauru and on Manus Island in Papua New Guinea (PNG); these locations, too, are remote and difficult to access from Australia. These centers were closed in 2007 but reopened in 2012 (Nethery and Holman 2016), and the regional processing center in Nauru currently remains open. In addition to their location, these offshore centers were governed according to a number of measures designed to minimize external scrutiny, including highly regulated travel and media access, with no visitor access, including family members. Staff were prohibited from publicly discussing detention conditions by legislation carrying imprisonment and fines for transgressions. These factors discouraged communication, engagement, and scrutiny by the wider community, and engendered a sense of isolation and disconnection among the detainees (Nethery and Holman 2016).

Although ostensibly anyone who arrived without prior authorization could be transferred offshore against their will, the process was selective. For example, out of more than 37,000 people who arrived in Australia in an unauthorized manner between 2012 and 2015, only approximately

1. The original decision was *Al-Kateb v Godwin*, HCA 37, (2004) 219 CLR 562, High Court (Australia), but in a recent landmark ruling on November 8, 2023, *NZYQ v. Minister for Immigration, Citizenship and Multicultural Affairs & Anor*, the High Court of Australia reversed this decision for those with no prospect of being returned.

4,100 were transferred and processed in Nauru or PNG, and about 140 people remain in those two countries as of 2025 (Asylum Seeker Resource Centre, 2025). Although most were transferred back to Australia for health-related reasons, they have nevertheless been deemed "transitory persons", forbidden by policy to ever settle in Australia. Some have been resettled in third countries, predominantly the US and New Zealand, and small numbers in Canada and some European countries. A proportion (955) have been returned, or "chose" to return, to their country of origin, despite many having been declared refugees (Refugee Council of Australia 2023). For many who returned to their country of origin, the primitive facilities, prison-like environment, hot and humid climate, limited education opportunities for children, loss of autonomy, and the indefinite nature of their situation in the Australian detention centers were powerful influences in their decision (Fleay and Hoffman 2014).

6.2 MENTAL AND PHYSICAL HEALTH IMPACTS OF OFFSHORE DETENTION ON ASYLUM SEEKERS AND REFUGEES

As noted above, the Australian-controlled centers in Nauru and PNG restricted external contact. However, limited scrutiny by authorized agencies does exist, including the United Nations High Commissioner for Refugees (UNHCR) and the Red Cross. This enabled some assessment of the physical and mental health of detainees, including a UNHCR-sponsored health survey in 2016 in the Manus Island detention center. This survey, conducted by two psychiatrists and a general practitioner, assessed about 180 detainees, or 20% of the center's population. They found high levels of mental illness, with 79% of people meeting diagnostic criteria for posttraumatic stress disorder (PTSD); 88% meeting criteria for a depressive or anxiety disorder; and 93% meeting criteria for either PTSD or a depressive or anxiety disorder (Sundram and Ventevogel 2017). These remarkable rates of mental illness attracted the interest of the Australian Parliament (UNHCR 2016).

Studies using publicly available records determined that the self-harm rate in the Nauru detention center was approximately 200 times that of the mainstream Australian population, at 260 episodes per 1,000 detainees, including young children (Hedrick et al. 2019). In addition, there have been nine recorded suicides and a number of deaths potentially preventable through more consistent and timely medical care (University of Oxford 2024).

Many of the detainees struggled in the hot and humid tropical conditions, which were compounded by the lack of air conditioning and inadequate ventilation, as well as limited access to water for bathing. There were high rates of skin irritations and infections, and renal and bladder calculi became a problem due to the mineral content of the available water. Moreover, the physical environment predisposed people to orthopedic injuries and, subsequently, to chronic pain (Sundram and Ventevogel 2017).

The aforementioned limited mental health data accord generally with extant data examining mental disorders in asylum seekers and refugees, albeit with greater illness severity in the PNG and Nauru cohorts (Turrini et al. 2017). This includes the rate of self-harm, including among young children, suggesting additional psychological factors were operating, such as the context of indefinite detention.

6.3 THE MENTAL HEALTH OF FORMER NAURUAN IMMIGRATION CENTER DETAINEES

A qualitative study by Passardi et al. (2022) attempted to capture these factors more fully in a small convenience sample of asylum seekers and refugees who had been exposed to indefinite immigration detention in Nauru prior to being transferred to Australia for medical treatment. The study comprised 13 participants (10 refugees and 3 asylum seekers) from six countries of origin. The average age was 37.9 ±13.5 years, and, with the exception of one individual, the length of time detained in Nauru prior to return to Australia was 6–36 months (15.3 ±10.9 months). All 13 participants temporarily resided in Australia; 12 were considered "transitory persons" who did not have permanent residency status in Australia and were therefore subject to being returned to Nauru.

Three main conclusions emerged from the data: (1) participants risked their lives on the journey to Australia, expecting safety; (2) they experienced deprivation, lack of agency, violence, and dehumanization after arrival, for which they held the Australian authorities responsible; and (3) these experiences led to their feeling irreparably damaged physically, mentally, spiritually, and morally.

With respect to the first conclusion, the narratives of forced migrants described an expectation of attaining safety in Australia, even among people who were not aware that Australia is a signatory to UN instruments and among those who had experienced human rights violations and/or threats to their moral or religious beliefs. Participants did not expect to experience harm in the process of seeking Australia's protection. The disconnect between their expectations given Australia's espoused social values and their actual experiences was perceived as a betrayal. This is underscored by symptoms cited by participants which extended beyond the circumscriptions of PTSD and mood and anxiety disorders. Simply put, people expected the worst of their suffering to be over once they arrived in Australia;

instead, their suffering became protracted and, like the conditions they fled, life-threatening.

Many contrasted their experiences of war and persecution in their home country with the reception they never anticipated but actually received. For example, in response to being asked if it was better to remain in their home country than come to Australia, one participant responded, "Yeah. Even if [the home country] is going through lots of problems like natural disasters or civil unrest."[2] Another stated, "When we [arrived] here we had hope to have freedom, to have a peaceful, quiet, nice life but it isn't. I feel I should [have stayed in Iran] and they put me in a jail, it [would have been] better because I had parents and I was my own [person]. Now I don't know who am I? I lost myself." (Passardi et al. 2022, 8).

A universal theme for participants was having experienced the opposite of what was expected upon arriving in Australia. Several expressed ongoing disbelief and bitterness. Many regretted coming to Australia, and some said they wished they had died on the boat journey (Passardi et al. 2022). Participants described the experience of extreme and dangerous conditions in the detention center in Nauru, such as living in tents in hot temperatures with high humidity, unhygienic facilities, and lack of privacy. They also reported excessive government control over their lives, including arbitrarily applied and enforced rules. Many described having to queue for long periods of time in harsh conditions; inadequate access to food, medication, clothing, and facilities, including phone and internet; and lack of schooling and play or educational materials for children (Passardi et al. 2022).

In addition, sanitation access was experienced as highly restricted and restrictive, and always inadequate; for example, there was not enough toilet paper or sanitary products and two-minute showers were enforced. Such practices were perceived by the forced migrants as intentionally punitive. Interviewees also noted that guards appeared to be trained to act inhumanely.

Several participants, strikingly, spoke about being raped or a family member being raped – either by members of the Nauruan community or by detention guards – and several female participants spoke about threats of sexual violence, stating that the detention center was not safe for women and citing sexual harassment by detention guards. Of note were two participants who had been raped in the Nauruan community who explicitly placed the responsibility on the Australian government rather than the local people (Passardi et al. 2022). For example, one of these women said, "I blame the Australian government instead of the Nauruan government. So, when

2. Uncited interview quotes were derived from unpublished raw data collected as part of the study reported in Passardi et al. (2022).

they attacked [raped] us, who can we blame? Australia. Because Australia promised us that they will give us a safe place. But it was not. Instead of giving us a safe place they gave us mental sickness, physical sickness. They put us somewhere where we will lose our hope, we will lose our dreams, we will lose our families." (Passardi et al. 2022, 7).

Violent transit experiences to and from Nauru were also central to participants' accounts: "They took my son. He was three months, he was a baby. And they took him. And because I didn't want to go, I was scared, they pulled me maybe one kilometer. They just hold my arm very hard and put me on a floor to get to the bus. . . . They took my son for 12 hours when he was breastfed. I didn't know what was going on. No one explained to me what was happening. Did I do something wrong?" (Passardi et al. 2022, 7).

A common thread in participants' accounts was the sense of having been stripped of their dignity. Many participants explicitly described "not being treated as a human being," (Passardi et al. 2022, 7) and many felt they were treated as, or less than, animals. Examples ranged from being denied information and explanations by doctors about their diagnosis and condition, to being verbally and physically abused by guards who used handcuffs and were present in excessive numbers for transfers. This culminated in participants questioning why they were treated like criminals in these detention centers (Passardi et al. 2022). The experience of dehumanization included the feeling of being a political pawn in an effort to "stop the boats" without regard for the human cost. It is noteworthy that participants distinguished between the Australian government and both Australian and Nauruan citizens, who were generally regarded by the detainees as "good people."

Another key loss was of physical and mental health. All participants who had spent at least six months in Nauru cited a slew of mental health problems, including anxiety, depression, irritability, fear, intrusive trauma symptoms, emotional numbness, sleep disturbance, obsessive-compulsive behaviors, and suicidal ideation and attempts. Psychiatric diagnostic interviews supported these self-evaluations and concurred with the aforementioned PNG study. In the Nauru sample, 84.6% (11/13) of people had one disorder (major depressive disorder [MDD] or PTSD), and 69.2% (9/13) had two or more disorders. Some felt haunted by feelings of guilt, questioning whether they had done something wrong to be treated so inhumanely. Self-harm was widespread, as described by one woman: "Everyone was hurting themselves, yeah, was harming themselves. Every day, every day, every day, that's what happened."[3]

3. Uncited interview quotes were derived from unpublished raw data collected as part of the study reported in Passardi et al. (2022).

The sustained and cumulative acts of omission and commission endured by asylum seekers and refugees held in Nauru also resulted in significant self-identified functional impairment and an even more profound characterological change. These included a feeling of "being completely destroyed—inside and out," (Passardi et al. 2022, Supplemental material). an erosion of trust in others, an inability to feel close to others, social alienation, and a negative view of themselves and the world. Individuals spoke of having lost the best years of their life and their sense of identity, along with the development of altered belief systems, as illustrated by the following: "It's changed me because I never think, in my entire life, I never think . . . there's a bad people or good people in this world. But now I know. Because I've been in Nauru. And I saw the way they treat you. . . . Our heart is different. Before I never know. I used to think everybody is innocent and everybody is nice. And I used to always smile for everybody. But now I'm scared to be close with anyone."[4] Another detainee said, "My whole life has changed. [I] Just don't feel really good about this world. Everything, I feel everything is devil. Everyone just think about their own benefit. There isn't much people that they're nice. I just feel that everyone just want to hurt each other"[5] (Passardi et al. 2022).

The destruction of faith in relationships with other people involved a loss of faith in social systems and a diminution of how much goodness was present in others. This emerged as anger and frustration toward representatives of powerful social systems, such as the detention guards and workers, as well as toward immigration officers. Moreover, this loss of faith made many participants question their own intrinsic value, resulting in a sense of despair.

Upon transfer to Australia, the practices of deprivation continued, with the precarity of visas needing to be reviewed and renewed every six months, restricted work opportunities, and exclusion from standard government welfare, including unemployment benefits, free public healthcare and subsidized medicines. This contrasted with the mainstream Australian population, including refugees who have access to national welfare schemes, universal free health care, and subsidized medicines.

6.4 THE EXPERIENCE BEYOND PSYCHIATRIC DIAGNOSES

The experience of the participants extended beyond the specific symptomatology of PTSD and MDD, to three general dimensions: betrayal, violence

4. Uncited interview quotes were derived from unpublished raw data collected as part of the study reported in Passardi et al. (2022).

5. ibid.

and brutalization, and deprivation. The psychological responses to these dimensions do not easily fit psychiatric nosology. One construct that potentially captures these dimensions and has been applied generally to the plight of forcibly displaced persons is "moral injury" (Nickerson et al. 2015).

The term moral injury as a "betrayal of what's right" was first conceptualized by Shay in 1991 to describe a psychological state in returned military personnel who were refractory to conventional PTSD and MDD treatment approaches. Shay conceptualized moral injury using the catastrophic failure of Agamemnon, Achilles, Odysseus, and Hector, each in his own way, to protect and care for those under their charge. This dereliction of doing what is right by someone with legitimate authority in a high-stakes situation is experienced by the affected individual as a betrayal resulting in moral injury (Shay 2014). Litz et al. (2009) expanded the concept to include the affected individual as the perpetrator of an act that violates their own moral framework. This has been termed "moral injury–self", and is distinguished from "moral injury–other" —the type of moral injury that is externally inflicted upon, or witnessed by, the individual (Houtsma et al. 2017). The potentiality of these acts, either inflicted by an external authority or perpetrated by the individual, to induce or not induce moral injury has led to their being labeled as potentially morally injurious events (PMIEs).

The recognition of the violation by the authority or by one's own self promotes in the individual negative moral emotions such as shame, guilt, disgust, anger, social withdrawal, self-condemnation, and difficulties in forgiveness (Griffin et al. 2019; Hall et al. 2022). These states of mind and emotion induced by PMIEs are proposed to engender psychological distress and mental disorder, where PTSD, MDD, and suicidality remain associated with PMIEs after controlling for sociodemographic characteristics, trauma history, and prior psychiatric diagnosis (Wisco et al. 2017).

However, the characteristics of moral injury are variously described to encompass features additional to symptoms of PTSD and MDD, including self-harming (such as non-suicidal self-injury), self-handicapping behaviors, demoralization (e.g., helplessness), ruptured social bonds (Nash et al. 2013), negative shifts in psychospiritual development (Harris et al. 2015), and other functional impairments (Farnsworth et al. 2017). Studies of PMIEs in military personnel demonstrate perceived or actual rejection by family or friends (Flipse Vargas et al. 2013), resentment due to feeling misunderstood by civilians (Ferrajão and Oliveira 2014, 2015, 2016; Worthen and Ahern 2014), and loss of trust in military command, romantic partners, government, or society in general (McCormack and Ell 2017). Similarly, in healthcare providers, alienation from colleagues and occupational guilds after exposure to work-related PMIEs (Gibbons et al. 2013; Haight et al. 2017) and distress due to guilt, shame, disgust, withdrawal, and self-condemnation have been described.

The saliency of this concept has seen burgeoning interest as it has been applied across a range of other groups, including refugees and asylum seekers (Nickerson et al. 2015). In diversifying its application, the specific concept has broadened, resulting in a variety of constructs grouped under the term "moral injury." With reference to refugees and asylum seekers, it can be easily perceived that pre-migration and migration events, such as human rights abuses that have compelled forcible displacement or have occurred in transit, may potentially be morally injurious. In addition, potentially morally injurious events in a post-migration setting in a settlement country, while not the focus here, could include discrimination, racism (Borges et al. 2022), and violence (Entorf and Lange 2023).

However, although there is substantive experiential comparability in the above descriptions, those with an immigration detention experience describe qualitatively different types of PMIE (Passardi et al. 2022). The descriptions of PMIE in the literature are of discrete, traumatic, and identifiable events; for example, Shay (2014) relates the experience of a soldier having to kill a baby used as a human-shield when shooting an enemy sniper. Although some former detainees experienced serious violence and trauma, all former immigration detainees describe a multitude of minor violations, indignities, and injustices regarding their detention experiences – such as being called by a number and not their name – and, as noted above, brief regulated showers and restricted access to sanitary products. This appears to undermine the applicability of the concept of moral injury as a response to a discrete, significant, and traumatic event. There are two clear exceptions to this generalization. The first are the descriptions of sexual assault and rape which have long been described as PMIEs (Hampton 1999) but in mainstream settings more commonly result in PTSD and depression (Lomax and Meyrick 2022) and which may of course result in both moral injury and mental illness.

The second relates to the expectation by detainees that Australia would provide a safe haven free from the persecutions they were fleeing. The betrayal of this expectation was noted, often bitterly, by many of the former detainees. It is not clear how this experience overlaps with the concept of betrayal as described in the moral injury literature, where the betraying or injuring entity is the authority that oversees or governs the individual in a direct relationship. For example, in initial formulations of moral injury the betrayal is by the leaders and system which have fiduciary responsibility toward the betrayed individual who has reciprocated with loyalty, such as a soldier in the army (Shay 2014). For the asylum seeker or refugee, the immigration system does not appear to accept fiduciary responsibility, and it would be difficult to envisage that the asylum seeker or refugee feels a sense of loyalty toward the immigration system. A lower level relationship does exist, however, where the asylum seeker expects the refugee determination process to operate in a fair and humane manner and the immigration system in detaining people has a duty of care toward them. In this lower level relationship the betrayal experienced by the asylum seeker may be due to the refugee determination process not being fair or humane and the immigration system not providing sufficient care.

Here the parallel concept of institutional betrayal may be more apposite (Smith and Freyd 2014). It describes the perpetration of wrongdoings on an individual, including the failure to prevent or respond to wrongdoings within the context of the institution. Examples here include church-based institutions not protecting children from sexual abuse perpetrated by the clergy, schools not protecting students from abuse by teachers, and workplaces not supporting injured workers (Smith and Freyd 2014). With regard to immigration detention, the impacts on the individual are the direct effects of the institution. In the Australian context, this institution is the Department of Home Affairs and Australian Border Force, and responsibility is ascribed by former detainees to these agencies and not to the individual staff. The relationship, though, is a duty of care rather than a fiduciary relationship, which is the nature of institutions such as churches and schools, which are the focus for Freyd. How this contextual difference in loyalty and responsibility – which are the hallmarks of moral injury and institutional betrayal – and the betrayal experience of the detained asylum seeker translate into psychological or psychiatric differences remains to be fully elucidated.

In summary, Australian immigration policies that utilize indefinite mandatory detention in offshore settings have had catastrophic impacts on the mental health of detainees. These include unprecedented rates of mental illness in those surveyed on Manus Island and in a small sample of former detainees in Nauru. Moreover, those who were in Nauru manifest a constellation of psychological harms with features analogous to moral injury and institutional betrayal. However, the characteristics of the traumas and violations, in particular the absence of a singular or specific traumatic incident for most, and anomalous psychological features – such as the general absence of guilt or disgust – argue against a direct equivalence between the experiences of former immigration detainees and the concepts of moral injury and institutional betrayal as described in the literature. The medium- to long-term consequences of the psychological harms inflicted on offshore immigration center detainees needs to be determined. Nevertheless, the short- to medium-term consequences are unequivocally profoundly damaging, and this must be prioritized by policymakers in considering such detention centers.

REFERENCES

Asylum Seeker Resource Centre. 2025. "Twelve years later, $13 billion, no plan: Offshore processing drags into its thirteenth year." https://asrc.org.au/2025/07/19/twelve-years-later-offshore-processing/.

Australian Human Rights Commission. "A Last Resort? National Inquiry into Children in Immigration Detention." Edited by Dr Sev Ozdowski. Sydney: Human Rights and Equal Opportunity Commission, 2004. https://humanrights.gov.au/our-work/asylum-seekers-and-refugees/publications/last-resort-national-inquiry-children-immigration.

Australian Human Rights Commission. 2013. "Human Rights Issues Raised by the Third Country Processing Regime." Australian Human Rights Commission.

Borges, Lauren M., Alisha Desai, Sean M. Barnes, and Jacob P. S. Johnson. 2022. "The Role of Social Determinants of Health in Moral Injury: Implications and Future Directions." [In eng]. *Current Treatment Options in Psychiatry* 9 (3): 202–214. https://doi.org/10.1007/s40501-022-00272-4.

Entorf, Horst, and Martin Lange. 2023. "Refugees Welcome? Understanding the Regional Heterogeneity of Anti-Refugee Hate Crime." *Regional Science and Urban Economics* 101: 103913. https://doi.org/https://doi.org/10.1016/j.regsciurbeco.2023.103913.

Farnsworth, Jacob K., Kent D. Drescher, Wyatt Evans, and Robyn D. Walser. 2017. "A Functional Approach to Understanding and Treating Military-Related Moral Injury." *Journal of Contextual Behavioral Science* 6 (4): 391–397. https://doi.org/10.1016/j.jcbs.2017.07.003.

Ferrajão, Paulo, and Rui Aragao Oliveira. 2014. "Self-Awareness of Mental States, Self-Integration of Personal Schemas, Perceived Social Support, Posttraumatic and Depression Levels, and Moral Injury: A Mixed-Method Study among Portuguese War Veterans." *Traumatology* 20: 277–285. https://doi.org/10.1037/trm0000016.

Ferrajão, Paulo Correia, and Rui Aragão Oliveira. 2015. "From Self-Integration in Personal Schemas of Morally Experiences to Self-Awareness of Mental States: A Qualitative Study among a Sample of Portuguese War Veterans." *Traumatology* 21 (1): 22–31. https://doi.org/10.1037/trm0000019.

Ferrajão, Paulo C., and Rui Aragão Oliveira. 2016. "Portuguese War Veterans: Moral Injury and Factors Related to Recovery from Ptsd." [In eng]. *Qualitative Health Research* 26 (2): 204–214. https://doi.org/10.1177/1049732315573012.

Fleay, Caroline, and Susan Hoffman. 2014. "Despair as a Governing Strategy: Australia and the Offshore Processing of Asylum-Seekers on Nauru." *Refugee Survey Quarterly* 33: 1–19. https://doi.org/10.1093/rsq/hdu004.

Vargas, Alison Flipse, Thomas Hanson, Douglas Kraus, Kent Drescher, and David Foy. 2013. "Moral Injury Themes in Combat Veterans 'Narrative Responses from the National Vietnam Veterans' Readjustment Study." *Traumatology* 19 (3): 243–250. https://doi.org/10.1177/1534765613476099.

Gibbons, Susanne W., Michaela Shafer, Edward J. Hickling, and Gloria Ramsey. "How Do Deployed Health Care Providers Experience Moral Injury?" [In eng].

Narrative Inquiry in Bioethics 3, no. 3 (Winter 2013): 247–259. https://doi.org/10.1353/nib.2013.0055.

Griffin, Brandon J., Natalie Purcell, Kristine Burkman, Brett T. Litz, Craig J. Bryan, Martha Schmitz, Claudia Villierme, Jessica Walsh, and Shira Maguen. 2019. "Moral Injury: An Integrative Review." [In eng]. *Journal of Traumatic Stress* 32 (3) (Jun 2019): 350–362. https://doi.org/10.1002/jts.22362.

Haight, Wendy, Erin Sugrue, Molly Calhoun, and James Black. 2017. "Everyday Coping with Moral Injury: The Perspectives of Professionals and Parents Involved with Child Protection Services." *Children and Youth Services Review* 82. https://doi.org/10.1016/j.childyouth.2017.09.025.

Hall, Nicole A., Adam T. Everson, Madison R. Billingsley, and Mary Beth Miller. "Moral Injury, Mental Health and Behavioural Health Outcomes: A Systematic Review of the Literature." [In eng]. Clinical Psychology and Psychotherapy 29, no. 1 (Jan 2022): 92–110. https://doi.org/10.1002/cpp.2607.

Hampton, Jean. 1999. "Defining Wrong and Defining Rape." In *A Most Detestable Crime: New Philosophical Essays on Rape* edited by Keith Burgess-Jackson: Oxford University Press.

Harris, Jeanette Irene, Crystal L. Park, Joseph Currier, Timothy Usset, and Cory Voecks. 2015. "Moral Injury and Psycho-Spiritual Development: Considering the Developmental Context." *Spirituality in Clinical Practice* 2: 256–266. https://doi.org/10.1037/scp0000045.

Hedrick, Kyli, Gregory Armstrong, and Rohan Borschmann. 2019. "Self-Harm among Asylum Seekers in Australian Immigration Detention." *The Lancet Public Health* 4 (12): e604. https://doi.org/10.1016/S2468-2667(19)30221-X.

Houtsma, Claire, Lauren R. Khazem, Bradley A. Green, and Michael D. Anestis. 2017. "Isolating Effects of Moral Injury and Low Post-Deployment Support within the U.S. Military." *Psychiatry Research* 247: 194–199. https://doi.org/https://doi.org/10.1016/j.psychres.2016.11.031.

Litz, Brett T., Nathan Stein, Eileen Delaney, Leslie Lebowitz, William P. Nash, Caroline Silva, and Shira Maguen. 2009. "Moral Injury and Moral Repair in War Veterans: A Preliminary Model and Intervention Strategy." [In eng]. *Clinical Psychology Review* 29 (8): 695–706. https://doi.org/10.1016/j.cpr.2009.07.003.

Lomax, Jane, and Jane Meyrick. 2022. "Systematic Review: Effectiveness of Psychosocial Interventions on Wellbeing Outcomes for Adolescent or Adult Victim/Survivors of Recent Rape or Sexual Assault." [In eng]. *Journal of Health Psychology* 27 (2): 305–331. https://doi.org/10.1177/1359105320950799.

McCormack, Lynne, and Linda Ell. 2017. "Complex Psychosocial Distress Post-Deployment in Veterans: Reintegration Identity Disruption and Challenged Moral Integrity." *Traumatology* 23: 240–249.

Meaney, Neville. 1995. "The End of 'White Australia' and Australia's Changing Perceptions of Asia, 1945–1990." *Australian Journal of International Affairs* 49 (2): 171–189. https://doi.org/10.1080/10357719508445155.

Nash, William P., Teresa L. Marino Carper, Mary Alice Mills, Teresa Au, Abigail Goldsmith, and Brett T. Litz. 2013. "Psychometric Evaluation of the Moral Injury Events Scale." [In eng]. *Military Medicine* 178 (6): 646–652. https://doi.org/10.7205/milmed-d-13-00017.

Nethery, Amy, and Rosa Holman. 2016. "Secrecy and Human Rights Abuse in Australia's Offshore Immigration Detention Centres." *The International Journal of Human Rights* 20 (7): 1018–1038. https://doi.org/10.1080/13642987.2016.1196903.

Nickerson, Angela, Ulrich Schnyder, Richard A. Bryant, Matthis Schick, Julia Mueller, and Naser Morina. 2015. "Moral Injury in Traumatized Refugees." [In eng]. *Psychotherapy and Psychosomatics* 84 (2): 122–123. https://doi.org/10.1159/000369353.

Passardi, Sandra, Debbie C. Hocking, Naser Morina, Suresh Sundram, and Eva Alisic. 2022. "Moral Injury Related to Immigration Detention on Nauru: A Qualitative Study." *European Journal of Psychotraumatology* 13 (1): 2029042. https://doi.org/10.1080/20008198.2022.2029042.

Refugee Council of Australia. 2020. "Australia's Detention Policies." https://www.refugeecouncil.org.au/detention-policies/2/.

Refugee Council of Australia. 2023. "Offshore Processing Statistics." https://www.refugeecouncil.org.au/operation-sovereign-borders-offshore-detention-statistics/.

Shay, Jonathan. 1991. "Learning about Combat Stress from Homer's Iliad." *Journal of Traumatic Stress* 4 (4): 561–579.

Shay, Jonathan. 2014. "Moral Injury." *Psychoanalytic Psychology* 31: 182–191.

Smith, Carly Parnitzke, and Jennifer J. Freyd. 2014. "Institutional Betrayal." *American Psychologist* 69 (6): 575–587. https://doi.org/10.1037/a0037564.

Sundram, Suresh, and Peter Ventevogel. 2017. "The Mental Health of Refugees and Asylum Seekers on Manus Island." *The Lancet* 390 (10112): 2534–2536. https://doi.org/10.1016/S0140-6736(17)33051-9.

The Conversation. 2025. "By sending non-visa-holders to Nauru, Australia is shifting its responsibilities." https://theconversation.com/by-sending-non-visa-holders-to-nauru-australia-is-shifting-its-responsibilities-264256.

Turrini, Giulia, Marianna Purgato, Francesca Ballette, Michela Nosè, Giovanni Ostuzzi, and Corrado Barbui. 2017. "Common Mental Disorders in Asylum Seekers and Refugees: Umbrella Review of Prevalence and Intervention Studies." [In eng]. *International Journal of Mental Health Systems* 11: 51. https://doi.org/10.1186/s13033-017-0156-0.

UN High Commissioner for Refugees. 2016. "Inquiry into the Serious Allegations of Abuse, Self-Harm and Neglect of Asylum-Seekers in Relation to the Nauru Regional Processing Centre, and Any Like Allegations in Relation to the Manus Regional Processing Centre." https://www.unhcr.org/au/media/submission-senate-legal-and-constitutional-affairs-committee-serious-allegations-abuse-self.

University of Oxford. 2024. "The Australian Border Deaths Database." https://www.law.ox.ac.uk/border-criminologies/australian-border-deaths-database.

Wisco, Blair E., Brian P. Marx, Casey L. May, Brenda Martini, John H. Krystal, Steven M. Southwick, and Robert H. Pietrzak. 2017. "Moral Injury in U.S. Combat Veterans: Results from the National Health and Resilience in Veterans Study." [In eng]. *Depression and Anxiety*. https://doi.org/10.1002/da.22614.

Worthen, Miranda, and Jennifer Ahern. 2014. "The Causes, Course, and Consequences of Anger Problems in Veterans Returning to Civilian Life." *Journal of Loss and Trauma* 19 (4): 355–363. https://doi.org/10.1080/15325024.2013.788945.

7

Toward a Pragmatic Solidarity with Refugees

THALIA ARAWI AND ANAS EL ZOUHBI

At a time when there are more refugees than ever, the rich world has turned its back on them. Our myths and religions are steeped in the lore of exile and yet we fail to treat the living examples of that condition as fully human.

—Ben Rawlence, *City of Thorns: Nine Lives in the World's Largest Refugee Camp*

7.1 INTRODUCTION

The world is witnessing an unprecedented global displacement crisis, reaching, according to the United Nations High Commissioner for Refugees (UNHCR), "more than 100 million forcibly displaced people including refugees, internally displaced persons and asylum seekers who have fled their homes to escape violence, conflict and persecution" (World Bank Group 2023). Among the plethora of displaced populations, refugees have the highest mortality and morbidity rate compared to their respective host communities. The ecology of refugee camps, which are marked by destroyed infrastructure and superstructure, contaminated water, lack of access to healthcare, epidemics on the rise, poverty, lack of education, and unemployment, to mention but a few perils, makes refugees prone to psychological troubles, chronic and communicable diseases, and social abdication. Most host countries look at these "guests" as a de trop package they are not willing to absorb, which in turn limits their access to their basic needs in general and healthcare in particular (Asgary and Segar 2011). This situation is poignant in the Global South in general and the Middle East in particular. With the increased number of crises faced by nations in the Middle East (such as Syria beginning 2011, Palestine since 1948, Lebanon in 2006 and

Thalia Arawi and Anas El Zouhbi, *Toward a Pragmatic Solidarity with Refugees*. In: *Forced Migration and Health Justice*. Edited by: Lisa A. Eckenwiler, Verina Wild, Anna Gotlib, Ryoa Chung, and Deborah Zion, Oxford University Press. © Oxford University Press (2026). DOI: 10.1093/oso/9780197795491.003.0007

2024), forced migration has taken its toll and placed even more limitations on healthcare access, leading to significant inequalities. This structural injustice, as Iris Marion Young (2011) defines it, produced by far-reaching social structures and practices that generate systemic disadvantages for large groups of persons, is exemplified, perhaps in its most extreme form, in the struggles faced by refugees, who are often positioned as stateless and dispensable, existing in what Giorgio Agamben (2005) calls a *state of exception*, that is, a situation where the normal legal order is suspended due to a crisis or emergency. Refugees leave their homeland in search of a better life for themselves and their families, risking almost everything in an attempt to escape hunger, poverty, and death. While the right to healthcare is considered a paramount right by international organizations and by many governments around the world, the following, often ignored question raised by Paul Farmer reverberates: "If access to healthcare is considered a human right, who is considered human enough to have that right?" (Farmer 2004).

This chapter addresses the plight faced by refugees in general, and those in the Middle East in particular, when it comes to accessing healthcare. We draw upon the work of Giorgio Agamben, along with Michel Foucault's notion of biopolitics, as well as Achille Mbembe's thinking on necropolitics, to help examine why this purported "right" is not recognized as belonging to refugees. We will start by providing you with a gaze that you can use to see the lived experience of refugees, offering a glimpse into the profound struggles they endure. By exploring the impact of displacement on their daily lives, we will highlight how a simple change in status can drastically alter their reality. From restricted mobility to the constant uncertainty of their future, the challenges are many. We will then shift our focus to the Middle East, examining key developments, statistics, and often overlooked issues that contribute to the complexities of the refugee crisis in the region. Finally, we will explore how these circumstances affect refugees' access to essential healthcare services, revealing the significant barriers they face in obtaining even the most basic medical care.

In his novel *Men in the Sun* (*Rijal fil al Shams*), Kanafani (1978) recounts the story of three refugees and their unsuccessful attempts to travel stealthily from country to country in search of a recovered life for themselves and their families. Their lives in refugee camps were harsh enough to push them into a risky journey. They hide inside an empty water tank and, while their smuggler is held up at the border, succumb to the unbearable heat. When the smuggler discovers their bodies, the novel ends with a poignant statement: "Why didn't you knock on the sides of the tank? Why didn't you say anything? Why?" (65).

Now, 41 years later and not too far from where Kanafani's heroes try to escape a bad fate, illegal immigration is on the rise in Tripoli, Lebanon's impoverished northern city, where, ironically, Lebanon's richest politicians live (MEMO 2022). A significant number of unemployed or impoverished families tried to escape their wrecked existence on board what came to be called "rescue" boats. Even when these "rescue" boats were filled beyond capacity, people attempted to take the hazardous trip to Europe just to flee from a painful situation where the simplest of human needs and rights are not met. Like Marwan in the novel the *Sea Prayer*, by Khaled Hosseini (2018)—a character fashioned after Syrian refugee Alan Kurdi, who drowned in the Mediterranean Sea while trying to migrate with his family to Europe in 2015—these immigrants are "a precious cargo" hoping to reach the shores of a country whose people live mostly unscathed by the trepidations of war and famine. We should see such stories as examples of structural injustice and, indeed, of Paul Farmer's thinking when he noted, "In this increasingly interconnected world, we must understand that what happens to poor people is never divorced from the actions of the powerful" (2003, p. 2020).

7.2 REFUGEES, STORIES, AND (IN)JUSTICE

A refugee is generally described as someone who has been forced to flee their country because of circumstances beyond their control, such as, though not limited to, persecution, war, or violence. The UNHCR (1951) Refugee Convention defines a refugee as someone who, "owing to well-founded fear of being persecuted for reasons of race, religion, nationality, membership of a particular social group or political opinion, is outside the country of his nationality and is unable or, owing to such fear, is unwilling to avail himself of the protection of that country; or who, not having a nationality and being outside the country of his former habitual residence as a result of such events, is unable or, owing to such fear, is unwilling to return to it" (UN Office of the High Commissioner for Human Rights 1950). Forced migrants can also be internally displaced persons (IDPs). The UN Office of the High Commissioner for Human Rights (n.d.) defines IDPs as "persons or groups of persons who have been forced or obliged to flee or to leave their homes or places of habitual residence, in particular as a result of or in order to avoid the effects of armed conflict, situations of generalized violence, violations of human rights or natural or human-made disasters, and who have not crossed an internationally recognized border."

However, the most moving and evocative accounts of what it means to be a refugee can be found in literature and the narratives of those who were exiled and became refugees. Palestinian political cartoonist Naji Al-Ali (1985) describes the iconic figure of Handala (a boy he invented who later became a symbol of resistance) as follows: "Handala is not a fat, happy, relaxed, or pampered child. He is barefooted like the refugee camp children." We see Dolores in Maalouf's (2020) novel *The Disoriented* lamenting the death of her boyfriend Adam, illustrating refugees as "condemned to deferral," living in a state of suspension, so to speak. In the preface of her *Baddawi*, Abdelrazaq (2015) describes Palestinian refugees as "born into a life of exile and persecution, indefinitely suspended in statelessness." Refugees are those who have no fixed address. They are the Ethiopians who live in London but "do not even furnish their flats. What possessions they acquire sit in their cardboard boxes ready for transport. The tower of boxes holding televisions, toaster ovens, microwaves, electric heaters teeters to the left of the door, ready to be shipped at a moment's notice. They commit to nothing. They float on the myth of return" (Gibb 2011, 29). "[C]aught between the ongoing war in Somalia and a world unwilling to welcome them, the refugees can only survive in the camp by imagining a life elsewhere. It is unsettling: neither the past, nor the present, nor the future is a safe place for a mind to linger for long" (Rawlence 2016, 5). They are people from Syria who live in *A Land of Permanent Goodbyes* (Abawi 2018). They are the Hamids and the Maryams of *All That's Left to You* (Kanafani 2004) living with a suppressed sense of abashment and blameworthiness among the refugees who eventually die. When one visits a graveyard one recognizes them, for there are no names on the tombstones, rather only numbers (Hosseini 2018). Perhaps it was Alsanousi (2015) who explained it best, simply though powerfully, when Jose, the protagonist of *The Bamboo Stalk*, speaks of yearning to be like a bamboo stalk taking root in whatever soil he plants his feet after leaving the Philippines. Jose admits that no matter how long he stayed in Kuwait, he was unable to feel at home: "I was more like a bamboo plant, which doesn't belong anywhere in particular. You can cut off a piece of the stalk and plant it without roots in any piece of ground. Before long the stalk sprouts new roots and starts to grow again in the new ground, with no past, no memory" (78).

Again, a refugee lives in a state of suspension, and, as noted by Schuilenburg, "[t]oday's refugees can be therefore labeled as 'margizens'; that is, individuals whose life is qualitatively distinct from that of the citizen" (2008, 363). A refugee is therefore someone whose identity and being are shaped by circumstances they have no control over—a being complex and shriveled, an outsider however hard they try, someone who suffers in silence, fights to stay alive and to move forward, someone whose basic needs are not always met and whose dignity stands in the way of asking for help. Many refugees are people whose roots keep pushing them toward a different destination, only to discover that the destination is a death that has no address.

7.3 REFUGEES IN THE MIDDLE EAST AND ACCESS TO CARE

Geopolitical wars and humanitarian disasters have long plagued the Middle East and forced millions of people to flee their homes and thus become refugees. Refugees' health and well-being are intricately linked to the larger issues that host communities and overburdened healthcare systems are dealing with as refugees seek safety and shelter. The Middle East refugee crisis and urgent need to treat the health needs of people who have been forcefully displaced presents complex problems compounded by the already existing and worsening socioeconomic crises that many host countries are facing; it is a crisis that requires the assistance and cooperation of the international community.

In September 2022, the *Middle East Monitor* reported continuous obstacles to patients' access to hospitals outside of the Gaza Strip due to political decisions, which resulted in five patients losing their lives. Data from 2018 show an unsettling reality about the transportation of patients by ambulance from various parts of the West Bank to Jerusalem. Surprisingly, patients had to be switched to another ambulance at checkpoints in 84% of the 1,462 documented ambulance transports before proceeding to Jerusalem. The requirement for ambulance-to-ambulance transfers at checkpoints significantly impedes timely and effective patient transportation, diverting critical healthcare resources and increasing delays in accessing critical medical treatments (World Health Organization [WHO] 2018).

Other issues faced by Palestinian refugees are chronic illnesses and the need for palliative care. When we first began writing this chapter, cancer care was largely provided in small oncology departments at Palestinian governmental hospitals in the West Bank, complemented by private institutions contracted by the Palestinian Ministry of Health. However, these facilities lack specialized pathology laboratories, advanced diagnostic and imaging capabilities, and radiation therapy. Patients who required radiation therapy or advanced diagnostic services at that time were typically sent to East Jerusalem or neighboring countries. Obtaining authorization and permits for these referrals is a convoluted and confusing process that leads to delays and denials that negatively affect patient outcomes. Consider one of the interview answers of a 54-year-old male in a study assessing the care for cancer patients in West Bank Palestine:

> By God, these permits are burdensome and taxing, burdensome and taxing. . . .Even though I have a commercial permit, they issued a permit for my son and they did not issue me a permit, not allowed. [With] my commercial permit, [I have to] go into the tunnel [a different crossing from his son's], they said let the boy in and I was not allowed. The Israeli soldier at the checkpoint said: you should go down and around to Bethlehem [in the south] to

> the checkpoint there, and the Israeli army checkpoint was so congested with workers [Palestinian workers wanting to cross to work in Israel] and I should have been there with my son at 7.30 am. (Mitwalli et al. 2023, Interview #7)

Moreover, lack of medication often accompanies the many other hardships faced by refugees. The absence of cancer treatment and pain medications reflects the lack of a proper palliative care program, which is an "essential and needed service within the definition of Universal Health Coverage" (Worldwide Hospice Palliative Care Alliance 2014). According to a UNICEF (2016) report, Yemen is experiencing an unparalleled humanitarian catastrophe, with around 12 million children without access to food, water, shelter, or healthcare: "Children are fighting an epidemic, a pandemic, famine, and a WAR all at the same time." Since the conflict that escalated in Yemen early 2015, more than 10,200 children have been injured or killed. Additional to the severe physical harms, a significant mental health disaster is taking place that will likely endure even after the war is ended. From the previous decade to the present, the Global South in general, and the Middle East in particular, have been disrupted by various types of wars and conflicts. Many people have abandoned their homes, while others have become refugees in their own countries (Table 7.1).

Syrians are the largest refugee population, 6.8 million displaced individuals, primarily hosted by Turkey, which shelters 3.7 million refugees. Venezuelans follow, at 3.9 million refugees, mostly in Jordan (3.0 million). Palestinians make up 3.4 million refugees, 1.5 million of whom are hosted by Uganda. Pakistan hosts 1.4 million of the 2.6 million Afghan refugees, and Lebanon provides refuge to 1.3 million of South Sudan's 2.3 million refugees (UNHCR 2022; World Population Review 2023).

It does not require a lot of research to realize that a huge number of migrants and refugees are being denied proper healthcare—and, at times, any form of healthcare. WHO's director of health and migration, Santino

Table 7.1. NUMBER OF REFUGEES BY ORIGIN AND BY HOST COUNTRY

Country of origin	Number of refugees (in millions)	Host country	Number of refugees hosted (in millions)
Syria	6.8	Turkey	3.7
Venezuela	3.9	Jordan	3.0
Palestine	3.4	Uganda	1.5
Afghanistan	2.6	Pakistan	1.4
South Sudan	2.3	Lebanon	1.3

Sources: United Nations High Commissioner for Refugees (UNHCR 2022), World Population Review (2023). The table shows those numbers that are most relevant to the chapter.

Severoni, pointed out that "[h]ealth does not begin or end at a country's border. Migratory status should therefore not be a discriminatory factor but a policy driver on which to build and strengthen healthcare" (Reuters 2022).

In January 2020, Médecins Sans Frontières (2020) reported that in the Moria camp located in Lesbos, Greece, the Greek government was "deliberately depriving at least 140 children with chronic, complex and life-threatening diseases of adequate medical care." The Syrian conflict of a decade ago led to Palestinian refugees being denied access to life-saving healthcare services and essential medicines. This is largely because the UN Relief and Works Agency for Palestine Refugees has either been disrupted or fully gone out of operation because of the bombardment. In the Palestinian Gaza Strip, IDPs have also been denied access to essential healthcare, often leading to permanent damage or death because of what is called the "political determinants of health" caused by decades of siege, physical impediments to movement, and a system of health permit travel that, by definition, challenges the very notion of healthcare as a human right (Dawes 2020; Abimbola 2023). Yemenis, including children and the elderly, have been denied access to healthcare to the point of death and food to the point of starvation. Perpetual attacks on hospitals and healthcare facilities in Taiz, Yemen, have damaged healthcare infrastructure.

Ghassan Abu-Sittah (personal communication, August 8, 2022), a surgeon who went to Yemen in 2020, describes the situation there:

> Even in South Yemen, which is the part of Yemen that's on the side of the coalition, the state of the healthcare system which is completely collapsed reflects the destruction of the state in the Arab world. Aden, which is ostensibly the capital of the area, and which is controlled by the government recognized by the Gulf states and the West, boasts a healthcare system that is dismal. The only functioning tertiary referral hospital was inaugurated by Princess Elizabeth when the British still controlled Aden in the 1960s. The government, including the health minister, is in Riyadh rather than in Aden and what is left of the remnants of the health system is divided between different factions within the government, rather than having a unified formulated health strategy.

As Abu-Sittah states, "We have fragmented health centers that answer to different political masters" (personal communication, August 8, 2022) He adds that the "destruction of the state and the arrival of different political elites for whom the provision of healthcare is not part of the state building project" is common in Syria, Lebanon, and Iraq. It is also manifest in the Palestine Authority, in the post-2023 Iraqi governments, and even in the discourse of the Syrian opposition (personal communication, August 8, 2022). He explains that "the provision of healthcare which was intrinsic to the state building project in the post-colonial period no longer occupies that central place," noting that one can see this "in Libya, in the recent civil war in Sudan, almost everywhere in the Arab world" (personal communication, August 8, 2022).

7.4 BIOPOWER, NECROPOLITICS, AND STRUCTURAL INJUSTICE

It is our contention that states no longer consider the provision of healthcare to all those living on their lands as a requirement of good governance. We even dare say that it is the deliberate withholding of healthcare from many, including refugees and IDPs, that is on states' agenda via an invisible biopolitical ideology meshing with Mbembian necropolitics—the political rendering of spaces and subjectivities somewhere between life and death. Settlements and plantation slavery have led to necropolitical practices that are promoted by white supremacy even to this day.

Who is to blame for the discrepancy embedded within healthcare systems that refuse some persons access to care? It seems impossible to assign blame to one distinct entity, let alone accuse any particular group of being entirely in the wrong. Instead we need to consider the larger scope of the issue by focusing on three factors: (1) structural injustice, (2) biopolitics and (3) the politics of space. Iris Marion Young discusses these in her book *Responsibility for Justice*:

> Structural injustice, then, exists when social processes put large groups of persons under systematic threat of domination or deprivation of the means to develop and exercise their capacities, while these processes enable others to dominate or to have a wide range of opportunities for developing and exercising capacities available to them. Structural injustice is a kind of moral wrong distinct from the wrongful action of an individual agent or the repressive policies of a state. Structural injustice occurs as a consequence of many individuals and institutions acting to pursue their particular goals and interests, for the most part within the limits of accepted rules and norms (2011,114).

The "docile bodies," colored and stateless, to borrow the words of the French thinker Michel Foucault (1977), are othered, dehumanized according to skin color, place of origin, and level of wealth, thus perpetuating a world that favors the few at the cost of the many. The many, as far as this chapter is concerned, are mainly refugees and IDPs. This brings us to the second element which helps us appreciate the bigger picture, namely, biopower and biopolitics. Under the guise and pretext of protection, governments are established, and, human nature being what it is, biopower emerges. The concept of biopower, usually attributed to Foucault's *The History of Sexuality* (1976), states that the biological health and well-being of the populace is entwined with the operations and functions of political power.

Foucault argues that biopower is a new form of social and political control that modern governments have produced by controlling life and subjugating populations through the medical, demographic, and biological sciences. This form of power entails healthcare as a commodity, statistics, and officialdom. We might add to that the hegemony of the dollar, the symbol of capitalism and neoliberalism. Thus modern powers get to decide who matters and who does not. Some populations (generally based on skin color, place of origin, and poverty level) are selected to be given life, while others are not, and the choice seems to be based on looking at the spectrum of worth and utility (with respect to capital) as interpreted by the government.

In his essay "Necropolitics," the Cameroonian thinker Achille Mbembe brought to light the idea of the conquest of life by the power of death: "The ultimate expression of sovereignty resides, to a large degree, in the power and the capacity to dictate who may live and who may die," which is incarnated in the modern political system of democracy (2003, 11). Mbembe refers to the Gaza Strip, where Israel is unilaterally exercising control over the mortality of Palestinian refugees, forced to leave their homes running from wars that threaten them and their families, crushed by necropower and the fear of death.

Death, we contend, is not only the loss of life. It has several other forms: psychological death, death of the future, hunger, and more. This is a perpetual death without the relief of final death, a "death in life," the best illustration of which are the Palestinian people living in the biggest open camp on earth: Gaza. Hasan Ahmed 'Abed al-Kharti, from the Deheisheh Refugee Camp near Bethlehem on the West Bank, suffered from tongue and throat cancer (Ministry of Health, Gaza 2021). He had received a medical referral for treatment at the al-Makassed Hospital in occupied East Jerusalem. On May 27, 2021, the Coordination and Liaison Department at the Ministry of Health applied for a travel permit for Hasan. The Israeli authorities refused his travel application, and Hasan died three days later. He was 62. Hasan is one of many Gazans who lived in the biggest open-space prison in the world, where hospitals are under siege and suffering serious damage to infrastructure and lack of access to medicines. Hasan is also one of the many refugees whose life and death depended on political power and biopolitics. It might be sufficient to take a quick look at the status of refugees around the world in general, and in the Middle East in particular, to appreciate the gravity of this issue. Some people are denied basic rights because they are viewed as "de trop," to use the words of the French philosopher Jean-Paul Sartre, meaning useless and disposable.

As described by Hashem Abushama in *On Refugee Agency, Bio-Politics, and a New World*, "Refugees are far from being bare lives; their bodies constitute sites onto which many 'bodily-spatial struggles' manifest: struggles with memory and remembrance; with the space of the camp, its expansion, its constant remaking; with narratives, humanitarian and nationalist, that aim to tell a unified story of suffering for the former and heroism for the latter; and, in some cases, such as Israel, French settler colonial Algeria, Canada, the United States, and Australia, with the settler colonial state and its racial apparatus" (2021, 35). As such, the struggles faced by refugees are beyond imaginable. Palestinian refugee camps in Lebanon, argues Hanafi (2013, 590), are treated "as a space of exception and an experimental laboratory for control and surveillance." Two telling examples of control and surveillance are (1) the "calorie count" strategy used by the state of Israel to limit Gaza food during the siege from 2007 to mid-2010, ensuring Gazans would neither starve to death nor live a reasonably healthy life, and (2) maiming the abled body to render it disabled, as became evident during the several Marches of Return in the Occupied Palestinian Territory (Hass 2012; Shehadeh 2015).

This so-called right to maim is one method employed by a sovereign power to control life or its lack. To quote Puar, "[A]s the inhabitants of the West Bank are suffering and resisting together with the collective punishment of the occupation, no one is constituted as an idealized able body" (2017, 158). Wars, which have been increasing during the past decades, particularly in the Middle East and the Global South, are a technique used to acquire more sovereign power and what is known as the "élan vital," Bergson's impulse for life, through the right to kill and subjugate (Butler 2006). Refugees are othered, constructed as less human, and ultimately reduced to the status of bare life, leading to the existence of a living dead: no rights, no acknowledgment, no healthcare. Some lives are deemed "livable," while others are deemed "unlivable"; similarly, certain bodies are deemed either "underdeveloped" or "undevelopable" (Weber 2016).

The international humanitarian laws, the Geneva Conventions, and their additional protocols set out laws to govern armed conflict (International Committee of the Red Cross, 1949). These laws are far too rarely observed by those in power, and one of the main tenets—proportionality—is often ignored in order to kill without accountability. One must use a different lens to view the effects of the recent wars in Yemen, Syria, Iraq, and Palestine to appreciate the gravity of the matter. With its power to give life or take it, biopower merges with necropower and biopolitics with necropolitics. Interestingly, in his *Biopolitics of the More-Than-Human*, Joseph Pugliese (2020) explores the notion of the biopolitical via a non-anthropocentric perspective. Scrutinizing the Occupied Palestinian Territory, Pakistan, Somalia, Yemen, and other countries, Pugliese criticizes the view of human exceptionalism by propounding the idea that it is not only humans who are victims of war and colonialism and who have claims of justice, and that these nonhuman entities are as subject to damaging biopolitical regimes as humans. Deciding who gets to live and who is allowed to die are based on predetermined inclusion/exclusion criteria that serve a *Lebensraum* (space thought to be essential to ensure growth and stability, particularly during the Nazi era), a geopolitical goal for territorial expansion.

Wars serve a political function and are "determined as an end and necessity not only in democracy but also in politics and in culture. War has become both remedy and poison—our *pharmakon*. Its transformation into the *pharmakon* of our time has, in turn, let loose gruesome passions that are increasingly pushing our societies to exit democracy and, as was the case under colonization, to transform into societies of enmity" (Mbembe 2019, 3). To Mbembe, domestic peace brings the notion of the politics of space.

Space is crucial for refugees and IDPs. It is about the right of human beings to move around a shared world, about other humans being forced to stay where they are even when in need of medical attention that requires travel, about others being forced to flee and live in exile. It is ultimately about freedom and confinement, which are often decided by sovereign power. One can even argue that superpowers gained their power by freely moving around the world, taking control of lands that are not theirs (e.g., Canada, the US, and Australia), colonizing others and making use of the natural resources of the countries they are colonizing, often industrializing the worlds they have occupied via slavery. This is a form of physical violence and spatial or geographical violence, which made the world we currently live in. While Locke and Hobbes divided life into two clear spaces, namely the state of nature and civil society with the help of the social contract, Mbembe makes one question this division and highlights a third dimension: slave plantations, refugee camps, colonies, large prisons like Alcatraz, Guantanamo Bay Prison, and others. What characterizes these is that they are neither in a state of nature nor in a civil society. They live suspended, stateless while under scrutiny and surveillance amid violence. Refugee camps are, ontologically, temporary spaces that people live in only to go back to where they were. Sovereign powers disagree: the very existence of the camps as permanent serves a political function. One need only examine modern history to realize that refugee camps have become the "new biopolitical nomos of the planet" (Agamben 1998), where each person is subjected to the risk of being considered *Homo sacer*, whose life can be freely taken with no accountability. "The West thus depends in large part on inflicting violence far away, on lighting up centers of atrocities, and on the fiefdom wars and other massacres that accompany the establishment of strongholds and trading posts around the four corners of the planet. . . . [T]he fulfillment of these new desires depended on institutionalizing a regime of inequality at the planetary scale" (Mbembe 2019, 19).

The so-called Arab Spring was a series of antigovernment protests, disturbances, and insurrections that took place throughout much of the Arab world in the early 2010s, when sovereign powers waged wars under the false justification of spreading democracy. The 2003 American invasion of Iraq is but one example. Mbembe's thoughts resonate: "The colony is not external to democracy and is not necessarily located outside its walls. Democracy bears the colony within it, just as colonialism bears democracy, often in the guise of a mask" (2019, 27). This explains the state-sponsored killings which characterize the politics of modern democracies: they reduce refugees to the status of *Homo sacer'* living in "states of exception" where laws need not apply because sovereigns simply decide to suspend the social contract, thereby obscuring the margins between life and death (Agamben 1998). Refugees become, in many ways, Fanon's "wretched of the earth" (Burke 1976). Thus space configures politics and makes sovereign power mightier by allowing it to choose who gets to live and who dies. The prevalence of camps forms a micro-representation of the dynamics of society in various contexts. Camps have existed throughout history, from colonial political economies to contemporary refugee camps and detention centers. Camps are described as a site of custody, care, and control, which often involve violence and function as a means of controlling and governing life. Claudio Minca (2015) discusses this further in "Geographies of the Camp," highlighting the connection between camps and colonialism, nationalism, and biopolitics, emphasizing the role of camps in shaping race, culture, and the sociopolitical body. Camps, Minca tells us, are part of a larger geography of fear and protective custody, and their presence in the 21st century demonstrates the pervasiveness of camp thought in politics and society. Minca highlights issues concerning the nature of the biopolitical body, human disposal, and the link between biosecurity, prophylactic interventions, and the protection and purity of the sociopolitical body. He also addresses the enduring role of camps in modern society, as well as their confluence with biosecurity and global health problems.

The three notions discussed earlier serve as a lens through which we suggest looking at the situation of refugees and access to, or denial of, healthcare. However, a statement of Edward Said must be borne in mind: biopolitics, or any other interpretation of the status of refugees, IDPs, and others, must not make one forget that "history does not get made without work, intention, resistance, effort, or conflict, and that none of these things is silently absorbable into micronetworks of power" (1983, 245).

Arguably, biopolitics, necropolitics, and the politics of space are not the only substantial or even viable interpretations of a racist (as Foucault 1977 notes) ideology of what we call the current *postcolonial refugee syndrome* (Perera and Pugliese 2018). Weheliye developed a conception of racializing accumulations within the dominion of modern politics that "constru[e] race not as a biological or cultural classification but as a set of sociopolitical processes that discipline humanity into full humans, not quite humans, and nonhumans" (2014, 4). His *habeas viscus* (you shall have the flesh) reveals new versions of individuals, those who exist, have dreams, wishes, and desires, but are not accepted as fully human in Western liberal conversations. Looking at the plight of refugees unable to access healthcare, Pelagia Soultatou presents an argument quite similar to the one we are presenting: that biopolitics "provides the grounds to understanding how market prevails over life at the expense of those in greater need, and how the state, serving *homo economicus*, intensifies instead of alleviating health vulnerabilities" (2021, 469).

In 1951, a convention was formed to discuss the rights and status of refugees, which was initially intended to protect European refugees after World War I; however, in 1967 a protocol amendment ensured broader coverage that included other refugees as well, in an effort to become a solution for the global refugee issue (UNHCR 2011). Unfortunately, refugees continue to carry the heaviest healthcare burden; despite all the advancements and milestones achieved in healthcare, its inaccessibility and unequal distribution remain core limitations for global health, not to mention its bioethical complications among others (Norredam et al. 2010; Langlois et al. 2016). Furthermore, given the rise in the number of refugees, increased demand for healthcare services is expected, which is one component of a complex equation leading to inequalities and disparities in the delivery of necessary healthcare services, with most of the damage and consequences falling on the shoulders of those who have been displaced (Langlois et al. 2016; Lebano et al. 2020). Healthcare is a commodity instead of a right; this is, we argue, the main premise from which governments operate in denying access to healthcare to refugees.

7.5 CONCLUSION

Humanitarian aid in times of crisis may seem critical and necessary to deal with a large influx of refugees, but it may also be the start of a large ripple effect and a progressively worsening spiral of larger corporations and international organizations taking advantage of those who have lost their homes, as well as refugees becoming too reliant on the humanitarian aid that they receive. Humanitarian aid provided to the refugees forms only a temporary solution that may cover up more basic problems, such as access to food and shelter; an inclusive and sustainable longer-term plan is needed in order to limit the dependency that the refugees may develop. While it may initially give a lifeline, it may also unintentionally develop a cycle of dependency and perpetuate immigrant marginalization; as such, international organizations should strive to empower refugees through the development of their skills and education, offering them the kinds of support that would allow them to eventually become more independent and self-reliant. By investing in the development of their skills and knowledge, refugees may become more resilient, autonomous, and self-sufficient. Training programs and educational efforts can provide refugees with the skills they need to rebuild their lives and positively contribute to their host communities.

Political, economic, and geopolitical considerations regularly impact aid distribution, which often leads to the politicization of humanitarian activities. In such cases, navigating the rough terrain of aid distribution, while keeping the primary focus on reducing human suffering and enhancing the well-being of people in need regardless of skin color, poverty level, and geography, becomes critical. Humanitarian aid becomes politicized when the distribution and allocation of relief resources are impacted by political agendas, self-interest, or power dynamics among interested organizations. As a result, rather than focusing purely on need, support may be directed toward certain individuals or regions depending on geopolitical factors. Conflicts of interest can arise when many parties compete for control of support resources, try to influence decision-making processes, or pursue their own interests. This is where regulation of humanitarian aid comes into play, because, as it stands today, no individual or organization is strictly *required* to provide any humanitarian aid. As described by Hugo Slim in his book *Humanitarian Ethics: A Guide to the Morality of Aid in War and Disaster*, "Humanitarian action is essentially voluntary and self-regulating. No party, whether donor, agency, local authority or recipient community, is under real external scrutiny to see if and how they are making the most of aid and are abiding by humanitarian law and principles in its application" (2015, 107). A parallel problem that arises, according to Slim, is the bias that exists when holding accountability, along with the pressures of politics, finances, and bureaucracy in carving and redirecting the guise of accountability to the donors rather than to the people whom agencies claim to help, in addition to the ongoing lack of regulation of the humanitarian sector. He argues that "no party, whether donor, agency, local authority or recipient community, is under real external scrutiny to see if and how they are making the most of aid and abiding by humanitarian law and principles in its application" (107). Had the accountability been placed in the hands of professionals or the recipients themselves, the risk of lost aid would diminish significantly. In a situation so complex, with numerous parties involved, where does one draw the line between humanitarian aid and conflicts of interest between the involved groups? In a world where one's misery can become another individual's opportunity, how can we control the politicization of humanitarian aid?

Writing about the ethics of intellectuals, Zreik noted that "the role of the intellectual in Said, as with the role of criticism, is in part to interrogate, question, investigate and to unsettle dominant modes of culture, hegemony, identity and power" (2021, 1). We tried, in this chapter, to raise the issue of refugee health and well-being from a different perspective than is normally assumed. Perhaps it is our way to knock on the side of the water tank. Farmer noted: "Medicine becomes pragmatic solidarity when it is delivered with dignity to the destitute sick. . . . By including social and economic rights in the struggle for human rights, we help to protect those most likely to suffer the insults of structural violence" (2003, 138). It is to that form of medicine, a medicine of pragmatic solidarity with refugees, that we turn, guided by Camus's "Je me révolte, donc nous sommes."

REFERENCES

Abawi, Atia. 2018. *A Land of Permanent Goodbyes*. Penguin Young Readers Group.

Abdelrazaq, Leila. 2015. *Baddawi*. Just World Books.

Abushama, Hashem. 2021. "On Refugee Agency, Bio-Politics, and a New World." *Refuge: Canada's Journal on Refugees/Refuge: Revue Canadienne sur les Réfugiés* 37 (2): 30–37. https://www.jstor.org/stable/48648250.

Abimbola, Seye. 2023. "Decolonizing Global Health." In *Oxford Research Encyclopedia of Global Public Health.*, edited by Bola O. Owolabi and Olugbenga J. Abimbola. Oxford University Press. https://doi.org/10.1093/acrefore/9780190632366.001.0001/acrefore-9780190632366-e-466.

Agamben, Giorgio. 2005. *State of Exception*. University of Chicago Press.

Agamben, Giorgio. 1998. *Homo Sacer: Sovereign Power and Bare Life*. Translated by D. Heller-Roazen. Stanford University Press.

Al-Ali, Naji. 1985. "Who Is Handala?" https://newint.org/blog/2013/05/16/handala-palestine-naji-al-ali.

Alsanousi, S. 2015. Translated by J. Wright. *The Bamboo Stalk*. Bloomsbury USA.

Asgary, Ramin, and N. Segar. 2011. "Barriers to Health Care Access Among Refugee Asylum-Seekers." *Journal of Health Care for the Poor and Underserved* 22 (2): 506–522. https://doi.org/10.1353/hpu.2011.0047.

Burke, Edmund. 1976. "Frantz Fanon's 'The Wretched of the Earth.'" *Daedalus* 105 (1): 127–135. http://www.jstor.org/stable/20024388.

Butler, Judith. 2006. "Violence, Non-Violence: Satre on Fanon." *Graduate Faculty Philosophy Journal* 27 (1): 3–24. https://doi.org/https://doi.org/10.5840/gfpj200627122.
Dawes, Daniel E. 2020. *The Political Determinants of Health*. Johns Hopkins University Press.
Farmer, Paul. 2003. *Pathologies of Power: Health, Human Rights, and the New War on the Poor*. University of California Press.
Foucault, Michel. 1977. *Discipline and Punish: The Birth of the Prison*. Pantheon Books.
Gibb, C. 2011. *Sweetness in the Belly*. Random House.
Hanafi, Sari. 2013. "Explaining Spacio-cide in the Palestinian Territory: Colonization, Separation, and State of Exception." *Current Sociology* 61 (2): 190–205. https://doi.org/10.1177/0011392112456505.
Hass, Amira. 2012. "2,279 Calories per Person: How Israel Made Sure Gaza Didn't Starve." *Haaretz*, October 17. https://www.haaretz.com/2012-10-17/ty-article/.premium/israels-gaza-quota-2-279-calories-a-day/0000017f-e0f2-d7b2-a77f-e3f755550000.
Hosseini, Khaled. 2018. *Sea Prayer*. Riverhead Books.
International Committee of the Red Cross. 1949. "International Humanitarian Law: The Geneva Conventions and Their Additional Protocols." https://www.icrc.org/en/law-and-policy/geneva-conventions-and-their-commentaries.
Kanafani, G. 2004. *All That's Left to You: A Novella and Short Stories*. Interlink.
Kanafani, Ghassan. 1978. *Men in the Sun*. Translated by Hilary Kilpatrick. Three Continents Press.
Langlois, Etienne V., Andy Haines, Goran Tomson, and Abdul Ghaffar. 2016. "Refugees: Towards Better Access to Healthcare Services." *The Lancet* 387 (10016): 319–321. https://doi.org/10.1016/s0140-6736(16)00101-x.
Lebano, A., S. Hamed, H. Bradby, et al. 2020. "Migrants' and Refugees' Health Status and Healthcare in Europe: A Scoping Literature Review." *BMC Public Health* 20 (1): 1039.
Locke, John. 1824. *Two Treatises of Government*. C. and J. Rivington.
Maalouf, A. 2020. *The Disoriented*. Translated by F. Wynne. World Editions.
Mbembe, Achille. 2019. *Necropolitics*. Duke University Press.
Mbembe, Achille. 2003. "Necropolitics." *Public Culture* 15 (1): 11–40.
Memo. 2022. "5 Gaza Patients Died in 2022 Due to Israel Travel Ban." *Middle East Monitor*, September 8. https://www.middleeastmonitor.com/20220908-5-gaza-patients-died-in-2022-due-to-israel-travel-ban/.
Minca, Claudio. 2015. "Geographies of the Camp." *Political Geography* 49: 74–83.
Mitwalli, Suzan, Weeam Hammoudeh, Rita Giacaman, and Richard Harding. 2023. "Access to Advanced Cancer Care Services in the West Bank–Occupied Palestinian Territory." *Frontiers in Oncology* 13: 1–10 https://doi.org/10.3389/fonc.2023.1120783.
Ministry of Health, Gaza. 2021. "MOH-Gaza Holds Conference Entitled 'Health Sector Challenges and Anticipations.'" https://www.moh.gov.ps/portal/moh-gaza-holds-conference-entitled-health-sector-challenges-and-anticipations/.
Médecins Sans Frontières. 2020. "Greece Denies Healthcare to Seriously Ill Refugee Children on Lesbos." https://www.msf.org/greece-denies-healthcare-seriously-ill-refugee-children-lesbos.
Norredam, Marie, Signe Nielsen, and Allen Krasnik. 2010. "Migrants' Utilization of Somatic Healthcare Services in Europe—A Systematic Review." *European Journal of Public Health* 20 (5): 555–563. https://doi.org/10.1093/eurpub/ckp195.

Perera, S., and J. Pugliese. 2018. "Sexual Violence and the Border: Colonial Genealogies of US and Australian Immigration Detention Regimes." *Social & Legal Studies* 30 (1): 66–79. https://doi.org/10.1177/0964663918767954.

Puar, Jasbir K. 2017. *The Right to Maim: Debility, Capacity, Disability*. Duke University Press.

Pugliese, Joseph. 2020. *Biopolitics of the More-Than-Human: A Forensic Ecologies of Violence*. Duke University Press.

Rawlence, Ben. 2016. *City of Thorns: Nine Lives in the World's Largest Refugee Camp*. Random House.

Reuters. 2022. "Denying Refugees and Migrants Healthcare Violates Rights, WHO Says." July 20. https://www.reuters.com/business/healthcare-pharmaceuticals/denying-refugees-migrants-healthcare-violates-rights-who-says-2022-07-20/#:~:text=%22Health%20does%20not%20begin%20or,migration%20said%20in%20a%20statement.

Sadek, Noreen, 2013. "The Palestinian boy who remains 10 years old." *The New Internationalists*. https://newint.org/blog/2013/05/16/handala-palestine-naji-al-ali.

Said, Edward W. 1983. *The World, the Text, and the Critic*. Harvard University Press.

Schuilenburg, Marc. 2008. "Citizenship Revisited—Denizens and Margizens." *Peace Review* 20 (3): 358–365.

Shehadeh, Said. 2015. "The 2014 War on Gaza: Engineering Trauma and Mass Torture to Break Palestinian Resilience." *International Journal of Applied Psychoanalytic Studies* 12 (3): 278–294. https://doi.org/https://doi.org/10.1002/aps.1457.

Slim, Hugo. 2015. *Humanitarian Ethics: A Guide to the Morality of Aid in War and Disaster*. Oxford University Press.

Soultatou, Pelagia. 2021. "Refugees as a Key Representation of Vulnerability: Politics and Biopolitics." *Journal of Humanities and Applied Social Sciences* 4 (5): 469–480. https://doi.org/10.1108/JHASS-10-2021-0169.

UNICEF. 2016. "Yemen: Children on the Brink." United Nations Children's Fund. https://www.unicef.org/yemen/reports/children-brink.

UNHCR. 1951. https://www.unhcr.org/about-unhcr/who-we-protect/refugees.

UNHCR. 2011. https://www.unhcr.org/about-unhcr/overview/1951-refugee-convention

UNHCR. 2022. "Global Trends Report 2022." https://www.unhcr.org/global-trends-report-2022.

UN Office of the High Commissioner for Human Rights. 1950. "Convention Relating to the Status of Refugees." https://www.ohchr.org/en/instruments-mechanisms/instruments/convention-relating-status-refugees.

UN Office of the High Commissioner for Human Rights. n.d. "About Internally Displaced Persons." Accessed July 11, 2023. https://www.ohchr.org/en/special-procedures/sr-internally-displaced-persons/about-internally-displaced-persons#:~:text=According%20to%20the%20Guiding%20Principles,avoid%20the%20effects%20of%20armed.

Weber, C. 2016. *Queer International Relations: Sovereignty, Sexuality and the Will to Knowledge*. Oxford University Press.

Weheliye, A. G. 2014. *Habeas Viscus: Racializing Assemblages, Biopolitics, and Black Feminist Theories of the Human*. Duke University Press.

World Health Organization. 2018. "Right to Health." https://www.emro.who.int/images/stories/palestine/documents/who_right_to_health_2018_web-final.pdf?ua=1.

World Population Review. 2023. "Refugees by Country." https://worldpopulationreview.com/country-rankings/refugees-by-country.
World Bank Group. 2023. "Forced Displacement." https://www.worldbank.org/en/topic/forced-displacement#:~:text=Globally%2C%20there%20are%20more%20than,displacement%20make%20these%20people%20vulnerable.
Worldwide Hospice Palliative Care Alliance. 2014. "Universal Health Coverage and Palliative Care." http://www.thewhpca.org/images/resources/publications-reports/Universal_health_coverage_report_final_2014.pdf.
Young, Iris Marion. 2011. *Responsibility for Justice*. Oxford University Press.
Zreik, Raef. 2021. "The Ethics of the Intellectual: Rereading Edward Said." *Philosophy & Social Criticism* 47 (1): 130–148. https://doi.org/10.1177/0191453720903479.

8

The Double-Edged Sword of Corporate Assistance to Humanitarian Work

The Case of Lebanon

JIHAD MAKHOUL AND CATHERINE EL ASHKAR

8.1 INTRODUCTION

The numerous emergency and crisis situations in the past few decades all over the world have resulted in a growing number of people who need varying types of assistance. Approximately 364.6 million people in 2023 were affected by such emergencies, the majority of which have occurred in low-income countries (Center for Disease Philanthropy 2024). In addition, the recent wars in Ukraine, Sudan, and Gaza have added approximately 12.7 million, 30.4 million, and 2 million people respectively to the number of people in need of assistance (United Nations Office for the Coordination of Humanitarian Affairs [OCHA] 2025a, 2025b; OCHA n.d.-a). OCHA reports 65,000 Palestinian fatalities and over 167,000 injuries in Gaza, and 3,384 fatalities between January and June 2025 in Sudan (OCHA 2025c; United Nations High Commissioner for Refugees [UNHCR] 2025a). In addition, other emergencies during the past few months have included armed conflicts in Yemen, Haiti, and Myanmar, and flooding in East Africa (OCHA 2024). Conflicts like the ones in Sudan and Gaza have led to mass displacement, with over 90% (2.1 million) of Gazans becoming internally displaced and over 12.8 million forcibly displaced in Sudan (OCHA n.d.-a; UNHCR 2025b). Other factors, such as the COVID-19 pandemic and climate change, have forced an estimated 100 million people to flee their homes (Center for Disease Philanthropy 2024).

The effects of these emergencies extend beyond geographical boundaries. If host or receiving countries are economically challenged or humanitarian

Jihad Makhoul and Catherine El Ashkar, *The Double-Edged Sword of Corporate Assistance to Humanitarian Work*. In: *Forced Migration and Health Justice*. Edited by: Lisa A. Eckenwiler, Verina Wild, Anna Gotlib, Ryoa Chung, and Deborah Zion, Oxford University Press.
DOI: 10.1093/oso/9780197795491.003.0008

assistance is insufficient or delayed, the health and well-being of affected forced migrant populations may be placed at risk. Although many types of organizations contribute to humanitarian assistance (Oloruntoba and Gray 2009; McGoldrick 2011), not all needs are adequately met. This chapter highlights the understudied implications of corporate assistance for humanitarian work, illustrated in particular by the case of Lebanon, a country in which multiple crises are taking place simultaneously—adjacent to other countries enduring crises—and where a consequent massive humanitarian predicament threatens both health and health justice.

8.2 FUNDING FOR HUMANITARIAN ASSISTANCE

With the growing number of protracted and new crises around the world, international funding for humanitarian assistance is inadequate (Development Initiatives 2023). For-profit corporations have stepped in to become major contributors to humanitarian aid, through financial or in-kind/non-monetary contributions (OCHA n.d.-b). The 2004 Indian Ocean tsunami served as a catalyst for increased corporate funding of relief services (Beamon and Kotleba 2006; Charles et al. 2010; Abidi et al. 2014). Sponsors such as Coca-Cola, the PepsiCo Foundation, Johnson and Johnson, and Nike have cooperated with non-governmental organizations (NGOs), such as CARE (n.d.), in their humanitarian aid programs.

The United Nations argues that the complex problems of today's world necessitate engagement of multiple actors and stakeholders, including businesses (OCHA n.d.-b). The business sector has been described as capable of contributing resources key to humanitarian efforts, such as knowledge, expertise, financing, access, and reach, which are often critical to advance UN goals, including solving international economic, social, cultural, and humanitarian problems (United Nations, n.d.). Initiatives such as the Connecting Business Initiative between OCHA, United Nations Development Program, and the private sector aim to engage corporations to respond to emergencies. In 2022, the Connecting Business Initiative reported that over US$7.2 million was distributed through its networks in response to earthquakes, typhoons, COVID-19, and more. This included cash assistance and corporate in-kind assistance, such as mobile phones, credit, meals, water, and cargo transportation (Connecting Business Initiative 2022). It is worth noting that this assistance offers corporations opportunities for tax reductions while increasing the public's faith in these corporations (Brisbois et al. 2016). Corporations further benefit by gaining opportunities for marketing (Charles et al. 2010; Jensen 2012). A closer look, with the lens of ethics, into the actors/stakeholders in the humanitarian assistance process identifies an imbalance of financial power and a divergence in objectives and accountability between corporations and humanitarian organizations.

8.3 COMMERCIAL DETERMINANTS OF HEALTH

Academic and in some cases government interest in the commercial sector's influence on public health has grown over the past three decades because of tangible and intangible conflicts of interest and corporate interference in social and public health policy, research, and practice. Examples of industries whose products and practices have been found to be harmful to health include the pharmaceutical, alcohol, food and beverage, tobacco, and arms industries (Baum and Anaf 2015; McKee and Stuckler 2018). Noncommunicable diseases, including cancer and diseases of the heart and vascular system, are the leading causes of mortality globally. The risk factors for these diseases include alcohol use, tobacco use, physical inactivity, and the consumption of highly processed foods. Corporations seek to make a profit from these commodities, using business practices to develop, produce, and sell their products. For example, one of these practices is the life course approach, which corporations use to target people from an early age to attract their attention and develop brand loyalty (Mialon 2020). Industries that produce health-harming products use strategies to appeal to youth, such as free products and sponsorship programs, all of which aim to create an exponential spread and uptake of these products, especially in low- and middle-income countries. These countries are particularly vulnerable to the spread of these commercial entities because of market globalization, lack of strong regulation to protect public health, and economic vulnerability (Abdalla et al. 2023).

8.4 ETHICAL DILEMMAS IN THE POLITICAL ECONOMY OF CORPORATE ASSISTANCE

Let us look at how corporations exploit and increase the vulnerabilities of disadvantaged communities. Low- and middle-income communities have been specifically targeted by food companies (Dia et al. 2021). The advertising for sugary foods and beverages, for example, was reported to be higher in less affluent areas and communities of color in northern England, especially in the areas where children are most likely to be present (Adams 2011). In the United States, outdoor advertisements for unhealthy products are more prevalent in minority and low-income communities, with Latino, Asian, and African American neighborhoods having 6 to 32 times more of these food advertisements compared to high-income white neighborhoods (Cassady et al. 2015). Indeed, this is generally common in industrialized countries. A study assessing 171 outdoor health-related advertisements in Sacramento, California, reported a dominance of advertising by fast-food restaurants and grocery stores, with four times more advertisements for unhealthy food and beverages compared to healthy options. The highest density of advertisements for unhealthy products was observed in low-income Latino and African American neighborhoods (Cassady et al. 2015). Similar findings were reported by a study in Newcastle upon Tyne in England, where advertisements of food products high in fat and/or sugar were more common in the least affluent areas (Adams et al. 2011). Interestingly, brand recognition is not exclusive to the food industry. For example, the Philip Morris International brand was recognized by more than 20% of five-year-old children in Brazil, India, Nigeria, Pakistan, China, and Russia (Collins et al. 2023).

Corporate assistance to humanitarian aid thus poses several ethical concerns. We focus on two in particular. First, when corporate products are health-harming, such as processed food and beverages, the principle of humanity, whose purpose is to protect life and health, is compromised. As noted, many of the companies providing resources are food and beverage corporations. Evidence clearly shows that the marketing of unhealthy foods and beverages has an impact on children's dietary preferences and purchasing requests and can contribute to childhood obesity (Dia et al. 2021). An increased intake of unhealthy food, particularly among children, was reported after exposure to advertisements for such foods (Boyland et al. 2016), which are part of the obesogenic environments promoting sedentary lifestyles and high intake of energy-dense foods (Adams et al. 2011; Boyland et al. 2016). This promotion of processed food, furthermore, can lead to its normalization, with potentially long-lasting health consequences (Adams et al. 2010).

Second, the humanitarian principle of independence, the requirement that assistance be autonomous and uninfluenced by objectives pursued by other actors, is also likely to be compromised (Makhoul et al. 2023). When corporations allocate funds or provide services to humanitarian organizations and corporate association increases visibility of humanitarian organizations, this challenges the humanitarian organizations' ability to contest corporate requests, thus unwittingly allowing corporations, rather than people's needs, to become the driving force in setting their agendas. This dynamic can compromise the humanitarian organization's original mission (Baur and Schmitz 2012). In addition, close relations between humanitarian organizations and corporations may enhance a positive image of these corporations among humanitarian agency staff, which may in turn increase the corporations' credibility among the populations served (Marks 2019). When populations are assisted in this way, loyalties to the involved corporate brands are more likely to develop, as intended by the corporate playbook marketing strategies, especially among the youth (Hotho and Girschik 2019).

Thus corporations indeed have an interest in penetrating new markets for their products and improving their image by supporting reputable humanitarian organizations under the pretense of corporate social responsibility (Baur and Schmitz 2012). It is shown that contributions to humanitarian efforts boost companies' reputations among stakeholders and consumers (Hotho and Girschik 2019). For example, consumers in France, Germany, Italy, and the US expressed their support for brands that offered educational or financial services to refugees or which provided corporate philanthropy to charities working with refugees (Erdem et al. n.d.-a, n.d.-b).

8.5 A DOUBLE-EDGED SWORD: THE CONTEXT OF LEBANON

Having laid out the ethical dilemmas in the political economy of humanitarian assistance, we will take a closer look at the case of Lebanon. After gaining its independence in 1943, the Lebanese state endorsed a laissez-faire economic system based on private enterprise combined with an income- and profit-tax-free environment (Research for Health in Conflict 2022). This enabled the private sector to flourish in the absence of a state-wide development plan. The disparities in the distribution of social and health services, historically favoring Mount Lebanon and Beirut, contributed to the current social and economic inequalities in the country (Research for Health in Conflict 2022). Since the 1975–1990 civil war, and in the absence of a functioning state, a number of NGOs have provided relief, health, and social services. After the war, an ambitious program of social and economic reconstruction entailed extensive renovation of the capital's port, airport, and downtown area at the expense of broader social development in the 1990s (Research for Health in Conflict 2022). This program placed the country in increasing internal and external governmental debt. Over the past 10 years, the country spent between 8% and 10% of its GDP on healthcare and treatment, concentrated in curative and high-tech, high-cost interventions in private hospitals which are inaccessible to a majority of the population (Research for Health in Conflict 2022) because there has been little political will to implement universal health coverage policies in Lebanon despite active advocacy. In addition, as an example of an ongoing conflict of interest for the industry, a cartel of medical suppliers which imports pharmaceutical products is believed to have made millions of dollars in profit, driven in part by government subsidiaries (Research for Health in Conflict 2022). At the same time, old and dilapidated water and sanitation systems and water privatization have created an inequitable environmental situation, which has exposed both refugees and the local population to risks of infectious disease outbreaks, most recently cholera (Department of Health Promotion and Community Health, University of Beirut 2022).

In the midst of these existing inequities, infrastructure issues, and profiteering, Lebanon also hosts the largest number of refugees per capita globally, including Palestinian, Ethiopian, Sudanese, Iraqi, and Syrian refugees (UN High Commissioner for Refugees 2022). Syrian refugees began to enter Lebanon in 2011, when the Syrian war began, which has placed substantial pressure on Lebanese education, health, and economic systems, already inadequate for the needs of the Lebanese (Washington Report on Middle East Affairs 2014). The COVID-19 pandemic, and then the massive August 2020 Beirut Port blast, exacerbated this existing instability (Abouzeid et al. 2020; CARE 2020; Amnesty International 2021). Since early 2021, in the absence of an effective government and without a president, the country has been facing a compounding debt crisis, which has exacerbated the already scarce resources and weak governance (Fund for Peace 2021).

The resulting humanitarian response has involved Lebanese civil society, as well as individual donors in the country and abroad, the UN, the European Union, and the World Bank (CARE 2020; OCHA 2021). Civil society includes the network of independent NGOs, community-based and advocacy groups, professional associations, and other organizations operating separately from the government. Ever since the civil war started in 1975, and in the absence of a strong equitable state, various civil society groups have provided various health, social, and environmental services to nationals as well as to migrants and refugees. Examples of their work include advocacy efforts for women, children, and refugees; improving urban settings; providing legal support; offering emergency medical and mental healthcare; responding to emergencies; providing vocational training; and creating and protecting public parks and natural reserves.

Against this background, corporations have been key sources of support for humanitarian aid in Lebanon. PepsiCo, for example, offers education scholarships to refugee youth in Lebanon through a local NGO. Coca-Cola Middle East has implemented the "Eradication of Hunger by 2020" initiative, which started in Lebanon and Jordan and expanded to other countries in the region; its aim is to assist Syrian refugees and disadvantaged families in Iraq (Food Banking Regional Network 2014). In a recent study by Makhoul et al. (2023), a majority of the interviewed humanitarian organizations serving refugees and other disadvantaged populations in Lebanon reported receiving money from for-profit corporations in varying amounts, as well as in-kind contributions from foundations linked to corporations, directly from multinational companies. Examples include contributions from Nestlé, PepsiCo, Procter & Gamble, and the local banking, automobile, and telecommunications sectors to support diverse projects such as rehabilitation of residential areas, university tuition fees, relief items, and COVID-19 protective materials.

The political economy of aid assistance reveals multiple ethical dilemmas everywhere in the world; however, in contexts of compounding crises such as Lebanon, these dilemmas are amplified. In recent years the absence of a strong state has created an opportunity for corporations to step in and aid local humanitarian organizations (Ayoub and Mahdi, 2018). Receiving funding and other incentives from corporations has been described by humanitarian organizations as a less laborious process with fewer requirements in comparison to applying to international and UN organizations (Makhoul et al. 2023).

The precise number of NGOs in Lebanon is unknown due to the absence of a centralized database, but estimates range from about 2,107 (Arab.org, n.d.) to over 8,500 (International Center for Non-Profit Law 2024). Among these, only 13 have signed onto the WANGO Code of Ethics and Conduct, as shown on its website, and these exclude those who participated in our study (World Association of Non-Governmental Organizations, n.d.). The principles cited therein, which are fundamental to humanitarian ethics, are not congruent with corporations' value systems, which are generally unfamiliar with the ethics of humanitarian work and have a different set of ethics that is limited to how their employees should interact with and gain trust of their consumers. The study found that the obvious health-harming industries, such as tobacco and alcohol, were described by six participants as unacceptable sources of humanitarian assistance, yet a number of other organizations were "flexible" and would consider assistance from these industries because of their need for financial support (Makhoul et al. 2023).

It is important to note that staff working for the humanitarian organizations interviewed by Makhoul et al. (2023) were unaware of the possibility of threats to ethical principles in the context of their collaborations with the private sector. None of the organizational representatives we interviewed, including those in charge of refugee health, reported experiencing any concerns raised by their collaborations with the corporations they worked for (Makhoul et al. 2023). This suggests that there may be opportunities for further study and ethics education.

8.6 CONCLUSION

In conclusion, we maintain that it is the responsibility of humanitarian organizations to reflect upon the ethical principles established to inform their work and, more specifically, to consider how these principles should guide their interactions with corporate sponsors. In addition, we argue that humanitarian organizations should consult existing pertinent guidelines, in particular the United Nations (n.d.) "Guidelines on a Principle-Based Approach to the Cooperation Between the United Nations and the Business Sector," and, consistent with their own mission and circumstances, develop their own guidelines accordingly in order to regulate their engagement with corporations, and especially to minimize potential harms to populations to whom they provide aid. To offer just one example, a due diligence process is needed to help the organizations vet requests from corporations so that these organizations may detect possible conflicts of interest and decide whether or not to engage, the extent of the engagement, and how to manage conflicts of interest if they arise. This is a matter of some urgency given the rise of conflicts around the world and the struggle among humanitarian organizations to procure needed resources.

REFERENCES

Abidi, Hella, Sander de Leeuw, and Matthias Klumpp. 2014. "Humanitarian Supply Chain Performance Management: A Systematic Literature Review." *Supply Chain Management* 19: 592–608. https://doi.org/10.1108/SCM-09-2013-0349.

Abouzeid, Marian, Rima R. Habib, Samer Jabbour, Ali H. Mokdad, and Iman Nuwayhid. 2020. "Lebanon's Humanitarian Crisis Escalates After the Beirut Blast." *The Lancet* 396 (10260): 1380–1382. https://doi.org/10.1016/s0140-6736(20)31908-5.

Adams, Jean, Ellie Ganiti, and Martin White. 2011. "Socio-Economic Differences in Outdoor Food Advertising in a City in Northern England." *Public Health Nutrition* 14 (6): 945–950. https://doi.org/10.1017/S1368980010003332.

Amnesty International. 2021. "Lebanon: One Year on from Devastating Beirut Explosion, Authorities Shamelessly Obstruct Justice." fahttps://www.amnesty.org/en/latest/news/2021/08/lebanon-one-year-on-from-beirut-explosion-authorities-shamelessly-obstruct-justice/.

Arab.org. n.d. "Information of Civil Society Organizations Operating In Lebanon." Accessed December 20, 2024. https://arab.org/countries/lebanon/.

Ayoub, Bachir, and Dima Mahdi. 2018. "Making Aid Work in Lebanon: Promoting Aid Effectiveness and Respect for Rights in Middle Income Countries Affected by Mass Displacement." Oxfam GB. https://www-cdn.oxfam.org/s3fs-public/file_attachments/bp-making-aid-work-lebanon-050418-en.pdf.

Baum, Frances E., and Julia M. Anaf. 2015. "Transnational Corporations and Health: A Research Agenda." *International Journal of Health Services* 45 (2): 353–362. https://doi.org/10.1177/0020731414568513.

Baur, Dorothea, and Hans Peter Schmitz. 2012. "Corporations and NGOs: When Accountability Leads to Co-optation." *Journal of Business Ethics* 106 (1): 9–21. https://doi.org/10.1007/s10551-011-1057-9.

Beamon, Benita M., and Stephen A. Kotleba. 2006. "Inventory Management Support Systems for Emergency Humanitarian Relief Operations in South Sudan." *International Journal of Logistics Management* 17: 187–212. https://doi.org/10.1108/09574090610689952.

Boyland, Emma J., Sarah Nolan, Bridget Kelly, et al. 2016. "Advertising as a Cue to Consume: A Systematic Review and Meta-Analysis of the Effects of Acute Exposure to Unhealthy Food and Nonalcoholic Beverage Advertising on Intake in Children and Adults." *American Journal of Clinical Nutrition* 103 (2): 519–533. https://doi.org/10.3945/ajcn.115.120022.

Brisbois, Ben W., Donald Cole, Colleen Davison, et al. 2016. "Corporate Sponsorship of Global Health Research: Questions to Promote Critical Thinking About Potential Funding Relationships." *Canadian Journal of Public Health* 107: e390–e392. https://doi.org/10.17269/CJPH.107.5653.

CARE. n.d. "Corporate Partnership." https://www.care.org/about-us/strategic-partners/corporate-partnerships/.

Care International. 2020. "Care International One of First International NGOs to Begin Vital Aid Assistance to Those Affected by Beirut Blast as Death Toll Continues to Rise." https://www.care-international.org/news/care-international-one-first-international-ngos-begin-vital-aid-assistance-those-affected.

Cassady, Diana L., Karen Liaw, and Lisa M. Soederberg Miller. 2015. "Disparities in Obesity-Related Outdoor Advertising by Neighborhood Income and Race." *Journal of Urban Health* 92 (5): 835–842. https://doi.org/10.1007/s11524-015-9980-1.

Center for Disease Philanthropy. 2024. "Complex Humanitarian Emergencies." https://disasterphilanthropy.org/resources/complex-humanitarian-emergencies/.

Charles, Aurelie, Matthieu Lauras, and Luk Van Wassenhove. 2010. "A Model to Define and Assess the Agility of Supply Chains: Building on Humanitarian Experience." *International Journal of Physical Distribution & Logistics Management* 40: 722–741. https://doi.org/10.1108/09600031011079355.

Collins, Tea E., Svetlana Akselrod, Lina Mahy, et al. 2023. "Engaging with the Private Sector for Noncommunicable Disease Prevention and Control: Is it Possible to Create 'Shared Value'?" *Annals of Global Health* 89 (1): 1–13.

Connecting Business Initiative. 2022. "CBI Annual Report 2021." https://www.connectingbusiness.org/publications/cbi-annual-report-2021.

Department of Health Promotion and Community Health, University of Beirut. 2022. "Cholera Spread: A Symptom of Structural Failures: A Vaccine Campaign Alone Will Not Solve the Outbreak." *Executive*, December 2. https://www.executive-magazine.com/last-word-2/cholera-spread-a-symptom-of-structural-failures.

Development Initiatives. 2023. "Global Humanitarian Assistance Report 2023." https://devinit.org/resources/global-humanitarian-assistance-report-2023/.

Dia, Oumy Erica Wie, Anne L. Løvhaug, Peter M. Rukundo, and Liv E. Torheim. 2021. "Mapping of Outdoor Food and Beverage Advertising Around Primary and Secondary Schools in Kampala City, Uganda." *BMC Public Health* 21 (1): 707.

Erdem, Tülin, Çağdaş Şirin, Vishal Singh, and Qianyun Zhang. n.d.-a. "How Helping Refugees Helps Brands." Accessed May 8, 2024. https://tent.org/wp-content/uploads/2021/09/TENT_HowHelpingRefugeesHelpsBrands_Report_FINAL.pdf.

Erdem, Tülin, Çağdaş Şirin, Vishal Singh, and Qianyun Zhang. n.d.-b. "How Helping Refugees Helps Brands: Europe." NYU Stern. Accessed May 8, 2024.

https://www.tent.org/resources/helping-refugees-helps-brands-europe/#:~:text=It%20reveals%20that%20business%20support,from%20brands%20that%20support%20refugees.

Food Banking Regional Network. 2014. "FBRN and Coca-Cola Middle East Protocol Signature on October 2014." https://foodbankingregionalnetwork.com/en/media-center/press-release/fbrn-coca-cola-middle-east-protocol-signature-on-october-2014-2.

Fund for Peace. 2021. "Searching for Hope in Lebanon's Compounding Crises." https://fragilestatesindex.org/2021/05/20/searching-for-hope-in-lebanons-compounding-crises/.

Hotho, Jasper J., and Verena Girschik. 2019. "Corporate Engagement in Humanitarian Action: Concepts, Challenges, and Areas for International Business Research." *Critical Perspectives on International Business* 15 (2–3): 201–218.

International Center for Non-Profit Law. 2024. "Lebanon." https://www.icnl.org/resources/civic-freedom-monitor/lebanon.

Jensen, L.-M. 2012. "Humanitarian Cluster Leads: Lessons from 4PLs." *Journal of Humanitarian Logistics and Supply Chain Management* 2: 148–160. https://doi.org/10.1108/20426741211260732.

Abdalla, Salma M., Leona Ofei, Nason Maani, and Sandro Galea. 2023. "Commercial Determinants of Health in Low-and Middle Income Countries." In *The Commercial Determinants of Health*, edited by Nason Maani, Mark Petticrew, and Sandro Galea. Oxford University Press.

Makhoul, Jihad, Catherine El Ashkar, Melissa Mialon, Anna Levy, Diana Sabbagh, and Rima Nakkash. 2023. "Benefits and Risks: Views of Humanitarian Organizations in Lebanon on Corporate Assistance." *PLoS Global Public Health* 3 (11): e0002291–e0002291.

Marks, Jonathan H. 2019. *The Perils of Partnership: Industry Influence, Institutional Integrity, and Public Health*. Oxford University Press.

McGoldrick, Claudia. 2011. "The Future of Humanitarian Action: An ICRC Perspective." *International Review of the Red Cross* (93): 965–991. https://doi.org/10.1017/S1816383112000306.

McKee, Martin, and David Stuckler. 2018. "Revisiting the Corporate and Commercial Determinants of Health." *American Journal of Public Health* 108 (9): 1167–1170. https://doi.org/10.2105/AJPH.2018.304510.

Mialon, Melissa. 2020. "An Overview of the Commercial Determinants of Health." *Globalization and Health* 16 (1): 74.

Oloruntoba, Richard, and Richard Gray. 2009. "Customer Service in Emergency Relief Chains." *International Journal of Physical Distribution & Logistics Management* 39: 486–505. https://doi.org/10.1108/09600030910985839.

Research for Health in Conflict. 2022. "How Politics Made a Nation Sick: The Political Economy of Health in Lebanon." Conflict & Health Research Group under R4HC-MENA Programme. https://r4hc-mena.org/wp1/wp-content/uploads/2022/01/The political-economy-of-health-in-Lebanon.pdf.

United Nations. n.d. "Guidelines on a Principle-Based Approach to the Cooperation Between the United Nations and the Business Sector." Accessed May 6, 2024. https://www.un.org/en/ethics/assets/pdfs/Guidelines-on-Cooperation-with-the-Business-Sector.pdf.

United Nations High Commissioner for Refugees. 2022. "Fact Sheet Lebanon." https://reporting.unhcr.org/document/1787.

United Nations High Commissioner for Refugees. 2025a. "Human Rights Situation in the Sudan 1 January to 30 June 2025." https://www.ohchr.org/sites/default/

files/documents/countries/sudan/ohchr-report-human-rights-situation-in-sudan-1-january-30-juin-2025.pdf.

United Nations High Commissioner for Refugees (UNHCR). 2025b. "Sudan Situation: UNHCR External Update #106 - 3 May 2025." https://data.unhcr.org/en/documents/details/116294.

United Nations Office for the Coordination of Humanitarian Affairs. n.d.-a. "Occupied Palestinian Territory". https://www.unocha.org/occupied-palestinian-territory.

United Nations Office for the Coordination of Humanitarian Affairs (OCHA). n.d.-b "Engagement with the Private Sector." Accessed May 26, 2024. https://www.unocha.org/engagement-private-sector.

United Nations Office for the Coordination of Humanitarian Affairs. 2021. "The Humanitarian Response to the Beirut Port Explosions: Lebanon 2020 Flash Appeal—End Report (30 April 2021)." https://reliefweb.int/report/lebanon/humanitarian-response-beirut-port-explosions-lebanon-2020-flash-appeal-end-report-30.

United Nations Office for the Coordination of Humanitarian Affairs. 2024. "Today's Top News: Occupied Palestinian Territory, Yemen, Eastern Africa, Haiti, Myanmar, Ukraine." https://www.unocha.org/news/todays-top-news-occupiedpalestinian-territory-yemen-eastern-africa-haiti-myanmar-ukraine.

United Nations Office for the Coordination of Humanitarian Affairs. 2025a. "Ukraine". https://www.unocha.org/ukraine.

United Nations Office for the Coordination of Humanitarian Affairs. 2025b. "Key facts and figures for the Sudan crisis (As of 30 September 2025". https://www.unocha.org/publications/report/sudan/key-facts-and-figures-sudan-crisis-30-september-2025).

United Nations Office for the Coordination of Humanitarian Affairs. 2025c. "Reported impact snapshot | Gaza Strip (24 September 2025)." https://www.ochaopt.org/content/reported-impact-snapshot-gaza-strip-24-september-2025.

Washington Report on Middle East Affairs. 2014. "ATFL Honors Americans of Lebanese Heritage." https://www.wrmea.org/014-june-july/arab-american-activism-atfl-honors-americans-of-lebanese-heritage.html.

World Association of Non-Governmental Organizations. n.d. "Guiding Principles." https://www.wango.org/codeofethics.aspx?page=2.

The Waiting Word

ALISON PHIPPS

The word is waiting.
The word is with me.
It lingers in my skin.
It plays my breastbone like a harp.
The word turns me to face the sunrise
moves my feet into the setting sun,
towards the melody
of morning light,
towards the dance.
The word.
The word is breath.
The word is breathing.
The word is promise.
The word is past.
The word hurts as it heals.
The word is laughter.
The word is old.
The word is strange
and praise.
The word humbles
and honors and holds.
The word.
The word suffers.
The word seeks.
The word rests in the heart space.
The word loves.

The word.
The word dwells.
The word is with us.
The word breathes.
The word waits.

PART THREE

"Host" Countries

The Wait

ANNA DZIUBAN

what is a head if not a laundry basket?
the white, the black, the delicate and rainbow,
they put us all in one big jolly casket,
with bullfight red smearing the care label

solved an escape room traced to Omicron,
I'm going home
barely exchanging masks for pacifiers
I'm doomed to be Sisyphus-suckling on,
should I not get somebody to atone
for what they deem a string of friendly fires,
conveniently tossing out the ashes,
painting the floor in lava where it's wretched
and counting down a nursery rhyme poem

my father called, delivering a lecture
on all the reasons I should not be going
home

when shepherds come, awaiting better omen,
we'll play "Reise nach Rom"
Trip to Jerusalem

a wolf dressed up like sheep still feeds on lamb

Vladimir V Putin, in brand new clothes,
5th term, good health, massage and heating throne.
they say it's better devil that you know,
invite to laugh it off against the odds
(last time my chair got nearly overthrown)

my laughter reads as a contagious cough
and when I smile, I show too many teeth
to an attention-hide-and-seeking Prof,
and at the entrance, I am mood-policed

a chair too few, somebody pulls the cable,
the music stops, I'm seeing Saraswati,
they pull another throne to their table
and eat the cake like it's a birthday party

I will be there—no need to be invited,
recruiting doves and mourners for my wake
and digging gutters blocking off the road.
I wonder what they've written on the cake,
and how much longer would the vaccine take,
and what's the waitlist for my final shot?

green zones, red lines, a vacant yellow sun
withholding blinking till all's good or gone

the night is young, the lion sleeps tonight
in May they could've, January they might

gray skin, black mask, a shivering old lock
ba-dum ba-dum awaiting knock-knock-knock

this Christmas
let the street lights stop the heart
so I don't have to watch things fall apart.

9

Phenomenologies of "Successful" Exile

Narratives of Displacement and Disorientation

ANNA GOTLIB

9.1 INTRODUCTION

Much of the work surrounding refugees tends to approach questions of their rights, their struggles against both the oppression they are leaving behind and the xenophobia and paternalism of their new home, and the arduous process of migration itself by considering their experiences from an outsider perspective. The focus is largely on worries about national, international, and nongovernmental organization policies; concerns about refugee health and well-being and how to improve both—all centering refugees as moral patients whose care is a matter of poorly prepared, and often morally suspect, institutions and systems. Although much remains to be said and done about the policies and procedures that govern the welfare of refugees and other exiles, what follows is not a policy paper, nor is it a philosophical argument about the failures of justice, care, and compassion. Instead I ask *what is it like* to be a refugee, centering the inquiry in a phenomenology of the displacement of "successful" refugees, where by "successful" I mean those who reached (ostensibly) safer shores, and by this particular dimension of "displacement" I mean what happens to their identity and sense of themselves once they have "succeeded."

My general claim is that both the external voices of powerful others in a refugee's adopted home, as well as her own internal narratives, implicate the role and significance of language and narratives in a refugee's well-being and sense of herself, casting significant shadows on how, and whether, she is able to successfully integrate. Because language is both said and heard, I center both the words used by powerful others as well as refugees' own written, spoken, and internal narratives, and suggest that

Anna Gotlib, *Phenomenologies of "Successful" Exile*. In: *Forced Migration and Health Justice*. Edited by: Lisa A. Eckenwiler, Verina Wild, Anna Gotlib, Ryoa Chung, and Deborah Zion, Oxford University Press.
 DOI: 10.1093/oso/9780197795491.003.0009

the threats to refugee identities—and often, lives—do not stop once they find themselves in their new home. First, I argue that, once the aid organizations, government officials, and others charged with refugee assistance, relocation, and care are no longer the center of an exile's world, a significant barrier to refugee well-being comes from how they are storied via master narratives of both the politically and socially powerful as well as those of the general public.[1] Second, I suggest that even as a refugee appears to assimilate into her new environment, her relationship to her new home can be grounded in a kind of internal disorientation, her acceptance of her circumstances ambivalent at best. Her sense of displacement is thus not lessened once migration itself recedes into the distance. The complexities of exile, I suggest, do not stop, but only begin, when a refugee is granted entry, the phenomena of displacement and disorientation persisting for decades after the initial flight from disaster.

9.2 REFUGEES AND DISORIENTATION (AND A CONFESSION)

First, a confession, and a clarification: My motivations for exploring these phenomenological aspects of migration are not mere academic curiosity. I myself am a refugee, having fled the USSR with my family, and as such I have been a recipient of geopolitically convenient goodwill from the West that welcomed Soviet refugees as brave escapees, renouncing the Iron Curtain through our flight. I am also a witness to the ongoing traumas of other "successful" refugees from the Eastern Bloc who nevertheless failed to adjust, to renegotiate their internal narratives about who they were, who they are, and who they might become. Thus my interest in the plight of refugees comes, at least in part, from firsthand experiences of not only the process of escape but also of being immersed in a number of refugee communities, of Eastern European origin as well as others. Perhaps I focus on the "successful" refugees because I was a child in the midst of the chaos, and my memory of migration is less clear than my recollections of what came after. Perhaps I also do so because I am especially moved by the drastically different experiences of other "successful" refugees whose presence was less geopolitically convenient for their adopted country. My desire to share all this is due to the worry that my focus on the external and internal disorientations that refugees experience might appear to neglect some of the crucial initial gatekeeping decisions made by host nations as well as by the international community. But I suggest that attention needs to be paid to what

1. For an insightful and powerful narrative of the various metaphors of "good" and bad" immigrants by Western governments, see Nayeri (2019).

takes place *after*, once permission to leave (or to enter) is granted, and one gains, *pace* Arendt (1968), some rights to action and to opinion. I argue that the struggles of refugees on foreign soil that follow transform into something more personal, less generalizable, and, in some cases, more internally disorienting and destructive.

Second, a few distinctions ought to be made for the sake of clarity. To begin, refugees differ from immigrants (and other migrants) in the sense that immigrants, for a number of reasons, choose to leave their home country and, in most cases, can return. Refugees, on the other hand, are directly or indirectly forced (by war and violence, economic deprivation, oppression, racism, and so on) to flee with no reasonable prospects of returning.[2] At the end of 2015, there were 21.3 million refugees worldwide (UN High Commissioner for Refugees 2016). Lacking a safe home to which they can return, they look to other nations, including the nations of the Global North, for asylum.

From the perspective of citizenship and national belonging, refugees are thus fundamentally homeless: they are no longer citizens, or indeed rightful claim-makers, of the home they left behind, but neither are they in a position to make rights-claims against a new location which has not accepted them as asylum seekers (Gotlib 2017b). As Hannah Arendt notes, "they are deprived of life, liberty, and the pursuit of happiness, or of equality before the law and freedom of opinion . . . but . . . they no longer belong to any community whatsoever. . . . They are deprived, not of the right to freedom, but of the right to action; not of the right to think whatever they please, but of the right to opinion" (1968, 474).

Yet, excepting cases in which it has been geopolitically or economically convenient, the homelessness and vulnerabilities of refugees have largely not moved the Global North to take the requisite measures—or, at least, they have not moved it sufficiently to offer assistance on the scale that is warranted. As Malkki argues, refugees thus find themselves in a kind of "structural invisibility" where they are everywhere yet "systematically invisible" (1995, 7; *see also* Malkki 1996). As I have argued previously (Gotlib 2017b, 2019), this is especially the case when the refugees are seeking entry from the Global South and when their race, religious beliefs, customs, and other markers of identity are storied as other, dangerous, threatening, or simply inconvenient for the host country. These policy-level decisions go a long way toward destabilizing and disorienting people who are already existentially threatened and politically liminal. The historical distinctions between how (some) European refugees have been welcomed while other

2. This is, of course, a general distinction, and the demarcation is not always this clear. In some cases, economic migrants flee destitution at a significant threat to their, and their families', lives. I am grateful to a referee for this clarification.

European and non-European refugees have been, and continue to be, turned away, is an injustice rooted in both political expediency and moral luck (Gotlib 2017b), and one which I will not address here.

So what is refugee disorientation? I suggest that there is a special kind of disorientation that is a part of many refugee experiences and that this disorientation makes refugees particularly vulnerable to master narratives that seek to define them in ways that further destabilize them as moral agents and as people. Becoming disoriented, as Ami Harbin tells us, means "losing our bearings in relation to others, environments, and life projects. . . . [D]isorientations are experiences that make it difficult to know how to go on" (2016, 13). These disorientations are ubiquitous, and can be mundane, such as an unpleasant encounter with someone previously trusted; they can also be world-destroying and reality-shifting, such as flight from a nation that no longer views one as fully human. "Such situations remove any protective layering we develop . . . that stabilise us and allow us to pursue individual, professional, or social paths in life" (Tarquinio 2020, 3, qtd. in Velasco et al. 2022). They create a schism between us and others, rendering us unable to locate ourselves as agents among other moral agents, or unable to do so with any confidence, choosing our words too carefully and defensively so as not to destabilize an already fragile sense of self. These kinds of schisms can, and do, lead to trauma.

Refugees find themselves in nations that might, or might not, want them there. Some are told that they "made it"; that they are "one of us"; that whatever it is they escaped is behind them, and their lives can start anew. Others are told that they are not welcome and that no matter how much they "succeed," they will never belong. In the former case, they doubt themselves when they cannot see any evidence of their own success, of "making it": when everything around them reminds them of their exile and of their inability to ever go home, despite triumphant public narratives that ignore their internal struggles and make the question of going on not only difficult but at times impossible to interpret. One might feel oneself a fraud: how can one so lucky now find oneself so hopeless, so rudderless, indeed so paralyzed by doubt and fear? In the case of those who are unwelcome no matter what, a refugee, perhaps even when experiencing all the trappings of economic success, steps into a brightly lit office building, fully aware that no matter how hard she tries to be a part of her new world, she is still marked as "other," only grudgingly allowed to share social spaces with those who actually belong.[3] Both of these cases are the same and different: the same with respect to the sense of disorientation and resulting trauma; different for the reasons these disorientations take place. My point is this: perhaps due

3. In fact, many kinds of migrants experience this kind of disorientation and liminality. I am grateful to a reviewer for this insight.

to the social norms and values within a number of countries of destination that, among other things, resist the "other," refugee stories do not necessarily find a satisfactory conclusion even when those in power, whether due to external pressures, internal calculations, or some other motivation, briefly open the door and allow them entry. After all, survival is relative—one can find one's way to a distant shore and still lose everything that matters. And the traumas of that kind of "successful" survival tend to last. Indeed, while some refugees view themselves as fortunate, being able to truly "move past" the dual traumas of their journeys and the difficult adjustments to alien worlds, some do not, remaining in psychological and emotional liminality: no longer belonging to the old, yet never quite feeling at home in the new. These kinds of refugee traumas can last a lifetime, becoming a totalizing force that unmakes the refugee's world, drawing sharp lines demarcated "before" and "after": the "before" a world and a self that she knew; the "after" marking the disorientation that remains.

These kinds of existential disorientations can lead to two specific kinds of "successful" refugee traumas. The first, which I call *external disorientation*, has to do with continuing public narratives of nonbelonging that a refugee encounters years after having settled in her new home. In addition to economic, professional, and social barriers that these narratives create, they also can induce ongoing anxiety about a lack of positive (or at least nonthreatening) relations with others, or indeed about how to go on. The externally disoriented refugee wonders, *What if they never stop seeing me as not one of them? What if they question my belonging? What if I really do not belong here—or anywhere?* The fact that these questions are too often met with official confirmation of xenophobia, suspicion, and discrimination only drives deeper the traumas of the "successful" refugee who happens to come from a disfavored part of the world or, whether as a result of ethnicity, religion, or culture, is marked as "other." Of course, external master narratives about unwanted refugees come in many forms. The flipside of agency-threatening hostility and mistrust is agency-destroying pity, grounded in stories of the "ideal refugee" as a pitiable moral patient, or else in demands that she be so in order to be recognizably and legitimately a refugee (rather than a scheming interloper, or worse). And thus, disoriented by the contradictory external messages that tell her to be resilient and tough while demanding that she surrender her agency, the refugee asks, *Who gets to speak for me—and why is it not me?*

The second kind of refugee trauma, which I call *internal disorientation*, has less to do with external narratives and more with the refugee's internal monologues, her sense of herself, and her relationship with her past. What this means is complicated: if, by the sheer moral luck of belonging to a "favored" refugee group, one does not encounter obvious contempt or unmistakable paternalism and pity from one's adopted home, internal battles, conflicts, and longings can nevertheless destabilize what on the outside appears to be a story of success, fortitude, and assimilation. Instead of wondering if one is truly "one of them," this refugee wonders, *Who am I now?* or *Who was I before?* Or she may be overcome by the thought that, unable to return, she is forever homeless. Finding no satisfactory answers, such a refugee can become liminal, trapped between severed connections with her past yet without having located herself as belonging in her present, or future.

These two kinds of "successful" refugee traumas—the traumas of external and internal disorientation—can lead to a kind of "undoing of the self," "a radical disruption of memory, a severing of past from present and, typically, an inability to envision a future" (Brison 1999, 39; *Also see* Brison 2002, 68). It can be experienced as helplessness before an overpowering and overwhelming force—of xenophobic master narratives, for example—that strips one's agency and capacity to imagine oneself otherwise. It forces a schism within one's sense of a previously coherent life, destroying one's narratives about oneself so dramatically that one can no longer see a connection to who, or what, one was before. And in the place of whatever was before, the trauma of refugee disorientation can offer stories that are frighteningly effective and efficient in filling up their narrative vacuum with tales of defeat, fear, loss of control, isolation, and worthlessness. To put it quite bluntly, refugee disorientation is not only a moral concern for all those engaged in the work of refugee justice but also a matter of refugee well-being and psychological health. I now turn to a closer examination of what these disorientations are and how they impact differently situated refugees.

9.3 REFUGEES, LANGUAGE, AND IDENTITY, OR, HOW TO GET EVERYTHING WRONG

9.3.1 External Disorientation or Refugees as "Other"

Refugees are faced with a number of damaging narratives that make the question of how to go on in their new home a matter not merely of concern but, at times, of existential despair. How does this take place? Certainly powerful voices from the far right (but not exclusively so) have made their mark by telegraphing their views on how refugees are to be perceived. But the problem does not lie solely with the powerful. Americans and other citizens of the Global North (and the more developed world more generally) have a long and storied history of, at best, ambivalence toward refugees and other exiles, which, at worst, is translated into outright nativism and suspicion of outsiders. Powerful voices capitalize on this ambivalence, often seeking to translate it into unsubtle xenophobia. In the UK, for example, asylum seekers have been described by politicians, social media, as well as by the deeply influential tabloid media as threatening "others" and as the chief sources of social unease—culturally, ethically, linguistically, morally. Indeed "[i]mmigrants are constructed as a homogeneous group that represents a threatening 'other' against which societal identity is constituted" (Innes 2010, 462). Indeed, David Cameron, at first embracing the language of "moral responsibility," subsequently announced, under substantial political pressure and growing xenophobia, that the UK could accept only 20,000 immigrants over a five-year period (Wintour 2015). And the UK Independence Party's Nigel Farage openly campaigned on a xenophobic and racist anti-refugee platform that so frightened the British public that a pro-Brexit vote followed (Forster 2016). To drive the point home, the Austrian government made plans to build a fence at its border with Italy to shield itself from the rising migrant numbers (BBC 2016). And in Australia refugees have been routinely described not only as a "problematic" but as a "deviant" population in relation to the integrity of the nation-state, race, and disease (Pickering 2001, 169 qtd. in Steimel 2010, 222). The United States, a standout in its history of selective anti-refugee policies, in the grip of its own decades-old anti refugee hysteria elected Donald Trump, who rose to power on narratives fueled by Islamophobic fear and mistrust of the other (Southern Poverty Law Center 2015). Indeed every major Republican presidential candidate has come out against admitting Syrian refugees into the United States while also expressing suspicion regarding those already here (Waldman 2015). Yet the sources of these destructive narratives do not lie solely in the more right-wing political factions. During the recession of 1993, Representative Anthony Beilenson, a liberal Democrat from Los Angeles, proposed a key change in the 14th Amendment in order to deny birthright citizenship of the US-born children of illegal immigrants. This proposal that was driven by the nativist fear of the growth of "non-native" populations—through the message that was conveyed to the general public via the 14th Amendment—centered narratives about "a growing number of pregnant women who come here for the precise purpose of having their 'American babies'" (Schrag 2010).

I suggest that this kind of speech is not a mere reflection of *some* anti-refugee sentiment in the US, EU, UK, and elsewhere. Indeed these public master narratives are not cherry-picked from otherwise normalized stories of migration, nor are they uncoordinated and unskilled expressions of overambitious politicians.[4] In fact, Chouliaraki and Zaborowski's 2017

4. Again, some of the trauma that I describe here also applies to many cases of economic migration, where the migrants lack an option to return to their homes. I am grateful to a reviewer for this insight.

analysis of over a thousand news articles on the European refugee crisis noted a remarkable organization, and clear intent, of anti-refugee narratives to other, marginalize, and dehumanize:

> The study showed that the "voices carried in the European press were not those of citizens or refugees but national politicians and EU officials" . . . whose "authoritative speech normalized the bordering practices, exerting the power to control and creating a structure of exclusions." . . . Three linguistic strategies were detected for consolidating authority and excluding others in the dominant narratives: 1) silencing, or the omission of voice altogether; 2) collectivization, or the incorporation of refugees into collective referents, such as nationality, in ways that eliminate their status as unique individuals; and 3) decontextualization, or the severing of individual lives from the historical conditions within which their requests to be hosted derive their legitimacy and justification. (Sahin-Mencutek 2020, 27)

But how does this speech (and the resulting policies) create refugee disorientation? Because refugees' mental health is to an important extent a function of their post-migration environment, I suggest that it is useful to consider official anti-refugee master narratives, which are likely to induce stress, anxiety, fear, and a sense of liminality, as partially constitutive of the social determinants of refugee mental health. In fact

> [t]he post-migration social conditions of refugees and asylum seekers often place them at the lower end of the social gradient. . . . This is partially due to the nature of forced migration, but is also a result of policies and public attitudes towards them, including their membership in groups that are stigmatized by the communities into which they migrate (e.g., as migrants, and/or as members of minority ethnic, racial, or religious groups). The result is often prolonged material deprivation, uncertainty, and social exclusion. Thus, many refugees and asylum seekers are at risk for poor mental health not only because of prior traumatic exposures, but also because of post-migration social determinants of health, and the impact of those determinants may increase over time. . . . Numerous studies suggest that the extent to which refugees feel welcomed or experience hostility has an impact on their mental health. Feeling accepted in one's country of settlement has had a significant impact on mood disorders among refugees from the former Yugoslavia. A large qualitative study with Colombian refugees in Ecuador found that regular experiences of discrimination and exclusion were associated with high levels of stress, anxiety and depression. (Hynie 2018, 299–300)

But perhaps an exile should speak for herself. Sharefa Daw, a refugee from Burma, writes, "We look like an American success story. But when we started hearing the anti-Muslim hate during the presidential election campaign, my husband said, 'My name is Haroon. Your name is Sharefa. Should we change our names?' He said, 'What if we have to leave the United States?' We had already given up our Burmese citizenship—this is our only home.

He was afraid people would know I was a Muslim refugee, and he said, 'Be careful wherever you go'" (Daw 2017).

9.3.2 Refugees as Sad Human-Interest Story

Narratives about refugee otherness are one thing. Stories about who they "really" are quite another. Aside from being unsubtly destabilized by hostile narratives, "successful" refugees also face a sense of displacement via dispiriting and demeaning stories about their ostensibly pitiable state. Because master narratives of frightening "otherness" are not exhaustive of how refugee identities are molded for public consumption, and perhaps because political speech is not the sole shaper of public image, public interest stories are a prominent refugee-defining lexicon. What these narratives sound like to refugees themselves is described quite vividly by Ece Temelkuran (2017), a Turkish journalist forced into having to flee:

> I was supposed to be writing about a refugee in Istanbul. Then she disappeared. . . . Then I had to disappear myself. So I am now the subject of this text. . . . I am now supposed to fill the shoes of this person called "the victim." Like a refugee waiting for a piece of bread with a stupid ticket in her hands, I should be ready to perform my victimhood whenever the act is called to the intellectual stage. I am now obliged to tell a story, but only the one particular story, the stupid story of my suffering that I hold like a ticket for my passage to the civilized world. . . . [W]hen a woman from the audience, holding her hands together with the graciousness of the Pope washing the feet of the poor, asks me, "So what CAN WE do for you?" I answer: "I feel like a baby panda that you're trying to adopt on a website!" The victim should be the victim but nothing else. Otherwise it becomes confusing for the audience. Be a number. Be a paragraph."

She continues:

> I remember this man from Somalia I met in a refugee camp on the Tunisian–Libyan border. . . . I was asking the same questions over and over again, "Do you have enough water to meet your daily needs?" "Do you have enough food to eat?" etc. . . . And this man, smiling the most sarcastic smile I've ever seen, asked me in perfect English, "I see it doesn't occur to you to ask me do I have a CV." Now I imitate the same smile to audiences when they are confused by my silly jokes, my defying the cliché of the suffering exile.

As Zahabi-Bekdash (2016) argues, these narratives—whether heroic, xenophobic, or victim-centered—"lump all refugees into one homogenous mass of 'people.' . . . We, citizens and governments, become ventriloquists for refugees, and strip them from the only things they still own: their stories, relationships, and experiences as human beings. We forget that there are as many refugee stories, experiences, and identities as there are refugees. We forget how complex identities are." As a result, we, as members of host nations, not only silence refugees but create spaces of liminality where refugees are unable to assert themselves not only as new citizens but as persons, for they are kept from those most powerful of moral spaces that make possible participation in identity-creation practices that individuate, that call on others to appropriately attend to one's rightful place in the moral universe. Indeed, these stories that—without their participation—paint refugees as broken and limited make them a blank canvas on which the host country's needs, anxieties, and political expediencies are projected. These stories give license to the powerful and force the powerless to forget that "[b]efore they became refugees, these people were parents, children, teachers, artisans, doctors and artists" (Zahabi-Bekdash 2016). Or, to put it in Harbin's (2016) terms, these narratives of refugee-as-sad-human-interest-story can lead refugees to lose not only their sense of who they are in relation to others in their new home but what life's projects are—indeed, who they are, outside of otherness and need. The disorientation that follows is just as Zahabi-Bekdash (2016) noted: stripped of their individualities and all the idiosyncrasies, stories, and passions of simply being human, refugees—now one indistinguishable mass—are not just physically dislocated but face an evisceration of their identity, the very identity that all through the traumas of escape and adjustment they have fiercely protected as their only locus of agency and control. Indeed the very identity that reminded them of the meanings and connections and understandings they carried with them the best way they could.

Some human-interest stories lack much of their humanity. Told for the benefit of sympathetic, but largely passive, local audiences, or else to eagerly echo the sentiments of outright hostile ones, both unmoved and repulsed by the struggles of those faceless masses, these sorts of stories can dehumanize with a few carefully placed words. In fact, "Goodman (2007) noted that media coverage of legislation on asylum-seeking families characterized them in terms usually used to describe animals breeding. . . . Hostility towards immigrants in the UK is also profound (Blackledge, 2005). Philo and Beattie (1999) observed that the coverage . . . in the British media used the terminology of a natural disaster, presenting Britain as the victim of 'floods,' even 'tidal waves' of immigrants. Lynn and Lea's (2003) analysis of readers' letters to newspapers showed that 'asylum seeker' now means 'bogus asylum seeker,' and genuine refugees are a rarity in the media" (Leudar et al. 2008, 188).

At the same time as refugees are dehumanized, their voices are silenced, and thus they are not among the storytellers. Indeed, in characterizing their plight, their voices are often largely, and I would suggest deliberately, missing, "rarely hav[ing] the opportunity to assert their identity in public"

(Leudar and Nekvapil 2000 qtd. in Leudar et al. 2008, 188). What is heard is a dehumanizing narrative designed either to other or to elicit pity—and I say "pity" and not "empathy" because empathy is something one can grant to another, imagining oneself in the other's place. This is not the case here, for these narratives are not about gaining insight into the experience of another, or are not offered, as Wittgenstein has said, with "an attitude towards a soul"(1953, 178). Instead these narratives of "invasions" and unindividuated masses offer no occasion for such an attitude, leaving the refugee without a non-liminal identity, story, or voice.

9.3.3 Refugees as "Good" and "Bad"

It would seem that once refugees' voices are taken away in the telling of their stories by others, nothing else remains to be said about how they are perceived or treated or, importantly, how these words are internalized. But narrative-creating is a complicated endeavor. Before considering the internal disorientation of refugees in the next section, I want to conclude with the problem of refugee curation and classification.

Let's begin with refugee story curation. Generally, while destination countries insist, despite much evidence to the contrary, that they indeed want to hear the voices of those who have made it to their shores, this invitation contains a number of caveats: these voices have to be of a particular kind, saying particular words, with the appropriate narrative arc so that some detail, some bit of phenomena, about refugee trauma is often encouraged in order to "move the audience." In fact "[i]n preparation for refugee events, some organisers send a list of prompt questions to refugee speakers about their life in their home country, their reasons for leaving, the challenges they have faced and how they have overcome them. There is an implicit narrative logic to the questions: 'tragedy' to 'success,' 'hell' to 'paradise'" (Tammas 2019).

Terms like "perseverance," "resilience," "devastation," and "hope" are urged in order to both inspire and move audiences who are distanced from these stories by the moral luck of privilege. The traumas of refugee journeys, put on maudlin exhibition, have the effect of oversimplifying and marginalizing complex human lives: *Tell us why you fled—was it awful there? Look at how terrible and different from us your lives were! Look at how you are trying to become just like us!* And thus refugee identities become a spectacle that both essentializes and "fixes" who they are (suffering heroes, objects of pity, with stories of resilience), packaging their complex phenomenologies into tidy soundbites for the consumption and inspiration of the listener. And witnessing these performative enactments of trauma and, importantly, gratitude, the listener walks away unmoved, or else convinced of the goodness of his "welcoming" nation. The refugees walk away, emotionally spent, re-marginalized, and, too often, re-traumatized.

I suggest that this tendency to curate refugee stories has its roots in the practice of refugee classification into "good" and "bad" refugees. Here I do not mean the official UN classifications of refugee versus immigrant versus migrant and so on. Instead, what I intend by refugee classification is what Liisa Malkki (1996) calls the privileged "universal humanitarian subject":

> Refugees were expected to behave in a certain way (for example: not to have a high standard of living) and to display characteristics that would justify the provision of aid, some of them being: poverty and passivity. Malkki argues that the most important aspects of social imagination of refugees are dehumanization and dehistoricization. Refugees are dehumanized when presented as devoid of agency, [a] speechless "sea of humanity" where individuals remain anonymous or sentimentalized (as the figures of refugee mothers with children). Dehumanization is reinforced by visual representation and photographic testimony of the media focused on showing tragedy, but also by humanitarian agencies which, in the visual materials for their fundraising campaigns show passivity and victimhood. (Szczepanik 2016, 31)

Thus, similar to the curation of refugee stories, the images and the background of a "good" refugee too often had to reflect helplessness, poverty, and, importantly, passive victimhood.[5] A good refugee is an object of pity, only a few days away from perishing without external aid, or else, lacking all agency, desperately waiting for enlightened assistance from those who know better. A good refugee, in other words, is only too grateful for crumbs from the tables of those who "know better." Victims of their (inferior) cultures, refugees ought to be nothing but grateful for the West's largesse and greater wisdom. For example, "Robins' (2003) analysis of American newspapers' coverage of the Sudanese 'Lost Boys' found that they were presented as coming from a situation beyond understanding and as vessels waiting to be filled by US material culture. Robins details the ways that common news descriptions like 'a child-man with glowing dark skin . . . who was clad only in tattered rags' . . . create an image of 'helpless' and destitute refugees in need of American protection" (Steimel 2010, 35).

Who, then, are the "bad" refugees? Frauds, driven by avarice and a desire for a free handout, intent on taking advantage of a generous host; men without families, whose only raison d'être is to threaten, rape, and steal. Emily

5. Although, as I have previously argued (Gotlib 2017b, 2019), for geopolitical purposes refugees can also be storied as decisive and brave rebels against oppressive systems, as many Eastern European Jewish refugees and others were during the decades of the Cold War.

Cousens (2015) has argued that one indication of this fictionalization of who refugees are, and why they have fled, stresses the numbers and features the photographs of women and children who have had to flee, emphasizing their innocence, vulnerability, and passive victimhood, in contrast to the threat posed by (especially younger) men.

And because in the EU, the UK, and the US the majority of local inhabitants do not directly converse with the refugees themselves, their ideas of who refugees are formed by the media, the government, aid organizations, and other third parties, who have already framed and curated the messages of the refugees. It is in this way that these classifications of "good" and "bad" refugees end up as the master narratives of how they should be perceived. The "good refugees" are dependent, victimized moral patients, eager to fit in. The "bad refugees" are agents of fear and chaos, coming into a nation without good cause, with the intent to subvert and destroy. In between these powerful and binary master narratives are actual people—frightened, hopeful, confused, and largely traumatized (Tammas 2019).

9.4 INTERNAL DISORIENTATION, OR THE PHENOMENOLOGIES OF EXILE

Thus far I have argued that external disorientation of "successful" refugees is grounded in harmful, destructive master narratives of powerful others. I would now like to conclude by suggesting that refugees face obstacles to their well-being that are functions of the traumas associated with both leaving the known and heading into the black box of migration. In this section, I will turn to territory personally much closer to home—the experiences of refugees who fled the Eastern Bloc to find themselves as liminal others in their new home. My intent here is not to argue that these internal disorientations impact only one subgroup of refugees, or that they are somehow more significant than the external disorientation experienced by so many others. Instead I want to share an experience that is fairly common among refugees who do not carry the stigma of otherness in the same way so many others do—the people whose experiences I share here (including my own) are perceived as white and educated and, importantly, were mostly welcomed by the West during the decades of the Cold War. My claim is that just because we were welcomed does not mean that all of us found a home.

The road to internal disorientation began at home. Even though often welcomed by Western nations for Cold War–era geopolitical reasons that I will not address here, for many leaving the Soviet Union and the Eastern Bloc, and especially for Jews fleeing rampant anti-Semitism, flight was a matter of hard-won official permission, or else of defection.[6] But once one's plans to leave became known (this was dangerous for social and political reasons, and was kept secret as long as possible), the reactions of one's compatriots were unforgiving:

> A former correspondent of *Literaturnaia Gazeta* . . . describes the hostility of his colleagues as soon as they learned that he had applied [to leave]. "No one in the office greeted me, no one bade me farewell. People with whom I had worked for years simply cut me." The correspondent's phone was bugged, he was followed and harassed by the KGB, and his application to leave was denied several times. The relatives, too . . . are adversely affected by their application to leave. One woman's father opposed her emigration. . . . As a result [of her emigration]. . . the father, a scholar employed by the Academy of Sciences, could no longer publish. An article of his was removed from a scholarly journal about to go to press. The editor of the journal told him, "you know, of course, we could have printed it but it was forbidden." (Gitelman 1982, 43)

Trauma was thus a motivator, as well as a central part, of the decision and the process of leaving. It did not abate during the arduous experience of the migration itself, which often took the refugees through several European countries where they did not speak the local languages, could not work, and had very little money. Once on American (or Canadian or other) shores, there was often a brief period of relief, or even the exhilaration of the newfound freedom to speak one's mind and, not unimportantly, to be able to buy the basic food items that in the 1970s through the early 1990s in Eastern Bloc countries were deemed luxuries and reserved for the most well-connected members of the Communist Party. The by now cliché image of the Soviet refugee passing out in an aisle of an average supermarket—think Robin Williams in *Moscow on the Hudson*— conveyed a fundamental truth: the "successful" Soviet refugees were often overcome by all that the West took for granted and spent their initial weeks and months taking in the abundance that both astounded and overwhelmed them.

But then came the later months, and years, and the newly arrived refugee was no longer so new—and neither were the shiny, formerly enticing promises of the West. It is here where their internal disorientation evolves further. In order to describe how this takes place, I want to make clear the assumptions about identities that I am using in making my claims. In several earlier papers, I argued that our personal identities are fundamentally a narrative in how they are created, understood, and evaluated, and that refugee identities are not an exception to the rule (Gotlib 2017a, 2017b, 2019). In those earlier works as well as here, I in part follow Paul Ricoeur

6. For a more in-depth examination of official narratives and policies defining Cold War–era refugees versus those defining refugees from elsewhere in the 2010s, please see Gotlib (2017b).

(1995), who noted that as a part of the narrative process of self-creation, we are capable of re-imagining and altering our identity. In *Oneself as Another*, he draws a distinction between two aspects of identity: *idem-identity* is identity understood as an immutable sameness of the self despite changes over time; *ipse-identity* is identity understood as a selfhood that is not fundamentally dependent on anything permanent and unchanging as it moves through time (Ricoeur 1995). I suggest that it is a tendency toward the extremes of both kinds of identity types that can become central to a refugee's conception of herself and which leads to a kind of epistemic and narrative disorientation that leaves her in a liminal state of nonbelonging either to the past or to the present. Here and elsewhere I also follow Andrea Deciu Ritivoi (2002), who suggested that it is the inflexibility of one's conception of oneself—whether in insisting on staying the same or on shedding one's "old self" entirely—that leads so many refugees to identity-annihilating destabilization in their life narratives and in their lives generally.

Among the number of various kinds of refugees, we can find rather polarized reactions, especially after a bit of time has passed since their arrival. Glossing over some differences for now, I will call the kind of refugee that tends to reject the new in favor of the old and familiar the "exile," and the kind that exists in a sort of event horizon where nothing before migration matters the "episodic." It is important to recall that refugees—especially the Eastern Bloc refugees I am centering here—escaped a dangerous, often unbearable situation at home, with no hope or possibility of return. Perhaps because of this sense of a permanently closed door, and perhaps due to much deep-seated (and justified) ill feeling toward their home countries, some episodics repudiated any good memories, or indeed any goodness whatsoever, of their country of origin (Lijtmaer 2001). This kind of "counterphobic assimilation," according to Akhtar (2011), can predominate when refugees "rapidly and fully take the dictates of the adopted country" (Akhtar 2011, 13 qtd. in Lijtmaer 2022, 309).

Others, the "exiles," can become "perennial mourners" (Volkan 1999, 173 qtd. in Lijtmaer 2022, 309). Indeed, some refugees—"especially those for whom home is invested with high ambivalence [engage in] pathological mourning" (Lijtmaer 2022, 309). The displacement that they experience destroys their sense of being rooted in a place, a culture, or a set of sense-making narratives. The break between their past and present disorients and existentially destabilizes these refugees in ways that echo throughout their whole experience of attempted acclimatization. Sometimes the acclimatization works only halfway, leaving the refugees in a state of constant negotiation about the moral, political, or emotional "acceptability" of their new location, leaving them half-exile, half-episodic. In other cases, the acclimatization largely fails, and the refugee is left as a permanent castaway, perhaps physically safe but psychologically, emotionally, and socially annihilated.

For a number of years, my mother was just such a liminal half-exile, half-episodic. Upon arriving in the United States, a well-educated, well-read, professional pianist who previously longed for the forbidden culture of the West, she quickly adopted the rejecting stance toward most things American. Specifically, although appreciative of the relative freedoms offered to her and her family, she kept a critical distance from what she perceived to be the uncultured, anti-intellectual, and coarse character of much of American life. In fact she invested a not insignificant amount of time and energy in making sure that I, old enough to be a culturally and linguistically fluent Russian yet young enough to be obsessed with becoming, as my mother would say with derision, a true *Amerikanka*, never forgot who I *really* was. She insisted that I remember which cultural heritage was *really* my own and which values and habits of mind I was to treasure and protect against the incursions of the flashy and loud static of my adopted home. "This is who you are," she would say approvingly, as I read Pushkin, listened to classical music, practiced the piano, and spent time with my parents and their refugee friends. She would sometimes shake her head with disappointment as I eagerly bought current rock albums, paid less and less attention to traditional holiday gatherings, expressed a preference for "fake" and "tasteless" American food, or used English with other Russians. "I don't even recognize who you are becoming," she would sigh. "You have changed—you are almost completely one of them." Although she eventually became more comfortable with, or perhaps more accustomed to, the US, to this day I don't think that my mother feels fully at home in a country in which she has spent more than half of her life.

A more extreme portrait of a true exile is found in the work of Ritivoi and the story of writer Vera Calin's journey from Romania to the United States. As a "successful" refugee but in all ways an "exile," Calin has made no attempt to acclimate or adapt to her new home:

> The formerly respected university professor does not brood over her inability to adjust to the New World, but records it as a personal triumph. She reminds herself constantly that she lives in a foreign universe, where nothing is or will be familiar and natural. . . . She perceives her new environment as the very opposite of the universe to which she is accustomed, and chooses the former over the latter precisely because the two are so different. The exile deems life in a foreign country an experience of non-belonging to the new milieu and cherishes it for that very reason. . . . In the alien environment, the exile aspires to test and certify her self-reliance, her independence from a particular social configuration. . . . To remember the old country, the old way of life, then, becomes a matter of commitment and responsibility toward the self, not toward a place. (Ritivoi 2002, 125)

Thus it seems that it was their *idem-identities* that Calin and, to some extent, my mother held dear in their dedication to the constancy of their "true," "original" selves which could not, and would not, change. Indeed, for Calin any move toward the "other" of her new surroundings would mean a fundamental betrayal of her sense of this self, her authenticity, and all that must never be violated by the shock and temptation of the new. This insistence that one must remain as "the one from before" is hard work (Ritivoi 2002, 129). Yet as one's own experiences begin to force their way into the narratives of daily life, the survival of the "one true self" becomes a desperate and all-consuming task: Ritivoi notes that Calin, in writing her memoir, shares facts about her life, yet "we do not find out who Vera Calin is, rather, we discover who she can no longer be. In matters of survival, the person who decides that survival has indeed taken place, the one who does the contrasts and comparisons, is the resulting self, the one-after, and not the one-before. 'Myself from before' is never present as an uncontestable term of comparison, but is always implicit, reconstructed, implied rather than referred to directly. The idem Calin so strenuously tries to preserve is a specter, a reminder of some obsolete identity formation. This idem is a souvenir" (Ritivoi 2002, 129).

Although my own mother has not written a memoir of her life as a refugee, she, too, for quite a while emphasized the discontinuity of her "old life" and "present situation," drawing a sharp distinction between an agential past self, which in however difficult circumstances, through dedication, effort, and endless striving, managed to make a life, and her current psychosocially liminal self in an anomic, constantly shifting world. Like Calin, between her "old life" and her "present situation," she insisted on the survival of the former, protecting and cherishing it like a precious object that cannot be marred or disfigured by any deep connections with the present. And thus one's identity is a souvenir, a precious and fragile thing that must be kept secluded on a shelf where the movement, the change—the life—taking place only a few feet away neither challenges nor in any way comes into contact with its splendid isolation.

The result is a kind of arid and, in the end, damaging alienation from both one's past and one's present that is truly disorienting. Because despite her rejection of its value and meaning, the exile must still live and experience life in a land she rejects while desperately trying to protect the idem-self of pre-migration; she becomes alienated from both—her unreachable and frozen pre-exile self, as well as her post-exile existence, which she rejects as not truly her own. Thus while Calin assured the authenticity of her "true" self by locating her presence "in the Far West" (Ritivoi 2002, 135), away from the self that matters, my mother surrounded herself with people and objects and cultivated the habits that she desperately hoped would allow "the before" to survive amid the untenable glare of "the now." It is perhaps only with the passage of time that it finally occurred to me just how vital it was for her that I remain a "genuinely Russian girl" and not turn into the dreaded "Amerikanka."

The post-migration disorientations of Calin and of my mother had similar symptoms but different outcomes. While my mother, weary of the social and psychological barriers of guarding her idem-identities, eventually rejected the purity of the pre-exile self and assumed the middle-ground position, Calin did not—or, at least, she did not do so soon enough. In quoting Calin's writing, Ritivoi chose a particularly telling passage: "Truth is, I don't have any holidays, that is, I don't have a mythology. . . . With no holidays and traditions, my life seems to unfold under the auspices of the ephemeral and an amorphous precariousness. I wish I could have for only a moment the awareness of duration, so New Englandly conveyed by Emily Dickinson" (Ritivoi 2002, 134).

Because her life in the present was one of eternal exile, disconnected from a storied past and unwilling to engage with the alien present, she could neither fully live within her memories nor create new ones through engagement. The result is an epistemic and social disorientation, a kind of inner liminality—a flat, gray landscape in which one goes through the requisite motions with only limited significance, for everything that mattered is necessarily in the past.

I suggest that this is not only destabilizing but tragic, traumatic, a kind of living death. If externally disoriented refugees could at least sometimes look beyond themselves in locating the sources of their suffering, those beset by these kinds of internal schism between the past and the present could not. While the externally disoriented refugees were dehumanized by master narratives that storied them as an undifferentiated mass of need, refugees like Calin convinced themselves of their own lack of a distinguishable self, their own lives narratively and agentially empty, hollowed out by the demands of backward-looking yearnings. As Ritivoi notes, "An uneventful life is a life with no memories: Nothing is worth recording because nothing is individualized . . . [but is] eternal, amorphous, present time, thus failing to create a new past" (2002, 135).

9.5 CONCLUSION

I began wondering about refugee disorientation before I knew the proper terms to describe it. Today I wonder if we are any closer to finding answers to the question of what to do about refugee well-being that reaches beyond political and socioeconomic reforms that are necessary but not sufficient.[7] There are indeed many reasons to worry. The current right-wing, xenophobic turn in so many Western nations signals troubling trends, including increased othering of refugees—especially of those whose ethnicity, religion, and cultural practices differ from their intended new homes. As a refugee who was privileged in ways that many are not, I cannot help but despair at the direction of policies and practices that await current and future generations of even the most "successful" of migrants. Who will get to tell their stories, and what will those stories say? And what can be done about those whose internal narratives are consumed by longings that cannot be satisfied by more humane migration policies? Can what Hilde Lindemann (2001) calls "counternarratives" be responsive to both external and internal disorientation experienced by refugees?

What would these counternarratives sound like? Ritivoi offers an account of the Polish refugee and writer Eva Hoffman, who, instead of falling into the traps of being either an exile or an episodic, set out to reconcile her Polish childhood with her new American realities. Ritivoi suggests that Hoffman's reconciliation of her plural identities allows for both a connection to her past as well as for an openness to the present and future. Her diary, for example, embraces her multiple selves—the Polish "Ewa" and the "Eva" of her post-migration self (Gotlib 2017a). Her own narratives about who she is thus resist the unyielding grip of her past without closing the door, creating fluid ambivalence regarding her refugee identity. She neither denies her disorientation nor allows it to swallow her whole, creating moral spaces for herself "as a constantly renewed and renewable process" (Ritivoi 2002, 170). Instead of signaling brokenness, Hoffman leaves for herself an opening to examine her divergent selves as versions of the same person, whose various incarnations do not necessarily have to serve as each other's faithful reflections or to add up to one (Gotlib 2017a).

As counterintuitive, and perhaps alarming, as this might sound to some, I do not think that refugee narratives have to center progress and assimilation or else sadness and loss. In fact they are not required to follow any kind of emplotment at all—to suggest otherwise would be to fall into the serious moral error of generalizing refugees into a collective, an unindividuated mass that bemoans its fate, praises its rescuers, or else tells simple stories of resilience and eventual triumph. As I argued earlier, this is fundamentally destructive to a refugee's well-being and sense of self.

So, then, let's consider who a "successful" refugee might be. Setting aside for the moment the clear need for sociopolitical, economic, and other

7. Access to community, to mental health services, and to other elements of distributive justice would indeed be necessary from a bottom-up, phenomenological perspective. I am grateful to an anonymous reviewer for this suggestion.

counternarratives that challenge a number of deficient and alienating social norms that are destructive to a refugee's well-being, I would like to conclude by focusing on the phenomenologies of the individual refugee herself. Perhaps she is just that person who, despite the trauma and the disorientation of migration, holds her nostalgias for the past, her uncertainty about the present, and the contingency of the future all at the same time, without feeling a need to choose or to declare allegiance to a single version of herself. Less of an exile without a past or future, she is more like Lugones's (1987) world-traveler, her lack of certainty of how to go on becoming more like an ongoing negotiation among the various selves that constitute her. And if this sounds odd or comes a bit too close to an embrace of internal chaos, I suggest that, for those of us who have endured migration, the normalization of this narrative fluidity—both external and internal—is perhaps what was needed all along.

REFERENCES

Akhtar, Salmam. 2011. *Immigration and Acculturation: Mourning, Adaptation, and the Next Generation*. Jason Aronson.

Arendt, Hannah. 1968. *The Origins of Totalitarianism*. Harcourt.

BBC. 2016. "Migrant Crisis: Austria Passes Controversial New Asylum Law."https://www.bbc.com/news/world-europe-36152927.

Blackledge, Adrian. 2005. *Discourse and Power in a Multilingual World*. Benjamins.

Brison, Susan J. 1999. "Trauma Narratives and the Remaking of the Self." *Acts of Memory: Cultural Recall in the Present*, edited by Mieke Bal, Jonathan Crewe, and Leo Spitzer, UP of New England.

Brison, Susan J. 2002. *Aftermath: Violence and the Remaking of a Self*. Princeton University Press.

Chouliaraki, Lilie, and Rafal Zaborowski. 2017. "Voice and Community in the 2015 Refugee Crisis: A Content Analysis of News Coverage in Eight European Countries." *International Communication Gazette* 79 (6–7): 613–635.

Cousens, Emily. 2015. "We Need to Stop Telling Ourselves That Women and Children Are the Only Refugees Who Matter." *The Independent*, September 9. http://www.independent.co.uk/voices/comment/we-need-to-stop-telling-ourselves-thatwomen-and-children-are-the-only-refugees-who-matter.

Daw, Sharefa. 2017. "I'm a Refugee. In America, I Felt Safe for the First Time. Now All I Feel Is Fear." ACLU, January 18. https://www.aclu.org/news/immigrants-rights/im-refugee-america-i-felt-safe-first-time-now-all-i-feel.

Forster, Katie. 2016. "Hate Crimes Soared by 41% After Brexit Vote, Official Figures Reveal." *The Independent*, October 13. http://www.independent.co.uk/news/uk/crime/brexit-hatecrimes-racism-eu-referendum-vote-attacks-increase-police-figures-official-a7358866.html.

Gitelman, Zvi. 1982. "Exiting from the Soviet Union: Emigrés or Refugees?" *Michigan Journal of International Law* 3: 43. https://repository.law.umich.edu/cgi/viewcontent.cgi?params=/context/mjil/article/1861/&path_info=.

Goodman, S. 2007. "Constructing Asylum Seeking Families." *Critical Approaches to Discourse Analysis Across Disciplines* 1: 35–49.
Gotlib, Anna. 2019. "I Am Not Your Canvas: Memory, Liminality, and the (Re)claiming of Refugee Voices." In *Refugees Now: Rethinking Borders, Hospitality, and Citizenship*, edited by Kelly Oliver, Lisa M. Madura, and Sabeen Ahmend. Rowman & Littlefield International.
Gotlib, Anna. 2017a. "Memory, Sadness and Longing: Exile Nostalgias as Attunement to Loss." In *The Moral Psychology of Sadness*, edited by Anna Gotlib. Rowman and Littlefield.
Gotlib, Anna. 2017b. "Refugees, Narratives, or How to Do Bad Things with Words." *Kennedy Institute of Ethics Journal* 27 (S2): 65–86.
Harbin, Ami. 2016. *Disorientation and Moral Life*. Oxford University Press.
Hynie, M. 2018. "The Social Determinants of Refugee Mental Health in the Post-Migration Context: A Critical Review." *Canadian Journal of Psychiatry* 63 (5): 297–303.
Innes, Alexandria J. 2010. "When the Threatened Become the Threat: The Construction of Asylum Seekers in British Media Narratives." *International Relations* 24 (4): 456–477.
Leudar, Ivan,J. Hayes,J. Nekvapil, and J. T. Baker. 2008. "Hostility Themes in Media, Community and Refugee Narratives." *Discourse & Society* 19 (2): 187–221. http://www.jstor.org/stable/42889189.
Leudar, I., and Nekvapil, J. 2000. "Presentations of Romanies in the Czech Category Work in Television Debates." *Discourse & Society* 11: 487–513.
Lindemann, Hilde. 2001. *Damaged Identities, Narrative Repair*. Cornell University Press.
Lijtmaer, Ruth. 2001. "Splitting and Nostalgia in Recent Immigrants: Psychodynamic Considerations." *Journal of the American Academy of Psychoanalysis and Dynamic Psychiatry* 29 (3): 427–438.
Lijtmaer, Ruth. 2022. "Social Trauma, Nostalgia and Mourning in the Immigration Experience." *American Journal of Psychoanalysis* 82 (2): 305–319.
Lugones, María, 1987. "Playfulness, 'World'-Travelling, and Loving Perception." *Hypatia* 2 (2): 3–19.
Lynn, N., and S. Lea. 2003. "'A Phantom Menace and the New Apartheid': Construction of Asylum-seekers in the United Kingdom." *Discourse & Society* 14 (4): 425–452.
Malkki, L. 1996. "Speechless Emissaries: Refugees, Humanitarianism, and Dehistoricization." *Cultural Anthropology* 11 (3). 377–404.
Malkki, L. 1995. *Purity and Exile: Violence, Memory, and National Cosmology Among Hutu Refugees in Tanzania*. University of Chicago Press.
Nayeri, Dina. 2019. *The Ungrateful Refugee: What Immigrants Never Tell You*. Catapult.
Philo, G., and Beattie, L., 1999. "Race, Migration and Media." In *Message Received*, edited by G. Philo. Addison Wesley Longman.
Pickering, S. 2001. "Common Sense and Original Deviancy: News Discourses and Asylum Seekers in Australia." *Journal of Refugee Studies* 14: 169–186.
Ricoeur, Paul. 1995. *Oneself as Another*. Translated by Kathleen Blamey. University of Chicago Press.
Ritivoi, Andreea Deciu. 2002. *Yesterday's Self: Nostalgia and the Immigrant Identity*. Rowman & Littlefield.
Robins, M. 2003. "'Lost Boys' and the Promised Land: US Newspaper Coverage of Sudanese Refugees." *Journalism* 4: 29–49.
Sahin-Mencutek, Zeynep. 2020. "Migration Narratives in Policy and Politics," *Working Paper* 17: 27.

Schrag, Peter. 2010. "Ambivalence About Newcomers." *New York Times*, August 16. https://www.nytimes.com/roomfordebate/2010/08/16/the-gop-and-birthright-citizenship/ambivalence-about-newcomers.

Southern Poverty Law Center. 2015. "American and European Radical Right Attacks Refugees Fueled Anti-Muslim Sentiment." October 6. https://www.splcenter.org/hatewatch/2015/10/06/american-and-european-radicalright%E2%80%99s-attacks-refugees-fueled-anti-muslim-sentiment.

Steimel, Sarah. 2010. "Refugees as People: The Portrayal of Refugees in American Human Interest Stories." *Papers in Communication Studies* 28: 219–237. https://digitalcommons.unl.edu/commstudiespapers/28.

Szczepanik, Marta. 2016. "The 'Good' and 'Bad' Refugees? Imagined Refugeehood(s) in the Media Coverage of the Migration Crisis." *Journal of Identity and Migration Studies* 10 (2): 23–33.

Tammas, Rifaie. 2019. "Refugee Stories Could Do More Harm Than Good." *Open Democracy*, November 1. https://www.opendemocracy.net/en/refugee-stories-could-do-more-harm-good/.

Tarquinio, C. 2020. "The Powerful Hold of COVID-19." *European Journal of Trauma & Dissociation* 4 (3): 100174. doi: 10.1016/j.ejtd.2020.100174.

Temelkuran, Ece. 2017. "We Want Our Refugees and Exiles to be Victims." Literary Hub, July 27. http://lithub.com/we-want-our-refugees-and-exiles-to-be-victims/.

UN High Commissioner for Refugees. 2016. "Forced Displacement in 2016." https://www.unhcr.org/statistics/unhcrstats/5943e8a34/global-trends-forced-displacement-2016.html.

Velasco, P. F., B. Perroy, U. Gurchani, and R. Casati. "Lost in Pandemic Time: A Phenomenological Analysis of Temporal Disorientation During the Covid-19 Crisis." *Phenomenoloy and the Cognitive Sciences* 2: 1–24. doi: 10.1007/s11097-022-09847-1.

Volkan, V. D. 1999. "Nostalgia as a Linking Phenomenon." *Journal of Applied Psychoanalytic Studies* 1 (2): 169–179.

Waldman, Paul. 2015. "The GOP's Despicable Rush to Demonize Refugees." *The Week*. https://theweek.com/articles/589927/gops-despicable-rush-demonize-refugees.

Wintour, Patrick. 2015. "UK to Take up to 20,000 Syrian Refugees over Five Years, David Cameron Confirms." *The Guardian*, September 7. https://www.theguardian.com/world/2015/sep/07/uk-will-accept-up-to-20000-syrian-refugees-david-cameron-confirms.

Wittgenstein, Ludwig. 1953. *Philosophical Investigations (Philosophische Untersuchungen)*. Translated by G. E. M. Anscombe. The Macmillan Company.

Zahabi-Bekdash, Lara. 2016. "Recreating the Refugees Narratives: From Sympathy to Dignity." *Huffington Post*, November 25. http://www.huffingtonpost.com/lara-zahabibekdash-md-phd/recreating-therefugees-n_b_8610422.html.

10

Disqualify, Disincentivize, and Dissonate

Immigration Law as a Barrier to Migrants' Healthcare Access

Y.Y. BRANDON CHEN

10.1 INTRODUCTION

Being able to access healthcare is crucial to migrants' integration into receiving communities. To the extent that healthcare access promotes good health, it facilitates migrants' active engagement in society (Ager and Strang 2008). Healthcare institutions can also function as a gateway that connects migrants with other resources and opportunities important for settlement (Martone et al. 2014). In countries where healthcare is purported to be universally available, having equal access thereto symbolizes migrants' inclusion, which may encourage their further integration (Penninx 2005).

However, studies from around the world reveal that migrants face a combination of barriers when seeking healthcare in receiving countries. Many migrants lack the financial means or health insurance to obtain the treatment they need (Gil-González et al. 2015). Such impediments are exacerbated by other expenses that migrants often must incur in order to access services, including those relating to transportation, child care, and time off from work (Hill et al. 2021; Tsai and Ghahari 2023). Even when affordability is not an issue, migrants' use of healthcare is frequently hampered by such obstacles as language barriers, health illiteracy, discrimination, and a lack of culturally appropriate services (Kacker et al. 2015; Dougherty et al. 2020; Galanis et al. 2022).

Y.Y. Brandon Chen, *Disqualify, Disincentivize, and Dissonate*. In: *Forced Migration and Health Justice*. Edited by: Lisa A. Eckenwiler, Verina Wild, Anna Gotlib, Ryoa Chung, and Deborah Zion, Oxford University Press.
 DOI: 10.1093/oso/9780197795491.003.0010

Law, "[b]y establishing the rules and frameworks that shape social and economic interactions" (Gostin et al. 2019, 1857), contributes to and reinforces these healthcare access barriers. Among other things, law defines migrants' entitlement to government benefits, structures migrants' encounters with healthcare providers, and dictates the extent to which migrants can avail themselves of socioeconomic resources like income and education (Chen 2017). Particularly immigration law, which governs one's ability to enter and remain in a country as well as the conditions of such entry and stay, acts as a significant determinant of migrants' access to healthcare. Research has repeatedly confirmed that "immigration policy is healthcare policy" (Pedraza et al. 2017, 926).

A scan of literature uncovers at least three ways that immigration law can modulate migrants' healthcare access. First, legal statuses and categories created by immigration law are regularly relied on to demarcate migrants' eligibility to publicly funded healthcare (Parmet 2020; Castellanos González 2022). Second, immigration law can deter or outright block migrants' healthcare use by subjecting them to screening and surveillance and by tying service access to adverse immigration consequences (Heyman et al. 2009; Pedraza et al. 2017). Third, restrictive immigration law stigmatizes migrants and can influence the extent to which providers see them as deserving (Grove and Zwi 2006). This in turn sours migrants' health-seeking experience and their perception of the healthcare system (Larchanché 2012; Castellanos González 2022).

In this chapter, I refer to these three permutations of the link between immigration law and migrants' healthcare access as disqualification, disincentivization, and dissonance, respectively. Using Canada as an example, this chapter aims to elaborate on these immigration law–related healthcare barriers in turn. In section 10.2, I explain how Canadian immigration law works in tandem with healthcare law to disqualify migrants from healthcare benefits both de jure and de facto. Next, in section 10.3, I identify several ways that immigration law discourages migrants from utilizing healthcare goods and services, including those that they are in principle entitled to receive. Section 10.4 shifts attention to immigration law's ability to generate dissonance between service providers' duty of care toward migrants and their other concerns, such as their views on migrants' healthcare deservingness and their role as immigration gatekeepers. Examples are provided to show how this dissonance can subsequently turn migrants away from the healthcare system. The chapter concludes with some reflections on the relationship between migrant health and justice, as well as the direction of necessary law reform to improve migrants' access to healthcare.

For the purpose of this chapter, "law" is broadly defined to encompass not only legislation and court decisions but also rules and practices adopted, both officially and informally, by such decision-makers as civil servants, hospital administrators, and healthcare practitioners when exercising their legally provided discretion. This broader conception of law reflects the reality of neoliberal governance that prevails in countries like Canada, where "authority for immigration control [is divested] from the state to a variety of non-state actors, transforming them into calculable and auditable sites" (Lehman et al. 2016, 45).

10.2 IMMIGRATION LAW AS DISQUALIFIER

Given the costly nature of many healthcare goods and services, accessing them typically requires government assistance. In Canada, such government support primarily takes the form of social insurance. One of the ways that immigration law obstructs migrants' healthcare access in Canada, therefore, is by rendering migrants ineligible for publicly funded health insurance.

According to the Canada Health Act (1985), Canadian provinces and territories must entitle all their residents to government health insurance plans. Failure to do so may cause provinces and territories to lose their annual healthcare funding from the federal government. A resident for this purpose, however, is not defined by physical presence alone. Rather, it refers to "a person lawfully entitled to be or to remain in Canada who makes [their] home and is ordinarily present in the province, but does not include a tourist, a transient or a visitor to the province" (Canada Health Act 1985, s. 2). The demand that an insured person be "lawfully entitled to be or to remain in Canada" and not be "a tourist, a transient or a visitor" has prompted corresponding provincial and territorial laws either to explicitly limit health insurance eligibility to those who possess certain citizenship or immigration statuses, or to be interpreted to the same effect (Health Canada 2025). As such, immigration rules around who is permitted to reside in Canada, and with which status, become embedded in healthcare law to deny public insurance coverage to some migrants.

In recent decades, migrants' healthcare entitlement in Canada has been in lockstep with the logic of neoliberal governance that grabs hold of Canada's immigration system. It valorizes "autonomous, flexible individuals open to risk-taking and aversion while barring the entry of those perceived as integrative risks or social burdens" (Walsh 2011, 872). Migrant workers, with their perceived entrepreneurialism and labor market engagement, are often regarded as an example of the former. Consequently they are awarded public health insurance coverage across the country, provided that their work permits are valid for the legislatively stipulated length, which is six months in some parts of Canada and 12 months in others (Chen 2017).

In contrast, asylum seekers—namely, those who have applied for refugee protection in Canada but whose status as a refugee is not yet confirmed—are frequently portrayed in policy discourse as a threat to national security and to the economy (Huot et al. 2016). They are disqualified from all provincial and territorial health insurance plans (Chen 2022). They must instead rely on the Interim Federal Health Program (IFHP) administered by the federal government for healthcare assistance, and their entitlement is not immune from the restrictive effects of immigration law either. Between 2012 and 2016, in the name of limiting government spending and combating fraud within the refugee system, healthcare benefits under the IFHP were stratified in favor of asylum seekers whose claim for protection was deemed more genuine. Asylum seekers from a list of Global North countries considered improbable to produce refugees, as well as people who received a negative first-instance decision on their asylum claim, had their healthcare coverage significantly reduced (Dhand and Diab 2015).

Canadian healthcare law is similarly unsympathetic toward migrants who lack any immigration status in the country. These migrants are excluded from both provincial and territorial health insurance, as well as the IFHP (*Toussaint v. Canada (AG)* 2011). For them, immigration law not only operates at the international borders to block their entry to Canada, but it also follows them even after they somehow find a way in, to impede their social integration by depriving them of healthcare entitlement. Notably some provinces and territories have extended such healthcare disentitlement beyond migrants themselves to encompass their Canadian-born children, who are Canadian citizens by birth. For instance, in Nova Scotia a government policy provides that children born in the province to non-citizen parents will not qualify for public health insurance unless their parents are legally deemed residents (Nova Scotia Department of Health and Wellness 2014). Relevant laws in British Columbia, Alberta, and, until recently, Quebec likewise tie the healthcare coverage of children born to migrants to the resident status of their parents (Rahimian 2020).

Besides manipulating who is considered a resident and who is a "genuine" asylum seeker, immigration law can affect migrants' healthcare eligibility by making it difficult for them to produce the necessary documents or meet other administrative requirements. This healthcare barrier can manifest either de facto or de jure. A de facto healthcare disqualification of this sort arises when access to healthcare goods and services is conditioned upon certain requirements not specified in the formal policy on healthcare eligibility, such as a need to present personal identification or proof of residency. As a case in point, when COVID-19 vaccine first became available, the government of Ontario assured that everyone in the province would qualify for it regardless of their citizenship and immigration statuses. Yet for a brief period after the vaccine was rolled out, some migrants could not book a vaccination appointment through the province's website because they had to enter a health insurance card number, which they did not have (Fox 2021). For migrants who were able to secure an appointment, some reported being turned away by service providers because they failed to show a provincial health insurance card when requested (O'Shea 2021). In both instances, as immigration status dictates whether a person is eligible for the requisite documentation, immigration law effectively acts as a healthcare disqualifier, albeit not at the stage of policymaking but at the point of service access.

For an example where immigration law draws on documentation requirements to deprive migrants of publicly funded healthcare de jure, consider the above-mentioned Nova Scotia policy. Pursuant to that policy, asylum seekers who have been granted protection in Canada are eligible for the province's health insurance program only if they have a letter from the federal immigration department confirming their application for permanent residence (Nova Scotia Department of Health and Wellness 2014). However, protected persons may be unable to immediately apply for permanent resident status for reasons ranging from unaffordability of the application fees to delay caused by the need to change names and/or gender markers first. Even if protected persons could submit their permanent residence application expeditiously, there is no guarantee that a letter from immigration authorities acknowledging this application will arrive quickly. All the while, asylum seekers will typically lose their IFHP benefits 90 days after being successfully recognized as people in need of protection (Government of Canada 2024). This means that the immigration-related documentation requirement in this case has the potential of leaving protected persons without any publicly funded healthcare, ironically rendering them worse off than before their asylum claim was accepted.

10.3 IMMIGRATION LAW AS DISINCENTIVE

Another way that immigration law hinders migrants' healthcare access is by limiting their ability or desire to seek out healthcare goods and services in the first place. Healthcare law in this situation, when compared with the role it plays when immigration law acts as a disqualifier, is less complicit in the obstruction of migrants' healthcare access. Rather than actively exploiting immigration categories and processes to circumscribe migrants' health insurance eligibility, when immigration law functions as a disincentive healthcare entitlement of the affected migrants is clearly provided. What immigration law does in such a scenario is cause migrants to refrain from using healthcare that they qualify for by linking healthcare utilization to some negative immigration consequences. As migrants strive against jeopardizing their ability to remain in or return to Canada, any healthcare entitlement they supposedly enjoy turns out to be illusory.

The disincentivizing effect of Canadian immigration law on migrants' healthcare access starts before one's arrival in the country. With a history of discrimination, Canada has long barred the admission of migrants who are suspected of imposing a burden on public resources (Hanes 2009). Today prospective migrants are found inadmissible to Canada if "their health condition . . . might reasonably be expected to cause excessive demand on health or social services" (Immigration and Refugee Protection Act 2001, s. 38(1)). This rule impedes migrants' access to healthcare in at least two ways. It physically keeps certain prospective migrants out of Canada and, by extension, prevents their utilization of Canadian healthcare goods and services. Moreover, insofar as the evaluation of excessive demand takes into account prospective migrants' past medical expenses, it discourages these migrants' healthcare use even before their seeking entry to Canada. For example, up until 2018 a federal policy deemed most HIV-positive immigration applicants who were on antiretroviral treatment inadmissible because of the therapy's high cost (Heywood et al. 2002). The only exception to this policy pertained to refugees and certain immigrants coming to Canada through family sponsorship (Immigration and Refugee Protection Act 2001). This raised concerns that some prospective migrants living with HIV who were aware of the policy might choose to postpone treatment in hope of circumventing a finding of excessive demand (Bisaillon 2022).

Even when migrants manage to enter Canada, the influence of immigration law as a disincentive to healthcare access proves inescapable. In particular, when migrants without legal status in the country are exceptionally made eligible for certain publicly funded healthcare, the risk of their being discovered by immigration authorities during the health-seeking process and subsequently removed from Canada poses a serious roadblock to healthcare access (Magalhaes et al. 2010). More than empty threats, detection and deportation of non-status migrants following healthcare use has been reported in the media (Britten 2016). In some Canadian jurisdictions, such as Ontario, the possibility of such immigration surveillance is aided by privacy legislation that authorizes immigration status collected in healthcare settings to be shared with law enforcement without the need for a warrant if the disclosure aims to assist with an investigation (Macnab 2021).

Outside the context of irregular migration, another well-documented example of Canadian immigration law acting as a healthcare deterrent concerns migrant agricultural workers. Each year the Seasonal Agricultural Worker Program (SAWP) brings in tens of thousands of migrants from Mexico and the Caribbean, who are desperate to earn a better living, to work in Canada's agri-food sector (Hennebry and Preibisch 2012). On paper, these migrant workers either enjoy provincial or territorial health insurance coverage or have private health insurance that employers are obligated to purchase on their behalf. They are also covered by provincial or territorial workplace safety and insurance regimes (MacIntosh 2018). In reality, however, many seasonal migrant workers do not seek healthcare or report work-related illnesses and injuries (Hennebry et al. 2016).

Although multiple factors contribute to seasonal migrant workers' underutilization of healthcare, a significant culprit is the extreme power imbalance created and reinforced by law between these migrants and their Canadian employers, which in turn places these migrants under constant fear of losing the ability to continue working in Canada, thus losing their income (MacIntosh 2018). Pursuant to the agreements reached between Canada and SAWP-participating countries, early cessation of seasonal migrant workers' employment contract is permitted in cases of workers' noncompliance, refusal to work, or for "any other sufficient reason" (Employment and Social Development Canada 2025a, s. 12.1; Employment and Social Development Canada 2025b, s. 10.2). In the absence of a clear definition of what constitutes "sufficient reason," Canadian employers have for years repatriated migrant workers prematurely with impunity when workers become sick, injured, or pregnant (Orkin et al. 2014). What is more, employers have the ability to request specific migrant workers' return in subsequent years, which ensures the named workers' continued participation in the SAWP (MacIntosh 2018). This naming system, coupled with the threat of early repatriation, exerts a coercive pressure on seasonal migrant workers to appear fit and to avoid healthcare use. Indeed, studies show that up to half of the seasonal migrant workers surveyed either have at one point decided to keep working while being ill or know a colleague who did so (Brem 2006; Hennebry et al. 2016).

Just as in circumstances where immigration law precipitates migrants' disqualification from public healthcare, when immigration law operates as a disincentive, its impact on healthcare access extends to migrants' Canadian-born children as well. The healthcare gap facing some newborns in Ontario offers an illustration of this spillover effect. Legally, any child born in Ontario, regardless of their parents' immigration status, is covered by the provincial health insurance so long as Ontario is their intended primary place of residence (R.R.O. 1990, Reg. 552). The health insurance registration process for newborns usually entails parents completing a simple mail-in registration form provided by either birthing hospitals or midwives. However, occasionally, hospital staff who have doubts about a newborn's residency in Ontario have opted to provide the parents with a "proof of birth" letter instead. The parents must then bring the letter to a government office to register their child for the provincial health insurance in person (Bates and Cheff 2018). This extra step imposes a burden on migrants, particularly those without legal status, who may have good reasons, as explained, to want to minimize direct interactions with government bureaucrats. And as a result of this hesitation, their Canadian-born children may end up with no public health insurance despite being eligible to register for it (Cheff and Bates 2018).

10.4 IMMIGRATION LAW AS DISSONANCE

In addition to disqualifying migrants from publicly funded healthcare and disincentivizing them from healthcare use, immigration law can come between migrants and their healthcare access by fueling stigma and discrimination toward migrants, thus pitting healthcare providers' patient-care responsibilities against certain other concerns. These other considerations may include, for example, healthcare practitioners' negative appraisal of migrants' healthcare deservingness and the immigration control function that healthcare providers are sometimes asked to assume. When these other considerations overshadow healthcare providers' duty of care toward migrants, the health-seeking experience of migrants often suffers. Sometimes migrants are denied healthcare by service providers outright, while at other times the health-seeking encounter proves so distressing that migrants end up choosing to disengage from the healthcare system.

Because its impact on migrants' healthcare access is mediated by migrants' unpleasant encounter with the healthcare system, immigration law, when acting as a source of dissonance, need not explicitly aim to inhibit migrants' healthcare use. In fact, immigration law in this situation may even have a stated purpose of bettering migrants' health. This distinguishes it from the two varieties of healthcare access challenges explored above, where immigration law is more openly hostile toward health-seeking migrants. Incidentally, this also gives rise to dissonance of another sort, between the law's supposedly health-promoting purpose and its health-impairing effects in actuality.

In particular, the dissonance generated and exacerbated by immigration law has had a profound impact on asylum seekers' healthcare access in Canada. Canadian immigration law has long contributed to the othering of asylum seekers (Olsen et al 2016). It does so, for example, by allowing asylum seekers who arrive in groups to be designated as irregular arrivals, who are subject to potentially lengthy detention as well as restrictions on their legal rights (Protecting Canada's Immigration System Act 2012). For a period of time, Canadian immigration law also targeted asylum seekers from certain countries that were considered "safe" by limiting their rights to appeal negative refugee determination decisions and to apply for alternative immigration pathways that may allow them to stay (Protecting Canada's Immigration System Act 2012). These immigration measures perpetuate the stereotype of asylum seekers as fraudsters who take advantage of the refugee system to bypass the usual immigration mechanisms (Huot et al. 2016). They cast suspicion on asylum seekers in the public discourse and paint asylum seekers as undeserving of social benefits (Jackson and Bauder 2014).

In the healthcare context, the influence of Canadian immigration law's othering effect on asylum seekers' deservingness is amplified by the setup of asylum seekers' healthcare in Canada. As described, asylum seekers receive publicly funded healthcare in Canada through the IFHP instead of provincial and territorial health insurance programs. The establishment of the IFHP circa 1995 was the federal government's response to successive decisions made by some provinces in preceding years to withdraw asylum seekers' coverage from their respective health insurance plans (Chen 2022). As such, the origin of the IFHP in itself exhibits the trappings of asylum seekers' othering, and the program stands as a constant reminder of asylum seekers' separation from the general populace.

Added to that, the IFHP operates on the basis of charity, and this opens asylum seekers' healthcare deservingness to greater scrutiny. On more than one occasion, coverage under the IFHP is characterized by the government as ex gratia, namely "a benevolent payment . . . made in the public interest . . . where the [government] has no obligation of any kind or has no legal liability or where the claimant has no right of payment or is not entitled to relief in any form" (*Canadian Doctors For Refugee Care v. Canada (AG)* 2014, para. 356). This representation contrasts with the typical characterization of provincial and territorial health insurance as an entitlement enjoyed equally by all residents. Seeing as charity is grounded in generosity as opposed to obligation, healthcare under a charitable approach "is always discretionary," where "the question of who should receive what kind of care is continuously negotiated and defined" (Huschke 2014, 353).

Given the logic of charity, asylum seekers' healthcare access under the IFHP hinges significantly on their perceived healthcare deservingness (Olsen et al. 2016). As the specter of "bogus refugees" conjured up by immigration law chips away at the socially constructed image of asylum seekers as vulnerable and in need of society's assistance, uncertainty about asylum seekers' deservingness grows (Vanthuyne et al. 2013). Research into patient experience under the IFHP has consistently identified access problems stemming from healthcare providers' hesitation to treat asylum seekers. Many healthcare practitioners never sign up to become service providers under the IFHP, and even when they do, some are known to have turned asylum seekers away either because they have not familiarized themselves with the program or because they find maneuvering the program too complex to be worth their effort (Chen et al. 2018; Leps et al. 2022). At times healthcare providers have charged asylum seekers for services or goods that are supposedly covered by the government, because they felt the government reimbursement process was too slow (Miedema et al. 2008). In short, asylum seekers' healthcare access under the IFHP is partly at the mercy of service providers' whim. Whereas immigration law shapes healthcare providers' calculus by raising doubts about asylum seekers' deservingness, the workings of the IFHP as charity normalizes providers' subsequent decision to refrain from caring for asylum seekers. After all, benefactors have no duty to keep giving if they no longer feel generous.

Although a conception of healthcare as charity rather than entitlement can help mobilize the dissonating effect of immigration law, it is not a precondition for this type of healthcare access barriers. To illustrate this point, I now turn to the impact of Canada's immigration medical exams on the healthcare access of some migrants living with HIV.

Besides the deterrence of fraud, another long-standing objective of the Canadian immigration system has been to mitigate the ostensible public health risk posed by migrants, which has its roots in another stereotype that views migrants as diseased bodies (Reitmanova et al. 2015). To that end, Canada's Immigration and Refugee Protection Act (2001) requires a large number of migrants to undergo medical exams as a part of their application for a visa, refugee protection, or permanent residency. Since 2002 these immigration medical exams have included mandatory HIV testing for all individuals age 15 and above (Bisaillon 2010). Migrants who test HIV-positive during this process are not automatically denied admission to Canada. However, as mentioned earlier, they may be found inadmissible on the ground that they are expected to pose excessive demands on Canada's healthcare system.

Studies reveal that "panel physicians," who are contracted by the government to perform the immigration medical exams, often conduct the HIV tests in a manner that falls short of professional ethics and internationally accepted medical standards (Bisaillon 2011). According to relevant guidelines published by the World Health Organization (2021), provision of pre-test information and post-test counseling is key to improving people's knowledge about HIV, reducing HIV-related stigma, and facilitating HIV-positive persons' linkage to care. Despite this, migrants who test positive for HIV during the Canadian immigration process have complained about panel physicians not adequately preparing them for the receipt of positive results, not offering them sufficient support to cope with the diagnosis, as well as not properly referring them to treatment and other resources (dela Cruz et al. 2022). Migrants have also raised concerns about potential breaches of confidentiality by panel physicians and their staff during and after the HIV testing process (Bisaillon and Ells 2014).

These troubling doctor-patient interactions have led commentators to conclude that the work of panel physicians when carrying out the immigration medical exams is "primarily focused on disease detecting and reporting[, thus] blurring the role of the doctor whose work in this setting is not about care as conventionally understood" (Bisaillon and Ells 2014, 294). In other words, panel physicians effectively function as immigration gatekeepers, and in that capacity their administrative responsibilities take precedence over their duty toward migrants as patients. To the extent that this dissonance between panel physicians' dual roles tarnishes migrants' perception of the Canadian healthcare system at large, it risks alienating migrants from the system and causing them to refrain from seeking care in the future (dela Cruz et al. 2022). In the HIV context, such a barrier to healthcare access is all the more problematic in light of the government's public health objective, given how important HIV treatment is to curbing the risk of HIV transmission (Cohen 2011).

10.5 CONCLUSION

In this chapter, I have used examples from Canada to illustrate how immigration law hampers migrants' access to healthcare through disqualification, disincentivization, and dissonance. Each of these healthcare access barriers results from a unique form of interplay between immigration and healthcare laws, whose respective intent to discourage migrants' healthcare use varies. First, immigration law and the various legal statuses it creates can feed into exclusionary healthcare law and serve as the bases for migrants to be disqualified from public healthcare programs. Second, in situations where healthcare law does furnish migrants with entitlement to publicly funded healthcare, immigration law can still disincentivize migrants' healthcare use by threatening them with adverse immigration consequences. Third, even when both immigration and healthcare laws do not outwardly aim to block migrants' healthcare access, immigration law can nevertheless achieve the same effect by causing healthcare providers to interact with migrants in ways that are dissonant from their patient-care responsibilities. As such, these three mechanisms together provide somewhat of a typology of immigration law–related impediments to migrants' healthcare access.

Although an in-depth comparative analysis is beyond the scope of this chapter, a cursory scan of literature suggests that the three-prong typology that I have advanced here also finds resonance in countries other than Canada. For instance, in the United States the disqualifying effect of immigration law is on display when migrants without legal status are excluded from an array of federally funded healthcare programs and are barred from purchasing affordable health insurance on the exchanges (Parmet 2020). Likewise, instances of American immigration law acting as a disincentive abound. Under a now-repealed rule introduced by the first Trump administration, access to certain healthcare benefits risked rendering migrants a "public charge" and inadmissible to the United States, and as a result it caused many migrants to forgo these benefits despite eligibility (Parmet 2020). Furthermore, insofar as medical screening is a mandatory component of migrants' application for permanent residency in the United States (Aptekar 2020), as in Canada, it seems reasonable to expect similar unpleasantries to arise when migrants encounter healthcare practitioners who place their role as immigration gatekeepers ahead of their patient-care responsibilities, thus causing migrants to become disengaged from the healthcare system. Indeed research from France corroborates such a possibility. It observes that physicians' involvement in the immigration process, such as being requested to provide a medical certificate attesting their migrant patients' need to remain in the country, could undermine the trust between them and these migrants (Cailhol et al. 2020).

At the same time, this typology does not purport to be exhaustive. To name but one example, immigration law is also known to interfere with migrants' access to healthcare by placing them in vulnerable socioeconomic circumstances, including financial hardship, precarious employment, social and/or geographical isolation, and more (Ahmed et al. 2016). However, seeing as migrants' health-seeking challenges in this case are mediated by other socioeconomic determinants of healthcare access (e.g., income, work conditions, social isolation), their link with immigration law is arguably less direct than when immigration law acts as a disqualifier, a disincentive, or a source of dissonance.

Imperfections notwithstanding, the typology developed in this chapter still offers important lessons on the obstacles that migrants face when accessing healthcare and what should be done to remedy them. For one, by identifying different ways that immigration law can thwart migrants' access to healthcare, the typology challenges the inevitability of the status quo and underscores the fact that migrant health is a matter of social justice (Vissandjée et al. 2017). That is, at least some aspects of migrants' health, relative to that of the general population, represent "avoidable health differences on which excluded or marginalized groups fare worse than socially better-off groups" (Paula Braveman et al. 2018, 4). Or, to quote Alicia Ely Yamin (2008, 47), the various legal dynamics unearthed and encapsulated by the typology "[force] us to see the suffering that is not the result of 'natural' biological causes but rather stems from human choices about policies, priorities, and cultural norms, about how we treat each other and what we owe each other." It follows that the betterment of migrant health will necessitate collective interventions to refashion sociolegal structures which prejudice and ostracize migrants (Wiley 2014).

Specifically, the typology draws attention to three areas of immigration law where a different collective choice needs to be made: Should immigration status inform one's eligibility for publicly funded healthcare? Should migrants' utilization of healthcare be shielded from border surveillance and delinked from immigration processes? And should immigration law continue to be organized around principles that stereotype migrants, including those depicting them as fraudulent and a public health threat? A complete strategy for improving migrants' healthcare access must involve legal reform on all these fronts. At minimum, this entails the establishment of firewalls between systems of immigration enforcement and healthcare provision, such that decisions about healthcare can be made without the undue influence of immigration controls. Beyond that, changes must also be made to immigration law more generally, even facets of it that do not appear to immediately concern healthcare. Among others, laws that provide for the differential treatment of migrants based on perceived self-sufficiency and contribution, as well as asylum seekers based on presumed genuineness, should be eliminated. The aim of this reform is to eradicate immigration law's stigmatization of migrants, which will have a positive signaling effect on migrants' healthcare deservingness. Migrants' well-being, as well as justice, demands nothing less.

REFERENCES

Ager, Alastair, and Alison Strang. 2008. "Understanding Integration: A Conceptual Framework." *Journal of Refugee Studies* 21 (2): 166–191. https://doi.org/10.1093/jrs/fen016.

Ahmed, Salim, Nusrat S. Shommu, Nahid Rumana, Gary R. S. Barron, Sonja Wicklum, and Tanvir C. Turin. 2016. "Barriers to Access of Primary Healthcare by Immigrant Populations in Canada: A Literature Review." *Journal of Immigrant and Minority Health* 18 (6): 1522–1540. https://doi.org/10.1007/s10903-015-0276-z.

Aptekar, Sofya. 2020. "Doctors as Migration Brokers in the Mandatory Medical Screenings of Immigrants to the United States." *Journal of Ethnic and Migration Studies* 46 (9): 1865–1885. https://doi.org/10.1080/1369183X.2018.1494545.

Bates, Lauren, and Rebecca Cheff. 2018. *Ensuring Equitable Access to OHIP Registration for Newborns*. Wellesley Institute.

Bisaillon, Laura M. 2010. "Human Rights Consequences of Mandatory HIV Screening Policy of Newcomers to Canada." *Health and Human Rights Journal* 12 (2): 119–134.

Bisaillon, Laura. 2011. "Mandatory HIV Screening Policy and Everyday Life: A Look Inside the Canadian Immigration Medical Examination." *Aporia* 3 (4): 5–14.

Bisaillon, Laura. 2022. *Screening Out: HIV Testing and the Canadian Immigration Experience*. UBC Press.

Bisaillon, Laura, and Carolyn Ells. 2014. "When Doctoring Is Not About Doctoring: An Ethical Analysis of Practices Associated with Canadian Immigration HIV Testing." *Public Health Ethics* 7 (3): 287–297. https://doi.org/10.1093/phe/phu036.

Braveman, Paula, Elaine Arkin, Tracy Orleans, Dwayne Proctor, Julia Acker, and Alonzo Plough. 2018. "What Is Health Equity?" *Behavioral Science & Policy* 4 (1): 1–14.

Brem, Maxwell, 2006. *Migrant Workers in Canada: A Review of the Canadian Seasonal Agricultural Workers Program*. North-South Institute.

Britten, Liam, 2016. "Undocumented Immigrants Who Fear Being Deported Need Health Care Says Advocate." CBC News, May 5. https://www.cbc.ca/news/canada/british-columbia/undocumented-immigrants-health-care-1.3567310.

Cailhol, Johann, Marie-Christine Lebon, and William Sherlaw. 2020. "Will My Patients Get Their Residence Permit? A Critical Analysis of the Ethical Dilemmas Involved in Writing Medical Certificates for Residence Permits in France." *BMC Medical Ethics* 21 (59): 1–10. https://doi.org/10.1186/s12910-020-00500-7.

Canada Health Act, R.S.C., 1985. c.C–6.

Canadian Doctors for Refugee Care v. Canada (AG), 2014 FC 651.

Castellanos González, Natalia. 2022. "United States Immigration Law as a Social Determinant of Health: A Mixed-Methods Systematic Review." *Public Health Theses* 2140. https://elischolar.library.yale.edu/ysphtdl/2140.

Cheff, Rebecca, and Lauren Bates. 2018. *Using the Law to Advance Health Equity: OHIP Eligibility of Ontario-Born Babies of Uninsured Parents*. Wellesley Institute.

Chen, Y.Y. Brandon. 2017. "Social Determinants and Marginalized Populations." In *Canadian Health Law and Policy*, 5th ed., edited by Joanna Erdman, Vanessa Gruben, and Erin Nelson. LexisNexis.

Chen, Y.Y. Brandon. 2022. "Citizenship as an Egg?" In *Citizenship as a Challenge: Dimensions of an Evolving Process*, edited by Tamara Nair and Maria Inês Amaro. Brill.

Chen, Y.Y. Brandon, Vanessa Gruben, and Jamie Chai Yun Liew. 2018. "'A Legacy of Confusion': An Exploratory Study of Service Provision Under the Reinstated Interim Federal Health Program." *Refuge* 34 (2): 94–102. https://doi.org/10.7202/1055580ar.

Cohen, Jon, 2011. "HIV Treatment as Prevention." *Science* 334 (6063): 1628. https://doi.org/10.1126/science.334.6063.1628.

Dela Cruz, Aniela M., Sithokozile Maposa, San Patten, et al. 2022. "'I Die Silently Inside': Qualitative Findings from a Study of People Living with HIV Who Migrate to and Settle in Canada." *Journal of Migration and Health* 5 (100088): 1–9. https://doi.org/10.1016/j.jmh.2022.100088.

Dhand, Ruby, and Robert Diab. 2015. "Canada's Refugee Health Law and Policy from a Comparative, Constitutional, and Human Rights Perspective." *Canadian Journal of Comparative and Contemporary Law* 1 (1): 351–406.

Dougherty, Louise, Jane Lloyd, Elizabeth Harris, Paula Caffrey, and Mark Harris. 2020. "Access to Appropriate Health Care for Non-English Speaking Migrant Families with a Newborn/Young Child: A Systematic Scoping Literature Review." *BMC Health Services Research* 20 (309): 1–12. https://doi.org/10.1186/s12913-020-05157-x.

Ely Yamin, Alicia. 2008. "Will We Take Suffering Seriously? Reflections on What Applying a Human Rights Framework to Health Means and Why We Should Care." *Health and Human Rights* 10 (1): 45–63.

Employment and Social Development Canada. 2025a. "Contract for the Employment in Canada of Commonwealth Caribbean Seasonal Agricultural Workers—2025." January 2. https://www.canada.ca/en/employment-social-development/services/foreign-workers/agricultural/seasonal-agricultural/requirements/caribbean.html.

Employment and Social Development Canada. 2025b. "Contract for the Employment in Canada of Seasonal Agricultural Workers from Mexico—2025." January 2. https://www.canada.ca/en/employment-social-development/services/foreign-workers/agricultural/seasonal-agricultural/requirements/mexico.html.

Fox, Chris. 2021. "'It's a Significant Barrier': Individuals Without OHIP Cards Told They Can't Book Vaccination Appointments at City Clinics." CP24.com, April 6. https://www.cp24.com/news/it-s-a-significant-barrier-individuals-without-ohip-cards-told-they-can-t-book-vaccination-appointments-at-city-clinics-1.5376632.

Galanis, Petros, Spyros Koureas, Olga Siskou, Olympia Konstantakopoulou, Georgios Angelopoulosm, and Daphne Kaitelidou. 2022. "Healthcare Services Access, Use, and Barriers Among Migrants in Europe: A Systematic Review." *International Journal of Caring Sciences* 15 (1): 28–47.

Gil-González, Diana, Mercedes Carrasco-Portiño, Carmen Vives-Cases, Andrés A. Agudelo-Suárez, Ramón Castejón Bolea, and Elena Ronda-Pérez. 2015. "Is Health a Right for All? An Umbrella Review of the Barriers to Health Care Access Faced by Migrants." *Ethnicity & Health* 20 (5): 523–541. https://doi.org/10.1080/13557858.2014.946473.

Gostin, Lawrence O., John T. Monahan, Jenny Kaldor, et al. 2019. "The Legal Determinants of Health: Harnessing the Power of Law for Global Health and Sustainable Development." *Lancet* 393 (10183): 1857–1910. http://dx.doi.org/10.1016/S0140-6736(19)30233-8.

Government of Canada. 2024. "When Does My Interim Federal Health Program Coverage Start and When Does It End?" June 10. https://www.cic.gc.ca/english/helpcentre/answer.asp?qnum=1275.

Grove, Natalie J., and Anthony B. Zwi. 2006. "Our Health and Theirs: Forced Migration, Othering, and Public Health." *Social Science & Medicine* 62 (8): 1931–1942. https://doi.org/10.1016/j.socscimed.2005.08.061.

Hanes, Roy. 2009. "None Is Still Too Many: An Historical Exploration of Canadian Immigration Legislation as It Pertains to People with Disabilities." *Developmental Disabilities Bulletin* 37 (1–2): 91–126.

Health Canada. 2025. *Canada Health Act Annual Report 2023–2024*. Health Canada. https://www.canada.ca/en/health-canada/services/publications/health-system-services/canada-health-act-annual-report-2023-2024.html.

Hennebry, Jenna, Janet McLaughlin, and Kerry Preibisch. 2016. "Out of the Loop: (In)access to Health Care for Migrant Workers in Canada." *Journal of International Migration and Integration* 17 (2): 521–538.

Hennebry, Jenna L., and Kerry Preibisch. 2012. "A Model for Managed Migration? Re-Examining Best Practices in Canada's Seasonal Agricultural Worker Program." *International Migration* 50 (1): e19–e40.

Heyman, Josiah McC., Guillermina Gina Núñez, and Victor Talavera. 2009. "Healthcare Access and Barriers for Unauthorized Immigrants in El Paso County, Texas." *Family & Community Health* 32 (1): 4–21.

Heywood, Neil, Kerry Kennedy, and Michel Lapointe. 2002. *Operational Processing Instruction 2002–2004: Medical Assessment of HIV Positive Applicants*. Citizenship and Immigration Canada.

Hill, Jessica, Darlene Xiomara Rodriguez, and Paul N. McDaniel. 2021. "Immigration Status as a Health Care Barrier in the USA During COVID-19." *Journal of Migration and Health* 4 (100036): 1–7. https://doi.org/10.1016/j.jmh.2021.100036.

Huot, Suzanne, Andrea Bobadilla, Antoine Bailliard, and Debbie Laliberte Rudman. 2016. "Constructing Undesirables: A Critical Discourse Analysis of 'Othering' Within the Protecting Canada's Immigration System Act." *International Migration* 54 (2): 131–143. https://doi.org/10.1111/imig.12210.

Huschke, Susann. 2014. "Performing Deservingness: Humanitarian Health Care Provision for Migrants in Germany." *Social Science & Medicine* 120 (November): 352–359. https://doi.org/10.1016/j.socscimed.2014.04.046.

Immigration and Refugee Protection Act, S.C. 2001, c. 27.

Jackson, Samantha, and Herald Bauder. 2014. "Neither Temporary, nor Permanent: The Precarious Employment Experiences of Refugee Claimants in Canada." *Journal of Refugee Studies* 27 (3): 360–381. https://doi-org.proxy.bib.uottawa.ca/10.1093/jrs/fet048.

Kacker, Karen, Maria Anies, Barbara L. Folb, and Leah Zallman. 2015. "Barriers to Health Care for Undocumented Immigrants: A Literature Review." *Risk Management and Healthcare Policy* 8: 175–183.

Larchanché, Stéphanie. 2012. "Intangible Obstacles: Health Implications of Stigmatization, Structural Violence, and Fear Among Undocumented Immigrants in France." *Social Science & Medicine* 74 (6): 858–863. https://doi.org/10.1016/j.socscimed.2011.08.016.

Lehman, Cheryl, Marcia Annisette, and Gloria Agyemang. 2016. "Immigration and Neoliberalism: Three Cases and Counter Accounts." *Accounting, Auditing & Accountability Journal* 29 (1): 43–79. http://dx.doi.org/10.1108/AAAJ-09-2013-1470.

Leps, Caroline, Jessica Monteiro, Tony Barozzino, et al. 2022. "Interim Federal Health Program: Survey of Access and Utilization by Paediatric Health Care Provider." *Paediatrics & Child Health* 27 (1): 19–24. https://doi.org/10.1093/pch/pxab045.

MacIntosh, Constance. 2018. "The Canadian Legal Regime for Providing Health Care Protection to Agricultural Migrant Workers." In *Health Law at the Frontier: Les rencontres en droit de la santé*, vol. 2, edited by Lara Khoury, Catherine Regis, and Robert Kouri. Éditions Yvon Blais.

Macnab, Aidan. 2021. "Feds Should Guarantee Health Information Will Not Be Shared with Immigration Authorities: Law Prof." *Law Times*, May 10. https://www.lawtimesnews.com/practice-areas/privacy-and-data/feds-should-guarantee-health-information-will-not-be-shared-with-immigration-authorities-law-prof/355842.

Magalhaes, Lilian, Christine Carrasco, and Denise Gastaldo. 2010. "Undocumented Migrants in Canada: A Scope Literature Review on Health, Access to Services, and Working Conditions." *Journal of Immigrant and Minority Health* 12 (1): 132–151. https://doi.org/10.1007/s10903-009-9280-5.

Martone, Jessica, Danielle Zimmerman, Maria Vidal de Haymes, and Lois Lorentzen. 2014. "Immigrant Integration Through Mediating Social institutions: Issues and Strategies." *Journal of Community Practice* 22 (3): 299–323. https://doi.org/10.1080/10705422.2014.929062.

Miedema, Baukje, Ryan Hamilton, and Julie Easley. 2008. "Climbing the Walls: Structural Barriers to Accessing Primary Care for Refugee Newcomers in Canada." *Canadian Family Physician* 54 (3): 335–336.

Nova Scotia Department of Health and Wellness. 2014. *Eligibility for Nova Scotia Health Insurance Program*. August 1. Nova Scotia Department of Health and Wellness.

O'Shea, Sean. 2021. "The Complications of Getting COVID-19 Vaccinations for Non-Residents in Ontario." *Global News*, April 25. https://globalnews.ca/news/7787849/covid-vaccinations-visitors-canada/.

Olsen, Christopher, Rowan El-Bialy, Mark Mckelvie, Peggy Rauman, and Fern Brunger. 2016. "'Other' Troubles: Deconstructing Perceptions and Changing Responses to Refugees in Canada." *Journal of Immigrant and Minority Health* 18 (1): 58–66. https://doi.org/10.1007/s10903-014-9983-0.

Orkin, Aaron M., Morgan Lay, Janet McLaughlin, Michael Schwandt, and Donald Cole. 2014. "Medical Repatriation of Migrant Farm Workers in Ontario: A Descriptive Analysis." *CAMJ Open* 2 (3): E192–E198. https://doi.org/10.9778/cmajo.20140014.

Parmet, Wendy E. 2020. "Immigration Law as a Social Determinant of Health." *Temple Law Review* 92 (4): 931–952.

Pedraza, Francisco I., Vanessa Cruz Nichols, and Alana M. W. LeBrón. 2017. "Cautious Citizenship: The Deterring Effect of Immigration Issue Salience on Health Care Use and Bureaucratic Interactions Among Latino US Citizens." *Journal of Health Politics, Policy and Law* 42 (5): 925–960.

Penninx, Rinus. 2005. "Integration of Migrants: Economic, Social, Cultural and Political Dimensions." In *The New Demographic Regime: Population Challenges and Policy Responses*, edited by Miroslav Macura, Alphonse L. MacDonald, and Werner Haug. United Nations Publication.

Protecting Canada's Immigration System Act, S.C. 2012, c. 17.

R.R.O. 1990, Reg. 552.

Rahimian, Tiran. 2020. "Parental Undocumented Status as an Analogous Ground of Discrimination." *Journal of Law & Equality* 16 (1): 93–132.

Reitmanova, Sylvia, Diana L. Gustafson, and Rukhsana Ahmed. 2015. "'Immigrants Can Be Deadly': Critical Discourse Analysis of Racialization of Immigrant Health in the Canadian Press and Public Health Policies." *Canadian Journal of Communication* 40 (3): 471–487. https://doi.org/10.22230/cjc.2015v40n3a2831.

Toussaint v. Canada (AG), 2011 FCA 213.

Tsai, Pei-Ling, and Setareh Ghahari. 2023. "Immigrants' Experience of Health Care Access in Canada: A Recent Scoping Review." *Journal of Immigrant and Minority Health* 25 (June): 712–727. https://doi.org/10.1007/s10903-023-01461-w.

Vanthuyne, Karine, Francesca Meloni, Monica Ruiz-Casares, Cécile Rousseau, Alexandra Ricard-Guay. 2013. "Health Workers' Perception of Access to Care for Children and Pregnant Women with Precarious Immigration Status: Health as a Right or a Privilege?" *Social Science & Medicine* 93 (September): 78–85. https://doi.org/10.1016/j.socscimed.2013.06.008.

Vissandjée, Bilkis, Wendy E. Short, and Karine Bates. 2017. "Health and Legal Literacy for Migrants: Twinned Strands Woven in the Cloth of Social Justice and the Human Right to Health Care." *BMC International Health and Human Rights* 17 (10): 1–12. https://doi.org/10.1186/s12914-017-0117-3.

Walsh, James P. 2011. "Quantifying Citizens: Neoliberal Restructuring and Immigrant Selection in Canada and Australia." *Citizenship Studies* 15 (6–7): 861–879. https://doi.org/10.1080/13621025.2011.600135.

Wiley, Lindsay F. 2014. "Health Law as Social Justice." *Cornell Journal of Law and Public Policy* 24 (1): 47–106.

World Health Organization. 2021. *Consolidated Guidelines on HIV Prevention, Testing, Treatment, Service Delivery and Monitoring: Recommendations for a Public Health Approach*. World Health Organization.

Hosts?

SYLVIA AGBIH

Yes, "we" in the global North grant asylum, according to our laws, according to our moral obligation to fend for human rights, according to the image we like of ourselves as rescuers, because of the suffering experienced by our grandparents and great-grandparents during the wars. We give some space and shelter—what kind of space? And we give carefully, so that it is not too much, not too good, not too attractive. And just for some time. It's just a short phase. Limited, limited space, limited time, limited movement, limited chances. Not too good, not too much, not too comfortable, not too attractive. We don't want to be a "welfare magnet". It's just passing, transit, they go back, go home—wherever that is. Do "we" want "them" to settle? Settle with "us"?

11

The Securitization of Migrants' Health and the Medicalization of Citizenship

RYOA CHUNG AND JOANNE LIU

11.1 INTRODUCTION

In this chapter, we argue that the medicalization of citizenship is worsening the plight of refugees. "The medicalization of citizenship" refers to the phenomenon whereby health considerations increasingly condition the admission of asylum seekers to other countries, especially the most affluent. Access to healthcare is an attribute of national citizenship. Although states provide healthcare services to their national populations to a greater or lesser extent, according to their political regime and corresponding to their more or less limited resources, their constituents have at least a normative claim to some degree of healthcare provision from their government. By contrast, refugees (as defined by the Geneva Convention), stateless people, and some of the world's most disadvantaged migrants fleeing extreme violence or poverty (forced migrants) who live in displacement camps exist in conditions of indigence and depend on humanitarian organizations to meet their primary healthcare needs when and if possible. The medicalization of citizenship exacerbates the recalcitrance of states to admit displaced people and asylum seekers, either because they are perceived as representing health risks to national security or because they are suspected of representing a public burden to health systems. For example, Title 42 Expulsion of the US Code was implemented in response to COVID-19 to accelerate the deportation of illegal immigrants, except for unaccompanied children. We argue that in every case where refugees, stateless people, or forced migrants are denied healthcare because they don't obtain national citizenship,

Ryoa Chung and Joanne Liu, *The Securitization of Migrants' Health and the Medicalization of Citizenship*. In: *Forced Migration and Health Justice*. Edited by: Lisa A. Eckenwiler, Verina Wild, Anna Gotlib, Ryoa Chung, and Deborah Zion, Oxford University Press. © Oxford University Press (2026). DOI: 10.1093/oso/9780197795491.003.0011 the international community fails to assume its shared responsibilities to protect the universal human right to health.[1]

The first part of the chapter explains how the *medicalization of citizenship* is a disquieting consequence of the contemporary phenomenon of the *securitization of health* in the name of national interests. The second part looks at the international community's responsibility toward asylum seekers in light of the concept of structural injustice, mainly according to the work of David Owen, Serena Parekh, and Iris Marion Young.

11.2 THE HEALTH OF FORCED MIGRANTS AND STATELESS HUMAN BEINGS

Even though the World Health Organization (WHO) proclaimed the universality of the human right to health at its founding in 1946, reality shows that access to healthcare is an attribute of national citizenship. Inequalities between states are reflected in the health inequities between individuals and those between populations. Some governments offer their citizens the most comprehensive range of healthcare. Some provide free care through complex financing mechanisms that vary according to the national system adopted. Others set up parallel systems of private and public healthcare, with some populations having access only to healthcare they can pay for, while others are left to fend for themselves and rely on nonprofit organizations to meet their primary healthcare needs. There are, of course, considerable economic and political differences between countries. The health status of individuals and populations varies according to their government's economic resources and political regime. National citizenship does not necessarily guarantee equitable access to healthcare for all constituents. However, when governments fail to meet the basic needs of their citizens for minimum security, subsistence, and political freedom, either due to immense poverty or armed conflict, the attributes of citizenship are so undermined that individuals and populations try to flee their home countries.

Migration trajectories forced by political persecution or destitution are often journeys through or into hell. Didier Fassin's ethnographic investigations bear witness to sexual, physical, and psychological violence that no

1. We are indebted to Verina Wild for her 2015 seminal article on these issues, "Universal Access to Health Care for Migrants: Applying Cosmopolitanism to the Domestic Realm." Although we take another angle to address our specific research questions in this chapter, we refer the readers to her work to know more about the philosophical foundations for arguing for a global responsibility to promote, provide, and protect the universal human right to health.

human being should ever have to experience (Fassin and Defossez 2024). The direct testimonies of refugees are overwhelming, such as that of Nujeen Mustafa, a young Syrian woman with cerebral palsy, who traveled 3,500 miles from Syria to Germany in a wheelchair with the help of her sister. Mustafa's extraordinary story captured the world's attention (Mustafa and Lamb 2017). However, most testimonies from Syrian refugees—a third of whom are disabled (Deutsche Welle 2023)—will never be heard, which constitutes a profound epistemic injustice. Indeed, the fact that these people don't have any political voice, are ignored or dismissed, contributes to testimonial injustice and to the abyssal gap of knowledge concerning their fate and health needs. Faced with the poverty and distress of our contemporaries, the indifference of the "international community" (driven by the selfish national interests of its member states) represents a moral aberration. According to the late Paul Farmer in his commentary following Bernard Kouchner's inaugural Jonathan Mann Memorial Lecture at the Harvard School of Public Health in 2003,[2] this will be the shame and guilt of our generation.

Stanley Hoffman (1983) described states as "cold monsters," which, according to the classical precepts of Hans Morgenthau's (1948) political realism in theories of international relations, seek to promote their national interests by any means necessary. However, a more nuanced understanding of political realism can also claim that *enlightened* self-interest projects a different light on the relation between means and ends, one that does not exclude solidarity with others in order to achieve one's self-interest. Cooperation between states, for example, can serve everyone's best interests more efficiently, according to contemporary realists. Nevertheless, the COVID-19 pandemic and the predatory race to obtain vaccines against SARS-CoV-2 once again demonstrate the shortcomings of serving exclusively one's self-interest in the face of transnational challenges. Confronted with climate change and global health crises, states seek to maximize their economic or political interests and health security according to a myopic vision that overvalues short-termism and electoral objectives; however, the illusion of autarky in an interdependent world is a gamble that will inevitably prove costly for the planet as a whole.

Populations crammed into refugee or displacement camps have limited access to healthcare and have been left to fend for themselves during the pandemic (United Nations High Commissioner for Refugees n.d.; Burki 2020). The condition of displaced people and asylum seekers is documented

2. Quote reported by Ryoa Chung, who attended the Jonathan Mann Inaugural Lecture, Harvard School of Public Health, March 6, 2003.

throughout this book. Our contribution is more specifically philosophical, but it unfolds against the backdrop of these empirical data.

11.3 HEALTH NATIONALISM: MORAL PARTIALITY AND PRIORITY FOR CO-NATIONALS

The predatory SARS-CoV-2 vaccine race revealed the lack of international cooperation that the WHO had hoped for with the implementation of COVAX. In consultation with major donors, including the Bill Gates Foundation, and key global health players such as GAVI, COVAX was supposed to facilitate the collaborative international distribution of vaccines to combat the pandemic. Instead, we have witnessed the frantic race of the wealthiest countries to stockpile vaccines for their populations and the refusal of the World Trade Organization's most powerful states to support the waiver of pharmaceutical patents requested by India and South Africa, supported by a hundred other countries and NGOs such as Médecins sans frontières (winner of the Nobel Peace Prize in 1999).

Many observers and researchers in the field of global health have decried *health nationalism*, which refers to the behavior of states that prioritize their country's national interests to the detriment of global cooperation. States' subjective, short-term perception of their national economic, political, electoral, or health interests can be countered by rational arguments and evidence justifying, on the contrary, the need for greater international solidarity regarding health and environmental crises. What we can learn about the second wave of mortality from SARS-CoV-2 that hit India in 2020, with the appearance of the Delta variant that spread around the world, is that unprotected pockets of world population represent greater risks of generating dangerous variants. Should another pandemic strike in the future, we must remember that the fair share of vaccines at the global level is not only morally warranted but is also a sound principle of collective prudence from an epidemiological point of view. Nevertheless, driven by instrumental rationality thwarted by short-term cost-benefit analysis, rich and powerful states, which have the means to survive containment policies and closed borders, have not hesitated to prioritize the health of their populations to the detriment of fairness and equitable sharing of vaccines on a global scale.

A certain amount of health nationalism is undoubtedly inevitable, perhaps even legitimate. Some contemporary philosophical analyses of nationalism describe it in terms of moral partiality toward co-nationals (MacIntyre 1984; Miller 1995). Liberal approaches to the social contract that gave rise to the philosophical justifications of Western democracies are based on the idea that special obligations exist between contracting members (Wellman 2001).[3] According to this liberal, contractarian tradition, the costs and benefits of social cooperation are borne by the citizens of a society delimited by geographical boundaries. These boundaries also delimit the nature and extent of the legal obligations to redistribute collective resources among the members of the society, which maintain the "basic structure" (as Rawls [1971] would say in his notorious work *Theory of Justice*) of political institutions that guarantee citizens' social rights and services. Citizens' access to healthcare and the functional organization of a public health system represent a country's most enviable sociopolitical successes. However, no society can devote all its resources or national budget to the health sector alone. According to the law philosopher Dworkin (1993), such an "isolationist" health system model is untenable since it would affect other important "spheres of justice"—to use Walzer's (1984) expression—such as education, national security, and the judicial system. Nevertheless, maintaining a public healthcare system that genuinely contributes to the population's quality of life represents substantial costs for all members of society who accept these sacrifices given the expected benefits.

From a consequentialist point of view, the global division of labor between all countries rests on a coherent, rational justification. Indeed, it seems more practical to urge all governments to take responsibility for their people. Even if we were to evacuate all the controversial questions attached to the identity, historical, cultural, linguistic, or religious components that define membership of different nations, the consequentialist division of tasks would still justify the distribution of these special obligations between countries, considered as purely instrumental entities of public management, in a world without world government.

In the context of the pandemic, special obligations of moral partiality have been invoked to justify the moral priority given to our compatriots. Emanuel et al. (2021) defend *vaccine nationalism* by arguing that a responsible government must first ensure the vaccination of its population to guarantee national protection so that global protection will be the sum of each country's immunity. Affluent countries have thrown themselves into merciless competition for access to the most significant volume of SARS-CoV-2 vaccines. In July 2021, for example, 75% of the Canadian population received the first dose of the SARS-CoV-2 vaccine, compared to only 1.1% in low-income countries (Our World in Data n.d.). Determining a national vaccination threshold based on epidemiological data may be

3. Other non-Western societies also promote special obligations toward their members; however, we are referring here to a specific literature and conceptual framework in contemporary political philosophy stemming from the liberal, contractualist tradition.

necessary for collective protection. However, ensuring the greatest possible immune protection beyond their own borders is also necessary. That said, it may be even better to propose distributing vaccines according to needs, based on epidemiological data for the populations most affected globally. An epidemic never affects everyone to the same degree. The problem is that states are unwilling to recognize the legitimate limits to moral partiality toward their compatriots. At some point, obligations towards non-nationals living elsewhere in the world have equal moral value, despite not sharing the same national citizenship, in the name of universal human rights, the cosmopolitan ideal of shared humanity, and corresponding principles of global justice. This moral egoism has a cost in the long term, insofar as the myopic obsession with immediate interests overshadows the disastrous collective environmental and health consequences. Everyone's health inevitably depends on the health of all in our interdependent world. The predatory race by the wealthiest countries to obtain SARS-CoV-2 vaccines at the expense of the poorest countries is a grotesque illustration of how moral partiality often becomes national selfishness.

11.4 THE SECURITIZATION OF HEALTH IN THE NAME OF NATIONAL INTERESTS

The notion of health securitization here refers to the phenomenon whereby health issues are elevated to high politics concerning state security (Elbe 2010). This notion has existed in international studies literature (Davies 2010; Youde and Rushton 2015) since the September 11 attacks in 2001 and must be distinguished from the UN notion of "human security," which, according to researchers at the United Nations Development Programme (1994),[4] encompasses health in a broader conception of the fundamental interests of every human being. Unfortunately, the phenomenon of the securitization of health in the name of national interests all too often leads to the subordination of fundamental human rights to states' rights, according to a problematic conception of state sovereignty. This phenomenon can be illustrated in at least three ways.

First, "securitization of health" is an expression that emerged in the wake of the attacks of September 11, 2001, as a means of placing the threat of bioterrorism and chemical weapons at the heart of national security considerations in the 21st century. Today's health security challenges include the threat of pandemics and future health crises. In a health emergency, health

4. On the distinction between health as one of the seven components of "human security" and the "securitization of health," see Chung and Liu (2023).

security policies can undermine people's rights or welfare, especially when international guidelines recommend containment and border closures. For instance, public health measures can limit individual rights to privacy or freedom of movement in the context of an emergency. Disadvantaged populations will probably suffer more from the economic impact of border closures.

The second illustration of the securitization of health refers to the instrumentalization of health issues in the context of armed conflict (Chung and Liu 2023). One of the most tragic modalities of this phenomenon refers to the attack on healthcare establishments and personnel as "soft targets" (i.e., targets that put up no military defense) to precipitate the collapse of the "enemy." The war in Syria, the attack on the pediatric hospital in the Ukrainian city of Mariupol, the American bombing of the Médecins sans frontières hospital in Kunduz, Afghanistan, the destruction of healthcare facilities in Gaza during the winter of 2023—there are numerous examples of this phenomenon. From a philosophical point of view, it is essential to remember that since the founding of the International Red Cross by Henry Dunant, international humanitarian law and the Geneva Conventions have condemned attacks on healthcare facilities and personnel, as well as noncombatant civilian populations in need of care, as violations of *jus in bello* principles—that is, such attacks are considered war crimes. From an ethical point of view, it is crucial to stress that these crimes constitute violations of fundamental human rights and to recall that the genesis of international humanitarian law is historically and philosophically rooted in the universal right to health.

The subject of this chapter is not a full-fledged political analysis of the Israel–Palestine conflict that has been unfolding before our eyes since the horrific hostage-taking, sexual violence, and murder of noncombatant civilians perpetrated in the name of Hamas on October 7, 2023. The historical context is undoubtedly complex and helps to explain the resistance movements in the occupied territories. However, all-out terrorism without any form of political discrimination between combatants and unarmed civilians must be condemned. Moreover, using the civilian population in Gaza as a human shield also constitutes a war crime.

Nevertheless, even if we acknowledge the right to self-defense against terrorist attacks, the monstrous excess of retaliation of the Netanyahu government has led to a catastrophic humanitarian tragedy. The Israeli military offensives violate all the tenets of humanitarian law, starting with the two fundamental criteria of *jus in bello*: respect for the immunity of noncombatants and the principle of proportionality. One of the most shocking aspects of the violent conflict is that, according to Médecins sans frontières and the International Committee of the Red Cross, health establishments and personnel, as well as hospitalized patients, have been the targets of deliberate attacks. As of September 2024, only 17 of the 36 hospitals are still partially functional, according to WHO (2023–2024). Al-Shifa Hospital, the central medical complex in the Gaza Strip, was utterly destroyed, according to observers from WHO (2024). The particularity of the situation in Gaza is that it is a rare conflict wherein the civilians under attack are prisoners within their own territory and cannot flee. In most conflicts, as in Ukraine, for example, despite the horrific challenges, people can escape, but not in Rafah.

The third case of the securitization of health in the name of national interests concerns migrants and the medicalization of citizenship. The phenomenon of forced migration—involving refugees, asylum seekers, and displaced people driven by social and economic distress—raises severe problems for the administration of healthcare, not least because the international community overlooks these populations as they fall into the no man's land between national borders. Rightly or wrongly, these migrant populations are seen as representing a threat of social and economic instability for national communities, which, in the eyes of some governments, justifies the erection of borders in the name of national security, including barbed wire fences and walls, as in Hungary (260 kilometers of barbed-wire and steel column fence), Belarus (180 kilometers of barbed wire; Rigby and Crisp n.d.) and the United States (727 kilometers; Giles 2021), just to name a few examples. Against the backdrop of Russia's invasion of Ukraine, Belarus has weaponized the threat of chaotic illegal migration by leading illegal migrants to the borders of Poland, the point of entry to the European Union. These migrants were thus stranded, in miserable conditions, in a forest between the two countries (Alboth 2021).

Among the selection criteria for new migrants or refugees, the criterion of "reasonable public charge to the health system" is invoked, more often than not, to reject the majority of asylum seekers with health problems or disabilities. The healthcare system is undoubtedly overloaded in numerous countries, where many citizens do not have access to primary care. Even in rich countries like Canada, the public healthcare system faces difficulties. However, this instrumentalization of health issues in the name of national security has always served to justify discriminatory and racist immigration policies, as witnessed in the history of Asian immigrants who were turned away from Angel Island in California and banned by the Chinese Immigration Act of 1923–1947 in Canada (Lee and Yung 2010). Canada's Conservative prime minister Stephen Harper substantially cut refugees' access to healthcare in 2012. This legislation was decried and fought in court by associations of physicians and lawyers defending the rights of refugees. "In a decision in July 2014 that strongly challenged Conservative leader's use of the term 'bogus' in justifying cuts to refugee health care, the Federal Court of Canada ruled that the cuts were unconstitutional and 'cruel and unusual treatment' that denied healthcare to more than 100,000 refugee claimants" (Webster 2015, 1436). Justin Trudeau's Canadian government overturned this legislation in 2016 by tripling the amount granted to refugee care, significantly relaxing the "public charge" criterion. Nonetheless, Harper's legislation, in one of the world's most enviable democracies, is an example of the medicalization of citizenship that warrants extensive academic research to address and, hopefully, curb this phenomenon.

In an age of pandemics, global warming (which will exacerbate the displacement of people), and the mobilization of xenophobic movements on an international scale, we must expect that the securitization of health will also determine national policies on the admission and, above all, exclusion of immigrants and refugees. From a philosophical point of view, we demonstrate in the following section that the principles of global health justice underpin the duties to welcome migrants and refugees and to guarantee their fundamental right not to be discriminated against on the grounds of their health status.

11.5 HUMANITARIAN MEDICAL ASSISTANCE AS A DUTY OF GLOBAL HEALTH JUSTICE

According to David Owen's enlightening book, *What Do We Owe to Refugees?* (2020), we certainly have duties toward refugees. Owen argues that the refugee concept must be understood according to the principles of state sovereignty that are coherent with human rights. The legitimacy of the international order is based on this crucial articulation between these two realms of rights. Should a state fail to protect the human rights of its constituent members, then the international community has a duty toward refugees to protect their fundamental rights. Owen's argument collapses if we do not support this normative foundation of the international community based on the mutual recognition of human rights and states' rights. However, the body of legal conventions and transnational institutions in the 21st century has grown out of this ethical foundation of the UN model, despite all the power plays, imperfections, and institutional failures that also plagued the history of the UN.

Echoing Serene Parekh's (2020) theses, if our international order creates "structural injustices" that endanger people without citizenship, the international community must correct the *global encampment regime for refugees*, which blatantly violates their fundamental human rights. Added to the problem of the abhorrent living conditions in refugee camps is the difficulty of gaining access to these shelters, however miserable they may be: "It is the cumulative effect of many different policies around refugee resettlement, refugee camps, humanitarian and development aid, immigration and border security enacted by countries around the world. The way these policies, laws, and norms interact create[s] the unjust outcome for refugees: their inability to access the minimum conditions of human dignity" (Parekh 2020, 159).

What do we mean by structural injustices? Parekh follows the work of feminist philosopher Iris Marion Young (2011), which she applies to the international sphere to better understand the harm done to refugees and the collective responsibility of states in the production and perpetuation of the global encampment regime. Young's concept of structural injustice, which is tied to the model of social connections, refers to the set of structures of collective interactions in which individuals participate without breaking any rules and without any explicit intention to harm others, but which maintain harmful social structures. One of the particularities of structural injustice is that it is challenging to identify upstream the specific actors responsible for these harms, since all agents involved in these complex interactions maintain social, economic, and political systems that produce morally unjustifiable inequalities. The notion of structural injustice thus also mobilizes a conception of individual and collective responsibility, which differs from the traditional model of direct liability. We argue that numerous global health inequities raise the need to interrogate the international statist order in terms of structural injustice.

There are other interpretations of structural injustice distinct from Young's concept. Powers and Faden (2020), for instance, are not interested in indirect social processes contributing to structural injustice. While acknowledging their existence, they argue that structural injustices are mainly produced and sustained by the deliberate and wrongful conduct of identifiable agents who profit from structural unfairness. Powers and Faden appropriately challenge Young's problematic aspects of her social connections model, which rests on a forward-looking (rather than backward-looking), somewhat ahistorical, and blameless account of collective responsibility. However, Young developed her work on structural injustice precisely to explore the idea of responsibility for cases that do not fit the classical model of direct accountability. She always acknowledged that injustices involve both direct and indirect causal responsibility. In this sense, Powers and Faden's position is close to Young's despite their criticisms.

Regarding the human rights of stateless migrants, asylum seekers, and refugees, the perspectives of Owen, Parekh, and Powers and Faden converge on the conclusion that our international order unjustly harms asylum seekers who have fled their native countries because of economic distress, social violence, or political persecution. These displaced people fall into the interstices of an international order that maintains a global regime of encampment that deprives them of fundamental freedoms, dimensions of well-being, and basic rights, including access to healthcare.

11.6 CONCLUSION: TOWARD A UNIVERSAL HEALTHCARE SYSTEM?

The genesis of humanitarian law and the creation of the WHO in 1946 are based on the defense of a universal right to health. The current situation of forced migrants and refugees is a clear violation of this fundamental right. We have shown that health nationalism, the securitization of health, and the medicalization of citizenship contribute to producing and maintaining this state of affairs. From a philosophical point of view nourished by the founding principles of contemporary international law and the UN model, the international community owes its legitimacy to the necessary articulation of human rights and the rights of sovereign states. When states fail in this commitment, the international community has a duty to protect the basic rights of stateless people.

What is the best model of global health governance for refugees? While it is impossible to explore these perspectives in depth here, three lines of research are worth pursuing. First, wealthier countries have an obligation to welcome displaced people and refugees to the best of their ability without discriminating against the health status of asylum seekers. Similar to Bill 83, which extends health coverage to all asylum seekers and their children in Quebec, all countries must provide for the health needs of asylum seekers within their borders.

Second, the universal health coverage (UHC) model must guide all global health governance efforts (Lal 2022). Currently the UHC model is limited to urging all countries to remove the financial barriers that impede access to healthcare for their nationals. More must be done to guarantee minimum access to healthcare for all, especially those without national citizenship. Improving living conditions in refugee camps should not be the goal of international mobilization but a necessary first step toward achieving UHC. The role of humanitarian international NGOs is crucial in this respect. Indeed, faced with states' moral bankruptcy and governments' failure to protect the basic human rights of populations victimized by violent conflict, economic distress, or natural disasters, international NGOs are sometimes perceived as essential players whose voice and agency can be decisive. In light of the crisis in the Middle East, we must salute the role played by international and national NGOs and the WHO, which have taken up the humanitarian defense of the fundamental rights of the people of Gaza. These groups have played an essential role in the face of political inertia by national governments. Could healthcare for refugees and displaced people worldwide be better provided under the coordination of the WHO and the various NGOs specializing in humanitarian medical assistance? If so, the UHC model must rethink how to support and finance these nonstate actors.

Third, it is crucial to emphasize that this argument does not absolve states and their governments of their responsibilities toward their populations. Neither the WHO nor NGOs can coordinate the long-term assistance of millions of people scattered across the planet. Local authorities and national governments must take action with humanity to protect and guarantee their population's human right to health. To ensure countries have equal abilities to provide basic social coverage to their constituents, the international community must find a way to reduce the abysmal inequalities that ultimately put everyone and future generations in danger in the face of global environmental and health crises.

At a time when the securitization of health in the name of national interests is reaching a paroxysm and health nationalism is exacerbating existing global inequalities, we must fear the medicalization of citizenship for those caught in an international no man's land. As we reach the 80th anniversary of the proclamation of the universal right to health, we hope to contribute to the mobilization of collective efforts to promote and protect the health of all human beings—first and foremost, those who suffer the greatest injustices in our troubled era.

REFERENCES

Alboth, Anna. 2021. "Helping Refugees Starving in Poland's Icy Border Forest Is Illegal—But It's Not the Real Crime." *The Guardian*, December 8. https://www.theguardian.com/global-development/2021/dec/08/helping-refugees-poland-belarus-border-forests-illegal.

Burki, Thala. 2020. "Covid-19: A Multifaceted Threat to Refugee Camps." *The Lancet* 1 (July): e110.

Chung, Ryoa, and Joanne Liu. 2023. "The Ethical Issues Raised by the Securitization of Health." In *Justice and Global Health: New Perspectives and Current Issues*, edited by H. Bhakuni and L. Miotto. Routledge.

Davies, Sarah E. 2010. *Global Politics of Health*. Polity Press.

Deutsche Welle. 2023. "Uncertain Futures: Syria's Hidden Crisis of Disabilities." *Frontline*, July 29. https://frontline.thehindu.com/news/uncertain-futures-syria-hidden-crisis-of-disabilities/article67134759.ece.

Dworkin, Ronald. 1993. "Justice in the Distribution of Healthcare." *McGill Law Journal Revue de droit de McGill* 38 (4): 883–888.

Elbe, Stefan. 2010. *Security and Global Health*. Polity Press.
Emanuel, Ezekiel J., Allen Buchanan, Shuk Ying Chan, et al. 2021. "The Ethics of Vaccine Nationalism: The Case for the Fair Priority for Residents Framework." *Ethics & International Affairs* 35 (4): 543–562.
Fassin, Didier, and Anne-Claire Defossez. 2024. *L'Exil Toujours Recommencé: Chronique de la Frontière*. Seuil.
Giles, Christopher. 2021. "Trump's Wall: How Much Has Been Built During His Term?" BBC, January 12. https://www.bbc.com/news/world-us-canada-46748492.
Hoffman, Stanley. 1983. *Une Morale pour les Monstres Froids: Pour une Éthique des Relations Internationales*. Boréal Express.
Lal, Arush, Salma M. Abdalla, Vijay Kumar Chattu, et al. 2022. "Pandemic Preparedness and Response: Exploring the Role of Universal Health Coverage Within the Global Health Security Architecture." *The Lancet* 10 (11): E1675–E1683 (November).
Lee, Erika, and Judy Yung. 2010. *Angel Island. Immigrant Gateway to America*. Oxford University Press.
MacIntyre, Alasdair. 1984. "Is Patriotism a Virtue?" The Lindley Lecture, University of Kansas, Department of Philosophy, March 26.
Miller, David. 1995. *On Nationality*. Oxford University Press.
Morgenthau, Hans. 1948. *Politics Among Nations*. Knopf.
Mustafa, Nujeen, and Christina Lamb. 2017. *The Girl from Aleppo: Nujeen's Escape from War to Freedom*. Harper Collins.
Owen, David. 2020. *What Do We Owe to Refugees?* Polity.
Our World in Data. n.d. "Coronavirus (COVID-19) Vaccinations." Accessed December 10, 2024. https://ourworldindata.org/covid-vaccinations.
Parekh, Serene. 2020. *No Refuge: Ethics and the Global Refugee Crisis*. Oxford University Press.
Powers, Madison, and Ruth Faden. 2020. *Structural Injustice*. Oxford University Press.
Rawls, John. 1971. *A Theory of Justice*. Belknap Press.
Rigby, Jennifer, and James Crisp. 2022. "Fortress Europe." *The Telegraph*. https://www.telegraph.co.uk/global-health/fortress-europe-borders-wall-fence-controls-eu-countries-migrants-crisis/.
United Nations Development Programme. 1994. "New Dimensions of Human Security." In *Human Development Report*, edited by Inge Kaul (Director of the UNDP Team). Oxford University Press.
United Nations High Commissioner for Refugees. n.d. *Covid-19 and Refugees*. Last Accessed December 10th, 2024. https://storymaps.arcgis.com/stories/95cc3b65d9264cf3b80fffef0daa0358.
Walzer, Michael. 1984. *Spheres of Justice: A Defense of Pluralism and Equality*. Basic Books.
Webster, Paul C. 2015. "Canada Criticised over Refugee Health-Care Restrictions." *The Lancet* 386(10002): P1436 (October).
Wellman, Christopher Heath. 2001. "Friends, Compatriots, and Special Political Obligations." *Political Theory* 29 (2): 217–236.
World Health Organization. 2023–2024. "Gaza Strip." OPT Emergency Situation Update, no. 46. https://www.emro.who.int/images/stories/Sitrep_46b.pdf?ua=1.
World Health Organization. 2024. "Six Months of War Leave Al-Shifa Hospital in Ruins." Mission Reports, April 6. https://www.who.int/news/item/06-04-2024-six-months-of-war-leave-al-shifa-hospital-in-ruins--who-mission-reports.

Wild, Verina. 2015. "Universal Access to Health Care for Migrants: Applying Cosmopolitanism to the Domestic Realm." *Public Health Ethics* 8 (2): 162–172.
Youde, J., and S. Rushton, eds. 2015. *Routledge Handbook of Global Health Security*. Routledge.
Young, Iris Marion. 2011. *Responsibility for Justice*. Oxford University Press.

12

Structural Health Vulnerabilities and Refugees with Disabilities in Canada

MONIKA NOBLE, MATHIEU SIMARD, LISA ECKENWILER, RYOA CHUNG, ROBYN MELLETT, AND MATTHEW HUNT

12.1 INTRODUCTION

Since 2013, the number of forcibly displaced people has increased each year, with the United Nations High Commissioner for Refugees ([UNHCR] 2023) reporting 108.4 million people displaced in 2022, including 35.3 million people who crossed international borders as refugees. Many refugees have some form of impairment which, in interaction with environmental, institutional, and attitudinal barriers, leads to disability impacting individual functioning and social participation. Some refugees have preexisting congenital impairments or impairments that developed earlier in life due to injury or illness. For others, impairments may be the result of or become exacerbated by the circumstances surrounding displacement and the migration process. While the World Health Organization (WHO) reports that 15% of the global population experiences some form of disability (WHO and World Bank 2011), Khan and Amatya (2017) estimated that as many as 66% of refugees experience mental health problems, and that 16% of refugees have a physical health problem which severely affects their daily life. While there is limited data on the prevalence of disability among refugees, it is clear that many refugees with disabilities go through immigration processes in countries around the world, including Canada.

Despite the significant number of refugees who experience some form of disability, there has been limited attention given to structural barriers that refugees with disabilities experience. These barriers are likely to be more extensive and greater than those faced by refugees in general. Considering how such barriers are manifested or addressed in the Canadian

Monika Noble et al., *Structural Health Vulnerabilities and Refugees with Disabilities in Canada*. In: *Forced Migration and Health Justice*. Edited by: Lisa A. Eckenwiler, Verina Wild, Anna Gotlib, Ryoa Chung, and Deborah Zion, Oxford University Press. © Oxford University Press (2026). DOI: 10.1093/oso/9780197795491.003.0012 context is important, as Canada is the country that received the highest number of "refugee resettlement arrivals" in recent years—that is, offering third-country resettlement "from countries of asylum who welcome large numbers of refugees" (UNHCR 2023). In this light, there is a pressing need to examine how social and institutional norms, processes, and structures could either undermine or support the immigration of refugees with disabilities to Canada. Such features could, in turn, threaten or reinforce health justice, which we interpret as the commitment to and creation of the conditions needed to support the capability of being healthy (Venkatapuram 2011).

We begin the chapter by providing an overview of the conceptual tool of *structural health vulnerabilities*, which is a useful analytical lens for examining Canada's immigration system and, in particular, structural barriers and facilitators for refugees with disabilities. Then we examine how specific features of this system may function as facilitators or as barriers that augment the vulnerability of refugees with disabilities to Canada and thus threaten health justice.

12.1.1 Terminology

Two terms that are used throughout this chapter are "barrier" and "facilitator". A barrier is a feature of the immigration system that increases a refugee's vulnerability to injustice, thereby hindering their immigration process. Conversely, facilitators include features of the immigration system such as persons, organizations, or procedures that may reduce or mitigate vulnerability to injustice.

Our definition of the term "disability" follows the United Nations Convention of the Rights of Persons with Disabilities. "Disability is an evolving concept that results from the interactions between persons with impairments and attitudinal and environmental barriers that hinder their full and effective participation in society on an equal basis with others" (United Nations Department of Economic and Social Affairs 2006). Instead of being viewed negatively, a person's impairments are a "neutral way of being" (Goering 2015). In this chapter, we use the term "disability" to encompass a wide spectrum of physical, mental, and sensory disabilities. We acknowledge, however, that there are debates within the disability community about terminology, including terms related to mental health and whether person-first or identity-first language should be used. We also acknowledge the significant variation of experiences among people with different forms of impairment and living in varying contexts.

12.1.2 Structural Health Vulnerability

To understand structural health vulnerabilities, it is useful to first discuss structural injustice. As described by Young, "persons suffer injustice by virtue of structural inequality when their group social positioning means that the operation of diverse institutions and practices conspire to limit their opportunities to achieve well-being" (2008, 82). When people experience structural injustice, or an injustice that has its origins in norms, assumptions, and processes, the causal responsibility is collective, which makes it more difficult to identify the injustice's source (Young 2008). Thus the underlying features which contribute to amplifying people's vulnerabilities are obscured, and only the immediate effects of these injustices receive attention, regardless of whether this is the intention. The underlying systemic causes are untouched, perpetuating the cycle of injustice. If structural injustices are continually ignored the resulting social inequalities can produce differences in a person's capacity to be healthy (Venkatapuram 2011).

A *structural health vulnerability* is an increased propensity to incur health risks directly related to social inequalities stemming from structural injustices that disproportionately affect an individual or a social group (Levine et al. 2004; Chung and Hunt 2012; Chung 2021). This form of vulnerability results in marginalization arising from "class-based economic exploitation and cultural, gender/sexual, and racialized discrimination" (Quesada et al. 2011, 339). The lens of structural health vulnerabilities draws attention to not just how people are vulnerable but how "they are made vulnerable", especially in regard to risks of worsened health outcomes (Ahmad et al. 2020, 1481). We will now consider how structural health vulnerabilities relate to aspects of the immigration process of refugees with disabilities.

12.2 A BRIEF OVERVIEW OF THE CANADIAN IMMIGRATION PROCESS

Our focus in this chapter is on the experience of refugees with disabilities once they have arrived in Canada and are moving through the stages of the immigration system. While barriers and facilitators are encountered by refugees with disabilities at other phases of their migration experience, they are outside this chapter's scope.

The immigration process of government-sponsored and privately sponsored (Convention) refugees begins long before they arrive in Canada. Privately sponsored refugees are supported by groups of individuals or organizations that support refugees for a minimum period of one year. Government-sponsored refugees are sponsored directly by the Government of Canada or the province of Quebec and must be referred by the UNHCR or a referral organization. Once a refugee is deemed to fit the UNHCR's (2018) definition of a refugee, their refugee claim is submitted to a host country such as Canada. They are then interviewed by a migration officer, who determines whether the applicant meets Canadian eligibility and admissibility criteria (UNHCR 2018). If they do, a medical exam is requested, and applicants must undergo criminality and security checks before they are granted entry to Canada (Immigration and Citizenship Canada 2025). When Convention refugees arrive in Canada, they already have permanent resident status.

Refugee claimants, on the other hand, apply for refugee status within the host country at a port of entry and apply for asylum after completing their basis-of-claim forms. They must then complete the Immigration Medical Exam and are interviewed by an Immigration Review Board member, who decides on their refugee claim. If their claim is approved, they are granted refugee status. If their claim is rejected, they can either appeal to the Refugee Appeal Division or they must leave the country. This is not the only form of removal that refugees may face; they may also be removed following an Admissibility Hearing (Immigration and Refugee Board of Canada 2022).

12.3 STRUCTURAL HEALTH VULNERABILITIES AND THE IMMIGRATION JOURNEY OF REFUGEES WITH DISABILITIES

The immigration journeys of refugees with disabilities present multiple aspects of structural health vulnerabilities and various potential facilitators and barriers. While many of these aspects overlap (such as how policy dictates access to medical care and how the legal process often depends on decisions regarding federal and provincial policies), the following sections highlight two distinct domains where issues related to structural health vulnerabilities arise: the legal domain and the medical and social services domain. More specifically, we highlight how sociocultural norms, economic and financial structures, and the organization of decision-making processes serve to either support or undermine the capability of being healthy for refugees with disabilities.

12.3.1 The Legal Domain

As noted earlier, refugees undergo an interview process with a migration officer for the purpose of verifying the identity and eligibility of applicants and the collection of a "detailed family composition and background information" (UNHCR 2022). Refugee claimants are interviewed by a member of the Immigration Review Board, who subsequently decides whether their claim should be accepted or rejected (Immigration and Refugee Board of Canada 2021a).

One barrier that refugees with disabilities may face in the legal process is access to legal support services. This is particularly concerning when trying to access a translator throughout the legal process. For people who are deaf, are hard of hearing, or use sign language, access to interpretation throughout the legal process is a necessity. One instruction from the Immigration and Refugee Board of Canada regarding the use of an accredited interpreter states that their use is "limited to interviews that have a significant impact on the client, such as in-Canada claims for refugee protection and eligibility interviews, interviews with individuals likely to be subject to a removal from Canada, pre-removal risk assessment hearings, interviews with victims of abuse" (Immigration, Refugees and Citizenship Canada 2023b). In these cases, a client can request an interpreter, and the officer in charge of the case "determines whether the application could have a significant impact on the client" (Immigration, Refugees and Citizenship Canada 2023b). If it is determined that the interview will not have a significant impact on the client and they still want an interpreter, then the client is responsible for finding their own interpreter. It is also stated that the officers who are involved in immigration cases should "allow for a degree of discretion when deciding to provide Immigration, Refugees and Citizenship Canada–funded interpretation services in other proceedings not included in this list" (Immigration, Refugees and Citizenship Canada 2023b). In this context, refugees with disabilities who require translation services are at a distinct disadvantage when these supports are not provided if they cannot effectively communicate with their legal counsel or the officials who are making decisions regarding their immigration or if they will incur substantial financial costs to secure translation. Communication difficulties and potential financial costs create barriers for refugees with disabilities when trying to navigate the immigration process. The communication challenges also exist for refugee claimants with learning and cognitive impairments. The recent Immigration and Refugee Board Accessibility Plan for 2023 to 2025 (Immigration and Refugee Board of Canada 2023c) has mandated that the Immigration and Refugee Board (IRB) produce easy-to-read documents and improve the accessibility of electronic documentation, questionnaires, and their website, after an internal review pointed to challenges in this area for accessibility of written communications.

Financial barriers and lack of accommodations for translation services are examples of how policies can contribute to structural health vulnerabilities for persons with disabilities. However, it is also possible to see where facilitators can help to reduce structural health vulnerabilities. For instance, the IRB has introduced sensitivity training for its members that includes attention to vulnerability and the need for accommodations. The "Chairperson's Guideline 8" pertains to vulnerable persons appearing before the IRB and aims to guide members toward better accommodating their specific needs. The guideline states that "the term vulnerability should be interpreted broadly, as the concept of vulnerability is difficult to define. The focus should be on whether an individual has any vulnerabilities that negatively impact their ability to fully participate at the IRB and to have a fair hearing" (Immigration and Refugee Board of Canada 2023a). The stated purpose of the guide is to "enhance access to justice at the IRB of Canada by providing guidance on granting procedural accommodations," specifically "identifying when they are legally required" as well as "encouraging the IRB to provide them when doing so would assist an individual even if there is no legal requirement to do so," and to promote "the use of appropriate language, avoiding myths and stereotypes, the principles of trauma-informed adjudication and intersectionality" (Immigration and Refugee Board of Canada 2023a). When the guidelines were updated, changes included removing the need to label individuals as vulnerable and for refugees to demonstrate that their capacity to present their case to the IRB was severely impaired in order to access accommodations. When immigration proceedings such as IRB hearings are conducted in a way that supports and accommodates various forms of disability, refugees with disabilities are more likely to be able to convey their experiences to the IRB and navigate the immigration process successfully. Although this chapter is unable to report on the effects of these guidelines, including the impact of the 2023 revisions, they do illustrate how changes are being made to policies to be more responsive to the needs of refugees with disabilities.

Another key facilitator for refugees with disabilities is the exemption of refugees and protected persons from the "excessive demands" criteria since 2000. These criteria state that an applicant may be refused if they have a health condition that might cause an excessive demand on health or social services, defined as costing more than three times the average Canadian's cost for these services annually (Immigration, Refugees and Citizenship Canada 2024). As of 2024, this limit is $131,100 over 5 years, or $26,220 per year (Immigration and Citizenship 2024). This updated policy still presents limitations, as it does not ensure that refugees with disabilities who require long-term financial assistance are exempt from future admissibility reviews. Figures are not available for the number of refugees with disabilities whose immigration applications were rejected before this exemption was applied in 2000. However, this exemption reduces the risks that refugees with disabilities are deemed ineligible because of healthcare costs.[1]

12.3.2 The Medical and Social Services Domain

A second component of the immigration system that raises questions related to structural health vulnerabilities is the accessibility of health and social services for refugees with disabilities. Resettled refugees and refugee claimants (including those with a disability) receive coverage under the Interim Federal Health Program (IFHP) of the Government of Canada. This plan is implemented by coverage under the Medavie Blue Cross, which is the IFHP claims administrator and provider for the federal government (Government of Canada 2022). Within Canada, the IFHP provides "limited, temporary coverage of healthcare benefits to people in the following groups who aren't eligible for provincial or territorial health insurance: resettled refugees, refugee claimants, in-Canada protected persons and certain other groups" for a given period of time (Immigration and Citizenship Canada, 2023). The plan provides coverage for basic and supplemental needs, prescription drug coverage, and the cost of the Immigration Medical Exam for those who require it (Immigration, Refugees and Citizenship Canada 2023a). For refugees with a disability going through the immigration process, the IFHP can help to defray part of the costs associated with assistive devices or professional health and social services (e.g., physician, social worker, physical therapist, psychologist). Partial expenses relating to mobility and hearing aids are also included under the supplemental coverage of the IFHP and subsequently help to reduce structural health vulnerabilities by covering various healthcare and social services that refugees with disabilities could require.

Despite this, barriers still result from the IFHP's limited coverage. To start, the benefits covered by the IFHP have certain limits, including the number of treatments and maximum financial contribution, meaning the fees reimbursed for certain services are well below the actual costs, or that treatment may be ended due to reaching the maximum number that are supported (Medavie Blue Cross 2022). For example, the IFHP provides

1. For temporary and permanent residency applicants, this figure amounted to 0.2% of the applicants being refused on medical admissibility grounds, resulting in a 0.1% decrease in potential cost to the public health system (Canadian Bar Association 2017), a small proportion that could support the potential to remove this additional barrier for applicants with disabilities.

$80 for an initial, simple orthopedic assessment in a physiotherapy clinic (Medavie Blue Cross 2022), yet clinics typically charge $115 to $130 for such an assessment in the province of Quebec. The reimbursement for physiotherapy therefore covers a portion of the costs for simple assessments in private clinics. However, such an assessment is likely to be insufficient for the assessment of persons requiring multidisciplinary care, including many people with disabilities. Some persons with disabilities require more specialized care in public healthcare settings, such as rehabilitation centers. In addition to the limited cost reimbursement of the IFHP, many refugees with disabilities face difficulties in knowing how to navigate the local health system and complex referral systems in the public healthcare sector. Once they successfully complete the application process, there are long waiting times and limited availability of such services.

The IFHP does cover interpretation and translation services, but only for psychiatry and psychotherapy/counseling (for initial assessment and treatments) or for post-arrival health assessment (Medavie Blue Cross 2022). Within the post-arrival health assessment, translation services are provided only to resettled refugees, and only for two hours (Medavie Blue Cross 2022). Even then, the cost covered is limited (e.g., $28.95/hour for translation services, which is approximately half of the typical cost for this service). This raises significant health and economic equity issues. Access to mobility aids (e.g., wheelchairs) is also limited by the IFHP's parameters. The IFHP covers a new wheelchair once every five years, and repairs to mobility aids require prior approval (Medavie Blue Cross 2022). This could result in refugees with disabilities facing significant wait times before they are able to access assistive devices or have them repaired. The IFHP will cover updates to custom wheelchair seating systems every two years for individuals who fit the criteria (Medavie Blue Cross 2022). These stipulations do not account for updating seating systems of individuals with degenerative conditions, those who are growing quickly (e.g., teenagers), or people who experience changes in their functional abilities, for whom these timeframes may be inadequate. These limitations decrease access to necessary aids and services, which can negatively impact the lives of refugees with disabilities, thus contributing to structural health vulnerabilities.

Interpretation services are not always available, and due to a lack of or incomplete coverage of health and social services in certain areas, refugees with disabilities covered by the IFHP face additional barriers when attempting to access healthcare. These barriers may impede access to health services.

12.4 HOW CAN BARRIERS BE ADDRESSED?

We have described both facilitators and barriers associated with the immigration process of refugees with disabilities. How these features impact a particular refugee with disability will vary based on individual and contextual factors, including the form of disability they experience, which in turn impacts the sort of actions that are required. Below we present pathways by which barriers may be reduced in relation to the legal domain, the healthcare and social services domain, and for the migration process overall.

Key barriers in the legal domain are related to legal support and translation, as well as financial costs. These challenges could be addressed by increasing the allocation for legal support and translation services throughout the entire process (not just for the IRB hearing). Additional support for sign language interpretation and ensuring accessible legal documents for guidance at the federal level (e.g., multiple sign languages, easy read, etc.).

Another suggestion is to clarify and limit the circumstances that can result in an admissibility hearing and potential rejection of a refugee claimant on the basis of a health condition or disability. The criterion that "health conditions (in some cases)" can necessitate an admissibility hearing should be removed or expressly state that disability is not considered a reason for initiating a hearing.

Persons with disabilities also experience more challenges to access to employment and present with a lower socioeconomic status than the general population. This compounds the barriers for legal and translation access, along with private health and social services provision. Since the refugees and their families need to demonstrate that they can have sufficient funds for self-support, a lower economic situation can also affect negatively their admissibility. This is not unique to refugees, since people with disabilities generally experience higher expenses along with lower income. Some facilitators for employment, such as access to orientation services within rehabilitation institutions, could be arranged prior to arrival in Canada. This step may decrease the time to gain the specific skills required for facilitating employment in Canada. Financial support systems could also be better adapted to the situation of persons with disabilities. Additionally, adapting the supplemental income allocated to refugees with disabilities would help to address this high-expense, low-income gap, in line with disability benefit provisions for Canadian citizens.

Accessible support services are also crucial for addressing barriers to healthcare and social services. A major challenge is ensuring access to a family physician, which may be necessary to access secondary and tertiary care services, obtain employment orientation services (e.g., public transport for persons with low vision, adapted electronic readers or speech production devices), and access physical mobility devices. Increasing the scope of what the IFHP covers will also decrease financial barriers to healthcare for refugees with disabilities, as well as increasing the awareness of health professionals in private and public settings regarding IFHP processes and eligibility. Additionally, ensuring the provision of sign language interpretation services throughout the immigration process for refugees with communication disabilities and providing information in formats that are accessible for refugees unfamiliar with legal and medical proceedings will facilitate access to healthcare services and legal aid.

Finally, effort should be directed toward ensuring that people working within the immigration system are aware of how structural features can give rise to health injustices for persons with disabilities. Providing trauma-informed and vulnerability sensitivity training will support IRB members who interact with refugees with disabilities to better understand how these refugees may experience structural health vulnerabilities. Greater appreciation for structural injustices and their implications for health can open new spaces for discussion about how the system can be improved in order to refine norms, processes, or structures to enhance health justice.

12.5 CONCLUSION

Our analysis has drawn primarily upon the concepts of structural injustice and structural health vulnerabilities. Before we conclude, we want to introduce an additional ethical concept and, indeed, a form of practice that we find pertinent here: care. Refugees, especially refugees with disabilities, are arguably among the most vulnerable groups globally. Even if we leave aside—and we do not believe we should—the ethical and policy matters of whether destination countries have obligations to welcome asylum seekers as long-term residents and perhaps, one day, citizens, these people deserve care as humans who have suffered. We do not mean that officials must demonstrate felt concern and compassion necessarily, though we believe this is in order. Rather our claim is that the social institutions charged with establishing and overseeing the processes involved in immigration and asylum seeking (and many other public functions) have responsibilities to not be indifferent or callous but rather more inclusive, attentive, and responsive to the needs of vulnerable groups and other persons of concern (Bourgault 2017, 2020).

While some facilitators that help enable the immigration of refugees with disabilities to Canada exist, there remain significant barriers. Through training for people involved in the immigration system, increasing the support services and healthcare refugees with disabilities can access, and creating more inclusive immigration policy, the immigration process for refugees with disabilities can be improved. Addressing these barriers in the immigration system is necessary to promote health justice.

REFERENCES

Ahmad, Ayesha, Ryoa Chung, Lisa Eckenwiler, et al. 2020. "What Does It Mean to Be Made Vulnerable in the Era of COVID-19?" *Lancet* 395 (10235): 1481–1482. https://doi.org/10.1016/S0140-6736(20)30979-X.

Bourgault, Sophie. 2017. "Prolegomena to a Caring Bureaucracy." *European Journal of Women's Studies* 24 (3): 202–217. https://doi.org/10.1177/1350506816643730.

Bourgault, Sophie. 2020. "Epistemic Injustice, Face-to-Face Encounters and Caring Institutions." *International Journal of Care and Caring* 4 (1): 91–107. https://doi.org/10.1332/239788219X15682725266696.

Canadian Bar Association. 2017. "Medical Inadmissibility of Immigrants." https://www.ourcommons.ca/Content/Committee/421/CIMM/Brief/BR9281090/br-external/CanadianBarAssociation-e.pdf.

Chung, Ryoa. 2021. "Structural Health Vulnerability: Health Inequalities, Structural and Epistemic Injustice." *Journal of Social Philosophy* 52 (2): 201–216. https://doi.org/10.1111/JOSP.12393.

Chung, Ryoa, and Matthew R. Hunt. 2012. "Justice and Health Inequalities in Humanitarian Crises: Structured Health Vulnerabilities and Natural Disasters." In *Health Inequalities and Global Justice*, edited by Patti Tamara Lenard and Christine Straehle. Edinburgh University Press. https://doi.org/10.3366/edinburgh/9780748646920.003.0012.

Global Affairs Canada. 2024. "The Citizenship and Immigration (CIC) Liaison Unit of the Office of Protocol: Clarification of Immigration Procedures and Suggested Contacts." https://www.international.gc.ca/protocol-protocole/immigration.aspx?lang=eng#:~:text=Foreign%20nationals%20are%20individuals%20who,for%20Canada%20or%20enter%20Canada.

Goering, Sara. 2015. "Rethinking Disability: The Social Model of Disability and Chronic Disease." *Current Reviews in Musculoskeletal Medicine* 8 (2): 134–138. https://doi.org/10.1007/s12178-015-9273-z.

Government of Canada. 2022. "Temporary Public Policy Regarding Excessive Demand on Health and Social Services—Canada.Ca." October 26. https://www.canada.ca/en/immigration-refugees-citizenship/corporate/mandate/policies-operational-instructions-agreements/excessive-demand-june-2018.html.

Immigration and Refugee Board of Canada. 2021b. "Resettle in Canada as a Refugee." https://www.canada.ca/en/immigration-refugees-citizenship/services/refugees/help-outside-canada.html.

Immigration and Refugee Board of Canada. 2022. "Admissibility Hearing Process." March 18. https://irb-cisr.gc.ca/en/legal-policy/procedures/Pages/ProcessAdmEnq.aspx.

Immigration and Refugee Board of Canada. 2023a. "Chairperson's Guideline 8: Accessibility to IRB Proceedings—Procedural Accommodations and Substantive Considerations." https://irb.gc.ca/en/legal-policy/policies/Pages/GuideDir08.aspx.

Immigration and Refugee Board of Canada. 2023b. "Interim Federal Health Program: What Is Covered." June 1. https://www.canada.ca/en/immigration-refugees-citizenship/services/refugees/help-within-canada/health-care/interim-federal-health-program/coverage-summary.html.

Immigration and Refugee Board of Canada. 2023c. "IRB Accessibility Plan 2023 to 2025." https://irb-cisr.gc.ca/en/transparency/accessibility/Pages/2023-2025-accessibility-plan.aspx.

Immigration, Refugees and Citizenship Canada. 2023a. "Interim Federal Health Program: Who Is Eligible." https://www.canada.ca/en/immigration-refugees-citizenship/services/refugees/help-within-canada/health-care/interim-federal-health-program/eligibility.html.

Immigration, Refugees and Citizenship Canada. 2023b. "Using the Services of an Accredited Interpreter." August 30. https://www.canada.ca/en/immigration-refugees-citizenship/corporate/publications-manuals/operational-bulletins-manuals/interview/interpreter/using-services.html.

Immigration, Refugees and Citizenship Canada. 2024. "Excessive Demand on Health Services and on Social Services." https://www.canada.ca/en/immigration-refugees-citizenship/corporate/publications-manuals/operational-bulletins-manuals/standard-requirements/medical-requirements/refusals-inadmissibility/excessive-demand-on-health-social-services.html#.

Immigration and Citizenship Canada. 2023. "Interim Federal Health Policy Program." https://www.canada.ca/en/immigration-refugees-citizenship/corporate/mandate/policies-operational-instructions-agreements/interim-federal-health-program-policy.html.

Immigration and Citizenship Canada. 2025. "How to Be Resettled in Canada as a Refugee." https://www.canada.ca/en/immigration-refugees-citizenship/services/refugees/resettle-refugee/eligibility.html.

Khan, Fary, and Bhasker Amatya. 2017. "Refugee Health and Rehabilitation: Challenges and Response." *Journal of Rehabilitation Medicine* 49 (5): 378–384. https://doi.org/10.2340/16501977-2223.

Levine, Carol, Ruth Faden, Christine Grady, et al. 2004. "The Limitations of 'Vulnerability' as a Protection for Human Research Participants." *American Journal of Bioethics* 4 (3): 44–49. https://doi.org/10.1080/15265160490497083.

Medavie Blue Cross. 2022. "IFHP Benefit Grid—Supplemental Coverage." https://ifhp-docs.medaviebc.ca/Benefit%20Grids/Supplemental%20Coverage%20-%20Eng/IFHP-Benefit-Grid-Supplemental-Coverage-EN.pdf.

Quesada, James, Laurie Kain Hart, and Philippe Bourgois. 2011. "Structural Vulnerability and Health: Latino Migrant Laborers in the United States." *Medical Anthropology* 30 (4): 339–362. https://doi.org/10.1080/01459740.2011.576725.

United Nations Department of Economic and Social Affairs. 2006. "Convention on the Rights of Persons with Disabilities." https://www.un.org/development/desa/disabilities/convention-on-the-rights-of-persons-with-disabilities/convention-on-the-rights-of-persons-with-disabilities-2.html.

United Nations High Commissioner for Refugees. 2018. "UNHCR Resettlement Handbook: Country Chapter—Canada." https://www.unhcr.org/media/unhcr-resettlement-handbook-country-chapter-canada.

United Nations High Commissioner for Refugees. 2023. "Global Trends: Forced Displacement in 2022." https://www.unhcr.org/sites/default/files/2023-06/global-trends-report-2022.pdf.

Venkatapuram, Sridhar. 2011. *Health Justice: An Argument from the Capabilities Approach*. Polity Press.

World Health Organization and World Bank. 2011. "World Report on Disability." https://www.who.int/publications/i/item/9789241564182.

Young, Iris Marion. 2008. "Structural Injustice and the Politics of Difference." In *Intersectionality and Beyond*, edited by Emily Grabham, Davina Cooper, Jane Krishnadas, and Didi Herman. Routledge-Cavendish. https://doi.org/10.4324/9780203890882-23.

PART FOUR

Responsibilities for Health Justice

I Heard You Say . . .

AYESHA AHMAD

I heard you say

I heard you say . . .
My asylum is
The cage
I
Thought would be
My home

My silence is
The voice
I
Used to shatter
My suffering

My invisibility is
The wing
I
Traveled with to
My heart

My persecution is
The scar
I
Unpicked to create
My personhood

My journey is
The prayer
I
Recited to reach
My world

My story is
The obituary
I
Lived to scribe
My headstone

My breath is
The sigh
I
Heard you say
To me

13

Culpability, Liability, Responsibility, and Self-Interest

Analyzing the Reasons for Our Duties to Refugees and Migrants

PETER WEST-ORAM

13.1 INTRODUCTION

National citizenship is often taken to form a deep and fundamental aspect of our personal identity and to be a feature of persons that shapes the core of who they are and how they relate to others (Rorty 1989, 192). However, global trade, rapid transport, and instantaneous electronic communication provide the means for people to be closely connected to the lives of distant others, rendering national boundaries increasingly porous and diluting the significance of nationality for personal identity (West-Oram and Buyx 2017; Shahvisi 2018). In so doing, they further solidify the global structures within which we all live and through which we are increasingly causally connected (Young 2003). Despite this, being of a particular nationality can have a profound impact on our sense of self, our place in the world, and the extent to which we establish, value, and prioritize different relationships with other people (Rorty 1989, 192). Citizenship is also widely taken to grant priority consideration over noncitizens for access to important public goods such as health and welfare services (Kymlicka 2015, 17; West-Oram 2018a).

In this chapter, I examine three categories of argument to reject this prioritization and the differential provision of healthcare it engenders. My goal is to provide an overview (rather than a full and comprehensive account) of these arguments and explain how they support, reinforce, and complement each other to collectively function as the basis for a more

Peter West-Oram, *Culpability, Liability, Responsibility, and Self-Interest*. In: *Forced Migration and Health Justice*. Edited by: Lisa A. Eckenwiler, Verina Wild, Anna Gotlib, Ryoa Chung, and Deborah Zion, Oxford University Press.
 DOI: 10.1093/oso/9780197795491.003.0013

comprehensive argument for wealthy nations to meet the healthcare needs of refugees and migrants. I note the challenges associated with assigning responsibility appropriately due to the structural nature of the harms associated with migration and the pursuit of refuge and of the interventions necessary to mitigate them (Young 2003; Dwyer 2020).

To achieve these objectives, I first provide an overview of the global health context of international movement, with reference to the rhetorical use of immigration in domestic politics in the UK and US. Second, I discuss each of the three types of arguments in favor of the provision of healthcare to refugees and migrants by wealthy nations: moral entitlement and responsibility, culpability and liability, and self-interest. In discussing these arguments, I note their interactions and their relationships to the structural factors which contribute to migration and the pursuit of refuge internationally. I conclude the chapter by explaining the interactions and overlaps between the arguments provided and discussing their limitations.

13.2 CONTEXT

As of the first of January 2022, there were 23.8 million non-EU migrants (including refugees) living in the European Union (Eurostat 2023). Correlatively, according to the United Nations High Commissioner for Refugees ([UNHCR] 2023a; Amnesty International 2023), at the end of 2021 there were approximately 27.1 million refugees worldwide, while a further 4.6 million people were seeking, though had not yet been granted, refugee status. While a number of international conventions affirm that refugees enjoy rights to certain important goods, including healthcare services (UN General Assembly 1948; UNHCR 2010), their efficacy is often limited in practice by domestic policy, which restricts access to care that wealthy nations have ostensibly promised to provide. In the UK, for example, those who seek or have been granted refuge are entitled to the same healthcare as British citizens. However, the British government has for years sought to deter people from seeking refuge in (or immigrating to) the UK, making it harder for them to successfully claim asylum and the rights it confers through its "hostile environment" strategy (Hiam et al. 2018; Uthayakumar-Cumarasamy 2020).

Equally, virtually all migrants to the UK must pay additional fees not levied against citizens to access healthcare services, even if legally resident in the UK long term and despite paying similar taxes as British citizens (Uthayakumar-Cumarasamy 2020, 133). Similarly, during the UK's recent Brexit referendum, the supposedly high cost to British citizens of immigration and the provision of refuge was a prominent part of the political messaging of the Campaign to Leave the EU (Bennett 2016; Dorling 2016; Virdee and McGeever 2018). Similar attitudes are pervasive in American politics, where President Donald Trump used explicitly xenophobic and nationalist language about migrants and asylum seekers throughout both presidential election campaigns and his presidency (Fullerton 2017, 327–328; Pierce and Selee 2017).

The term "migrant" is an umbrella category, "reflecting the common lay understanding of a person who moves away from his or her place of usual residence, whether within a country or across an international border, temporarily or permanently, and for a variety of reasons" (International Organisation for Migration 2023). The category "refugee" is therefore a subcategory of this broader group (Amnesty International 2023) and refers to people "who have been forced to flee their homes and have crossed an international border to find safety in another country" (UNHCR 2023a). Consequently, while all refugees are migrants, not all migrants are refugees, and the legal status, vulnerabilities, motivations, experiences, and needs of people in different categories can vary significantly (Boise et al. 2013; Rechel et al. 2013; Hebebrand et al. 2016). Even acknowledging the meaningful differences between those classified as refugees and as migrants, many of the same arguments for (or indeed against) the provision of healthcare to one group will apply, at least to some degree, to people in the other category as well. In the following section, when outlining each of the three arguments, I note how well each applies to different categories of migrant/refugee.

13.3 THREE ARGUMENTS

13.3.1 Moral Duties

In this section I outline a moral argument for the provision of healthcare to refugees and migrants by wealthy countries. I focus on the most basic or narrow understanding of a moral argument—that which is derived purely from the moral status of the agents involved. In this way, a moral argument for the provision of healthcare to refugees and migrants by wealthy destination countries is very simple, since it focuses only on the moral status of refugees and migrants as sources of moral claims and on the power of wealthy countries to satisfy those claims.

A right to health or healthcare, the fulfillment of which is argued to be owed to all people everywhere, including refugees and migrants, is endorsed by a wide range of institutions and theorists (UN General Assembly 1948, art. 25; Wolff 2012; Shue 1996, 13, 18). The range of arguments given for this right is similarly broad (West-Oram 2016, 108–110): health and access to healthcare are argued to be essential for living "even a minimally decent human life" (West-Oram 2016, 109), while deprivations of it are painful, damaging, and extremely limiting to our ability to enjoy any other rights (Shue 1996, 24–25). Health is also seen as fundamental to many other important human functions; Nussbaum argues that "bodily health" is a fundamentally necessary human capability (2003, 41–42). Brock suggests that physical and mental health are necessary for human agency (2009, 66). David Owen has proposed that public health services which safeguard and promote individual health are necessary for individuals to participate "as equals in social and political life" (2016, 176). Correlatively, various theorists have argued that agents have duties to provide assistance or aid to others when doing so will not be excessively costly (Singer 1972, 231; Scanlon 2000, 224–228; Ho 2005, 59–60). Consequently, the argument that wealthy countries should guarantee refugees and migrants equitable access to healthcare on moral grounds may seem to some prima facie relatively straightforward and compelling.[1] Refugees and migrants are people with rights to healthcare, so someone has an obligation to fulfill that right, and it may seem appropriate to assign responsibility for doing so to the countries in which they reside.

However, in the absence of further contextual detail, this argument is insufficient to provide a comprehensive justification for wealthy countries to guarantee access to healthcare, even if the basic premise of the existence of moral claims is accepted. While the simplicity of the moral argument seems compelling, it can be objected that it provides justification at best to the claim that *someone* should ensure that refugees and migrants enjoy access to healthcare, but not that specific countries of residence should do so, given potentially high costs. It is not necessarily the case, for instance, that ensuring equitable access to healthcare will meet the "no excessive or unreasonable costs" standard, and given that most refugees are not resident in wealthy countries, this simple argument may inadvertently ignore the needs of many refugees (many of whom are resident in countries with limited resources to care for existing residents and citizens; Rawlence 2016; Parekh 2020) or make it impossible for destination countries to adequately meet the needs of their existing residents, as discussed in section 13.3.3 (UNHCR 2023b).

1. This is obviously a major simplification (for the sake of brevity) of a much more complex argument. It is, however, sufficient for my goal to provide an overview of the various arguments surrounding the fulfillment of migrant rights to healthcare. In a chapter of this length, more detailed analysis is not possible. I should also note that even in this simplified and abbreviated form, this argument is the one that I think should be sufficient to motivate wealthy nations to provide equitable access to healthcare to refugees and migrants.

Accepting that guaranteeing equitable access to healthcare could be highly expensive, it could therefore be argued that while refugees should be provided with access to care by their countries of residence at no cost, at least some additional costs can fairly be imposed on voluntary migrants. This is because, although they may contribute through taxation to the costs of care in the same manner as citizens following their arrival in their country of residence, they did not do so prior to their arrival, meaning that citizens will have made more contributions than migrants. However, not all citizens pay the same amount in taxes (and some migrants may ultimately pay more tax than some citizens), and in most wealthy countries access to healthcare is not contingent upon making a threshold number of tax payments, nor is the care which one receives proportional to the amount of tax one pays.[2] What matters is official recognition of having the moral status of being entitled to healthcare, not how much tax one pays or how long one has been a resident of a particular jurisdiction. This, then, returns us to the problem of moral recognition, and there may be reasons, convincing to some, that citizens should hold higher status and thus take priority over migrants (voluntary or otherwise). In the following section, I consider this claim and note one way of responding to the asserted moral priority of citizens over migrants and refugees.

13.3.2 Culpability and Compensation

Guaranteed, equitable access to healthcare for refugees and migrants is sometimes argued to be a "pull factor" which incentivizes people to migrate or seek refuge in a particular country (Shahvisi 2018). Ascertaining the accuracy of this claim is beyond the scope of this chapter, but it is worth noting that while pull factors may contribute to the motivation of some people to migrate to or seek refuge in one country rather than another, there are a wide range of reasons which also motivate people to leave or flee their original country of nationality (Souter 2014). In this section, I argue that when wealthy countries contribute to factors such as war, famine, and poverty (Plange 1979; Tan 2007; Mayblin 2017; Tadei 2018) which often serve as push factors in motivating migration, they harm the people forced to leave their homes as a result, and therefore have duties to compensate those who leave or flee their original country of nationality. Further, I argue that guaranteeing access to healthcare is a reasonable part of this compensation because many of the harms caused are directly related to

2. Ignoring for the moment the highly inequitable and inaccessible nature of the health insurance system in the US.

health. This argument is based on norms of tort liability and compensation (Coleman 1992) and the idea of reparations as a way of rectifying harm (Souter 2014, 326).

Indeed we do sometimes treat nations as responsible for the consequences of their actions and thereby liable for compensating their victims (Miller 2008; Tan 2008; Souter 2014). To illustrate, the British government has paid substantial compensation to Iraqi victims of "cruel and inhumane treatment, arbitrary detention or assault" by members of the British military during the invasion and occupation of Iraq by the US-led "coalition of the willing" in 2003 (Meyer and Zdrada 2006; Sabbagh 2021). In 2005, the United Nations adopted General Assembly Resolution 60/147, which states that victims of "gross violations of international human rights law and serious violations of international humanitarian law" (sec. VII. 11) are entitled to "[a]dequate, effective and prompt reparation for harm suffered" (sec. VII. 11. (b)). There are, therefore, existing norms which assert expectations that when nations (or those representing or acting on their behalf) act in ways that cause harm, they have liability-based obligations to compensate their victims.

These expectations are relatively clear in relation to those displaced by recent conflicts—there are specific harms (injuries, illness, trauma, displacement itself, etc.), identifiable agents (nation-states) that caused (and potentially benefited from) those harms, and specific actions which could be taken to moderate, ameliorate, or compensate for those harms (e.g., the provision of asylum and healthcare to treat injuries and ill health). Consequently, the argument that destination countries should provide equitable access to healthcare for refugees and migrants who were displaced by their actions is correspondingly clear—this particular country has specific responsibility to care for the needs of these particular people because of the special relationship created between them by the harm inflicted on the latter by the former. This argument can also be extended to refugees not resident in the country responsible for their displacement since the same causal relationship exists between them. Indeed, General Assembly Resolution 60/147 states that liable parties should either "provide reparation to the victim or compensate the State if the State has already provided reparation to the victim" (United Nations General Assembly 2005, sec. IX. 15), implying a continuation of state responsibility to refugees outside of their own borders.

The argument from liability becomes less clear, however, when the causal link between inciting state action and displacement is less obvious or immediate (Souter 2014, 339) or, as discussed by Iris Marion Young (2003, 9), when harmful actions were not strictly voluntary or were performed under conditions of ignorance. In such contexts, Young argues, responsibility for the harm caused is often "mitigated if not dissolved" (9). Climate change provides a useful illustration of these limitations of a strict liability model (Murtaugh and Schlax 2009; Sharma 2011; West-Oram and Widdows 2012, 4; Dwyer 2020). As the product of systemic factors as much as the aggregation of many individual actions, responsibility for the consequences of climate change is shared among a wide range of people, some of whom may not be equally culpable. It is difficult, therefore, to identify the specific agents responsible for the displacements caused by climate change (Dwyer 2020, 566–567).

Unlike cases where displacement is the result of military aggression, we cannot specify which carbon emissions from which country (much less, which person) contributed to the specific effects of climate change which led to the displacement of specific people, and thus cannot assign responsibility for providing compensation to specific parties accordingly. Further, it is possible that many people who directly contributed to climate change did so without knowing that their actions would cause harm, given the high levels of emissions prior to their impact becoming common knowledge.

The liability argument is further challenged when we acknowledge that many factors contributing to climate change, and subsequently to migration, are fundamentally built into the structures and institutions of the societies in which they occur (Young 2003, 6). Hence they may not easily be avoided by those who would be held responsible under a strict liability model (Hillier et al. 2009; Mayers et al. 2015; Beno 2021; Doğan and Dalkılıç 2023). To illustrate, in the absence of reliable public transport, the use of high-emission personal vehicles to commute to work becomes somewhat less than fully voluntary. To assign responsibility for compensating for the forced migration caused by climate change to individuals or their government[3] may seem unfair or implausible when there is uncertainty over which emissions caused which migrations and when certain emissions are simply necessary for participation in society.

However, while a liability model does have limitations (Young 2003, 10), it can provide an argument for the provision of aid in circumstances applicable to a high number of refugees given its proximity to existing norms of liability and compensation in widely accepted civic and legal norms. Viewing the provision of equitable access to healthcare to refugees as the equivalent of compensation in civic liability cases highlights the connection between the needs of certain refugees and the role in creating those needs by specific countries or groups of countries. Having to migrate or seek asylum because

3. Given that any costs required of governments or states found to be liable for the displacement of migrants will be met by residents of those states.

of the actions of other people is to be harmed by those people (Parekh 2014). This initial harm is often exacerbated by the increased vulnerability to deprivations of health experienced by refugees and caused by displacement (Boise et al. 2013; Hebebrand et al. 2016). This harm occurs regardless of the intent of the parties that caused it, which, having done so, should acquire moral responsibilities to compensate their victims (Miller 2008). It is important and appropriate to frame at least part of this compensation in terms of equitable access to healthcare because of the noted deprivations of health often endured by refugees—it is a specific, urgent need which wealthy, destination countries can address. Given that wealthy countries have historically emitted significantly higher levels of carbon than poorer countries (Dwyer 2020, 566), it can be argued that they have at least proportionally greater collective responsibility to provide support to climate refugees and migrants. These nations collectively contributed more to displacing these people, so they should collectively contribute proportionally more to meet their health needs (Souter 2014, 340).

In this section, I have outlined the argument that, according to the extent that wealthy countries create the push factors which make people seek asylum or residence internationally, they should provide access to care to those affected as a form of reparations for harms caused (Dwyer 2020). In this way, this argument responds to the pull factor, location of residency, and specificity problems identified in the previous section. It does not, however, apply to refugees and migrants who were not motivated to migrate by the harmful actions of wealthy nations.

13.3.3 Self-Interest and Reciprocity

Concern over the perceived high cost of immigration and asylum to destination countries (Hebebrand et al. 2016; Boise et al. 2013) has been described by Will Kymlicka (2015) as the "progressive's dilemma." Kymlicka argues that this dilemma arises from a tension between two commitments of progressive cosmopolitanism: first, to respect the rights to freedom of movement and to seek refuge and welfare support; second, to ensure that vulnerable people in destination countries retain access to important welfare services. According to Kymlicka, these commitments may be in competition with each other, or even be incompatible, given the potentially high costs of simultaneously fulfilling both adequately. At the core of this tension is the concern that mass migration or the provision of refuge may place unanswerable costs on health and welfare systems.

Central to Kymlicka's idea of the progressive's dilemma is the assumption, noted above, that there is at least some validity to the idea that citizens should take priority over migrants and refugees in accessing health and welfare services, and that this may seem a compelling reason to deny migrants and refugees equitable access to healthcare in their country of residence. In this section, I argue that doing so is at odds with the interests of destination countries and their citizens, for both economic and epidemiological reasons. I draw on earlier work noting the economic benefits gained by destination countries from migration as well as the epidemiological risks of failing to provide adequate healthcare to all residents of a nation (West-Oram and Buyx 2017).

First, in many contexts immigration has been shown to provide significant economic benefits to destination countries as a result of the taxes paid by migrants and their consumer spending. For example, a study on the economic impact of migrants in the UK found that between 2001 and 2011 the net positive contribution of migrants was roughly £20 billion (Dustmann and Frattini 2014). Similarly, immigration to the UK by highly educated people was estimated to save the country approximately £18 billion in training costs met by exit countries, which did not subsequently benefit from the presence of those departing (Taylor et al. 2011; Shahvisi 2018). While refugees may not initially contribute as effectively as migrants, it has been shown that when enabled to do so, through language training and the provision of healthcare, for instance, refugees do make significant economic contributions to their new country of residence (Legrain 2016, 7).

It has also been shown that in some contexts, denying access to care can be more costly than providing full access (Bozorgmehr and Razum 2015, 10. This is caused by the high costs of administering a second, more restrictive care pathway for refugees and migrants, and of policy decisions which delay care and prioritize the provision of only (typically less cost-effective) acute care rather than preventative measures (Bozorgmehr and Razum 2015). It is worth noting that guaranteeing migrants and refugees access to prophylactic and therapeutic services, such as vaccination and treatment for infectious diseases, also benefits citizens by limiting the spread of infectious disease (though this is not specific to migrants and refugees and applies to any underserved social group). Vaccination programs can generate herd immunity, for example, only if there is mass community participation, facilitated by universal accessibility to the program (Widdows and Marway 2015). Correlatively, ensuring equitable access to care can contribute to limiting the evolution of drug resistance by reducing the frequency of infections, increasing the likelihood that infections are appropriately managed and limiting opportunities for antimicrobial resistance to evolve (West-Oram 2013, 240; Battin et al. 2009, 142).

While the examples given here may not reflect the inevitable or universal outcome of guaranteeing equitable access, they do provide evidence for the argument that expanding access to healthcare systems can be in the interests of destination countries. Indeed it might be argued that there may be good reasons for wealthy countries to actively encourage immigration, given the economic benefits noted in this section.

A strength of this category of argument is that it does not rely on any shared recognition of the moral claims of refugees and migrants, and it responds directly to concerns about the cost of equitable care for migrants and refugees. However, in relying on empirical claims about the economic and epidemiological benefits of providing equitable healthcare to refugees and migrants, the argument is vulnerable to changes in circumstance. If it becomes apparent that it is no longer the case that the provision of healthcare services does provide economic benefits to wealthy nations, or if there is a way to limit epidemiological risk more effectively, by closing borders and deporting people, for example (West-Oram 2018a, 348), then the argument from self-interest loses (some of) its force. Equally, the epidemiological strand of the argument has limited applicability to noninfectious diseases or other sources of health deprivation (West-Oram 2018b, 583 n.74).

In the following section, I summarize the three types of argument for motivating the provision of guaranteed access to healthcare for refugees and migrants and discuss the ways they may overlap and function together to provide a comprehensive justification for such provision.

13.4 A HOLISTIC APPROACH: INTERACTION AND OVERLAP

My goal in this chapter has been to outline the foundations of three categories of argument for the provision of equitable healthcare to refugees and migrants by wealthy nations: the argument from moral status, the argument from liability, and the argument from self-interest. The first of these arguments is the simplest but lacks detail. It may not be convincing to those who have strongly nationalist, rather than cosmopolitan, intuitions about the people to whom duties are owed, or those who are concerned about the cost of providing equitable access to healthcare to refugees and migrants (the challenge at the heart of Kymlicka's "progressive's dilemma").

The second argument retains a focus on the entitlements of refugees and migrants but may be more convincing for some people since it draws on widely acknowledged legal norms of liability and compensation. However, it does not apply at all to refugees and migrants whose reasons for migration are not connected to the actions of other nations (but given the scale and impact of colonialism, for instance, may apply to more people than is immediately obvious; Plange 1979; Tan 2007). Importantly, it also fails to fully acknowledge the structural nature of many factors which motivate migration (Dwyer 2020), and in so doing may assign excessive liability to agents who may not have been able to act otherwise, and not enough to those whose actions were less obviously direct but more actively harmful (Young 2003, 9).

The third argument does not make any appeal to the moral or (quasi/pseudo-)legal entitlements held by refugees and migrants, and instead emphasizes the benefits which accrue to destination countries of providing healthcare to noncitizens. This argument is therefore intended to fill a rhetorical gap left by the first and second categories of argument and to appeal to those who remain unconvinced by their claims. It is, however, limited by the fact that it is based on context-dependent empirical data, meaning that if the context changes and data shows that it is no longer in the interest of wealthy destination countries, the argument loses its force.

The three categories of argument presented here should not be viewed as options from which to pick one optimal response to opposition to the provision of healthcare to refugees and migrants. Instead, my goal in this chapter has been to present an overview of a set of complementary, mutually reinforcing components of a comprehensive argument which can be refined according to distinct circumstances. My goal in framing the chapter in this way has been to acknowledge and respond to the reality that in different contexts, different arguments will have greater or lesser force and/or relevance. Further, given that the causes and consequences of migration and the pursuit of asylum/refuge are both systemic and multifactorial, an overly narrow argument cannot provide a comprehensive justification for the provision of healthcare to refugees and migrants in all circumstances. Thus, while each category may be individually applicable in specific circumstances, or more or less convincing to a particular audience, as noted, individually they are each subject to various limitations. However, considered collectively the three categories serve to provide a more detailed argument than they do alone, apply to a correspondingly wider range of circumstances, and better respond to the complexities arising from the structural nature of the injustices driving migration and the pursuit of refuge. Concern about high costs may be alleviated by reference to empirical data on the economic benefits of equitable healthcare provision, while the moral argument may be strengthened with reference to legal norms of liability and compensation.

REFERENCES

Amnesty International. 2023. “Who Is a Refugee, a Migrant or an Asylum Seeker?” https://www.amnesty.org/en/what-we-do/refugees-asylum-seekers-and-migrants/.

Battin, Margaret P., L. P. Francis, J. A. Jacobson, and C. B. Smith. 2009. *The Patient as Victim and Vector: Ethics and Infectious Disease*. Oxford University Press.

Bennett, Asa. 2016. "Did Britain Really Vote Brexit to Cut Immigration?" *The Telegraph*, June 29. https://www.telegraph.co.uk/news/2016/06/29/did-britain-really-vote-brexit-to-cut-immigration/.

Beno, Michal. 2021. "Face-to-Display Working: Decarbonisation Potential of Not Commuting to Work Before Covid-19 and During and After Lockdowns." *Academic Journal of Interdisciplinary Studies* 10 (3): 17–24.

Boise, Linda, Anais Tuepker, Teresa Gipson, Yves Vigmenon, Isabelle Soule, Sade Onadeko. 2013. "African Refugee and Immigrant Health Needs: Report from a Community-Based House Meeting Project." *Progress in Community Health Partnerships: Research, Education, and Action* 7: 369–378.

Bozorgmehr, Kayvan, and Oliver Razum. 2015. "Effect of Restricting Access to Health Care on Health Expenditures Among Asylum-Seekers in Germany." *European Journal of Public Health* 25 (3): 19. https://doi.org/10.1093/eurpub/ckv171.102.

Brock, Gillian. 2009. *Global Justice: A Cosmopolitan Account*. Oxford University Press.

Coleman, Jules L. 1992. "Tort Law and the Demands of Corrective Justice." *Indiana Law Review* 67: 349–379.

Doğan, Nezahat, and İbrahim Dalkılıç. 2023. "Environmental Footprint of Hollywood Film Industry: Myths vs Facts." *Environmental Science and Pollution Research* 30: 75029–75040. https://doi.org/10.1007/s11356-023-27643-5.

Dorling, Danny. 2016. "Brexit: The Decision of a Divided Country." *British Medical Journal* 354: i3697. https://doi.org/10.1136/bmj.i3697.

Dustmann, Christian, and Tommaso Frattini. 2014. "The Fiscal Effects of Immigration to the UK." *Economic Journal* 124: F593–F643. https://doi.org/10.1111/ecoj.12181.

Dwyer, James. 2020. "Environmental Migrants, Structural Injustice, and Moral Responsibility." *Bioethics* 34 (6): 562–569. https://doi.org/10.1111/bioe.12738.

Eurostat. 2023. "Migration and Migrant Population Statistics." Intergovernmental Organisation Data, Eurostat: Statistics Explained, August 7. https://ec.europa.eu/eurostat/statisticsexplained/index.php?title=Migration_and_migrant_population_statistics.

Fullerton, Maryellen. 2017. "Trump, Turmoil, and Terrorism: The US Immigration and Refugee Ban" *International Journal of Refugee Law* 29: 327–338. https://doi.org/10.1093/ijrl/eex021.

Hebebrand, Johannes, Dimitris Anagnostopoulos, Stephan Eliez, Henk Linse, Milica Pejovic-Milovancevic, and Henrikje Klasen. 2016. "A First Assessment of the Needs of Young Refugees Arriving in Europe: What Mental Health Professionals Need to Know." *European Child & Adolescent Psychiatry* 25: 1–6. https://doi.org/10.1007/s00787-015-0807-0.

Hiam, Lucinda, Sarah Steele, and Martin McKee. 2018. "Creating a 'Hostile Environment for Migrants': The British Government's Use of Health Service Data to Restrict Immigration Is a Very Bad Idea." *Health Economics, Policy and Law* 13 (2): 107–117. https://doi.org/10.1017/S1744133117000251.

Hillier, Jonathan, Cathy Hawes, Geoff Squire, Alex Hilton, Stuart Wale, and Pete Smith. 2009. "The Carbon Footprints of Food Crop Production." *International Journal of Agricultural Sustainability* 7: 107–118. https://doi.org/10.3763/ijas.2009.0419.

Ho, Anita. 2005. "Pharmaceutical Corporations and the Duty to Aid in HIV/AIDS Epidemic." *Business & Professional Ethics Journal* 24: 51–81. https://doi.org/10.2307/27801397.

International Organisation for Migration. 2023. "Who Is a Migrant?" https://www.iom.int/who-migrant-0.

Kymlicka, Will. 2015. "Solidarity in Diverse Societies: Beyond Neoliberal Multiculturalism and Welfare Chauvinism." *Comparative Migration Studies* 3 (17): 1–19. https://doi.org/10.1186/s40878-015-0017-4.

Legrain, P. 2016. *Refugees Work: A Humanitarian Investment That Yields Economic Dividends*. Tent Foundation.

Mayblin, Lucy. 2017. *Asylum After Empire: Colonial Legacies in the Politics of Asylum Seeking*. Rowman & Littlefield.

Mayers, Kieren, Jonathan Koomey, Rebecca Hall, Maria Bauer, Chris France, Amanda Webb. 2015. "The Carbon Footprint of Games Distribution." *Journal of Industrial Ecology* 19: 402–415. https://doi.org/10.1111/jiec.12181.

Meyer, Christoph O., and Adrian Zdrada. 2006. "Unpacking the 'Coalition of the Willing': A Comparative Analysis of Norms in British and Polish Press Debates on the Iraq Invasion." *European Security* 15: 23–45. https://doi.org/10.1080/09662830600776686

Miller, David. 2008. "National Responsibility and Global Justice." *Critical Review of International Social and Political Philosophy* 11: 383–399.

Murtaugh, Paul A., and Michael G. Schlax. 2009. "Reproduction and the Carbon Legacies of Individuals." *Global Environmental Change* 19: 14–20. https://doi.org/10.1016/j.gloenvcha.2008.10.007.

Nussbaum, Martha. 2003. "Capabilities as Fundamental Entitlements: Sen and Social Justice." *Feminist Economics* 9 (2–3): 33–59.

Parekh, Serena. 2014. "Beyond the Ethics of Admission: Stateless People, Refugee Camps and Moral Obligations." *Philosophy & Social Criticism* 40: 645–663.

Parekh, Serena. 2020. *No Refuge: Ethics and the Global Refugee Crisis*. Oxford University Press.

Pierce, Sarah, and Andrew Selee. 2017. "Immigration Under Trump: A Review of Policy Shifts in the Year Since the Election." Migration Policy Institute. https://www.migrationpolicy.org/research/immigration-under-trump-review-policy-shifts.

Plange, Nii-K. 1979. "Underdevelopment in Northern Ghana: Natural Causes or Colonial Capitalism?" *Review of African Political Economy* 6: 4–14. https://doi.org/10.1080/03056247908703393.

Rawlence, Ben. 2016. *City of Thorns: Nine Lives in the World's Largest Refugee Camp*. Picador.

Rechel, Bernd, Philipa Mladovsky, David Ingleby, Johan P. Mackenbach, and Martin McKee. 2013. "Migration and Health in an Increasingly Diverse Europe." *The Lancet* 381: 1235–1245. https://doi.org/10.1016/S0140-6736(12)62086-8.

Rorty, Richard. 1989. *Contingency, Irony, and Solidarity*. Cambridge University Press.

Owen, David. 2016. "Right, Well-Being and the Republic of Health: A Response to Jennings." *Public Health Ethics* 9 (2): 178–179. https://doi.org/10.1093/phe/phw009.

Sabbagh, Dan. 2021. "MoD Has Settled 417 Iraq War Compensation Claims This Year." *The Observer*, November 6. https://www.theguardian.com/uk-news/2021/nov/06/mod-has-settled-417-iraq-war-compensation-claims-this-year.

Scanlon, Thomas. 2000. *What We Owe to Each Other*. Harvard University Press.

Shahvisi, Arianne. 2018. "Health Worker Migration and Migrant Healthcare: Seeking Cosmopolitanism in the NHS." *Bioethics* 32 (6): 334–342. https://doi.org/10.1111/bioe.12432.

Sharma, Susan Sunila. 2011. "Determinants of Carbon Dioxide Emissions: Empirical Evidence from 69 Countries." *Applied Energy* 88: 376–382. https://doi.org/10.1016/j.apenergy.2010.07.022.

Shue, Henry. 1996. *Basic Rights: Subsistence, Affluence, and U.S. Foreign Policy*. Princeton University Press.

Singer, Peter. 1972. "Famine, Affluence, and Morality." *Philosophy and Public Affairs* 1: 229–243.

Souter, James. 2014. "Towards a Theory of Asylum as Reparation for Past Injustice." *Political Studies* 62: 326–342. https://doi.org/10.1111/1467-9248.12019.

Tadei, Federico. 2018. "The Long-Term Effects of Extractive Institutions: Evidence from Trade Policies in Colonial French Africa." *Economic History of Developing Regions* 33: 183–208. https://doi.org/10.1080/20780389.2018.1527685.

Tan, Kok-Chor. 2007. "Colonialism, Reparations and Global Justice." In *Reparations: Interdisciplinary Inquiries*, edited by Jon Miller and Rahul Kumar. Oxford University Press.

Tan, Kok-Chor. 2008. "National Responsibility, Reparations and Distributive Justice." *Critical Review of International Social and Political Philosophy* 11: 449–464. https://doi.org/10.1080/13698230802415912.

Taylor, Allyn L., Lenias Hwenda, Bjørn-Inge Larsen, and Nils Daulaire. 2011. "Stemming the Brain Drain—A WHO Global Code of Practice on International Recruitment of Health Personnel." *New England Journal of Medicine* 365: 2348–2351. https://doi.org/10.1056/NEJMp1108658.

United Nations General Assembly. 1948. "The Universal Declaration of Human Rights." https://www.un.org/en/about-us/universal-declaration-of-human-rights.

United Nations General Assembly. 2005. "Basic Principles and Guidelines on the Right to a Remedy and Reparation for Victims of Gross Violations of International Human Rights Law and Serious Violations of International Humanitarian Law." Resolution 60/147. https://www.ohchr.org/en/instruments-mechanisms/instruments/basic-principles-and-guidelines-right-remedy-and-reparation.

United Nations High Commissioner for Refugees. 2010. "Convention and Protocol Relating to the Status of Refugees." https://www.unhcr.org/protection/basic/3b66c2aa10/convention-protocol-relating-status-refugees.html.

United Nations High Commissioner for Refugees. 2023a. "Figures at a Glance." June 14. https://www.unhcr.org/figures-at-a-glance.html.

United Nations High Commissioner for Refugees. 2023b. "What Is a Refugee?" https://www.unhcr.org/what-refugee.

Uthayakumar-Cumarasamy, Amaran. 2020. "The 'Hostile Environment' and the Weaponization of the UK Health System." *Medicine, Conflict and Survival* 36 (2): 132–136. https://doi.org/10.1080/13623699.2020.1766792.

Virdee, Satnam, and Brendan McGeever. 2018. "Racism, Crisis, Brexit." *Ethnic and Racial Studies* 41: 1802–1819. https://doi.org/10.1080/01419870.2017.1361544.

West-Oram, Peter G. N. 2013. "Freedom of Conscience and Health Care in the United States of America: The Conflict Between Public Health and Religious Liberty in the Patient Protection and Affordable Care Act." *Health Care Analysis* 21: 237–247. https://doi.org/10.1007/s10728-013-0251-6.

West-Oram, Peter G. N. 2016. "Three Approaches to Global Health Care Justice: Rejecting the Positive/Negative Rights Distinction." In *International Development and Human Aid: Principles, Norms and Institutions for the Global Sphere*, edited by Gabriele De Angelis and Paulo Barcelos. Edinburgh University Press. https://edinburghuniversitypress.com/book-international-development-and-human-aid.html.

West-Oram, Peter G. N. 2018a. "From Self-Interest to Solidarity: One Path Towards Delivering Refugee Health." *Bioethics* 32 (6): 343–352. https://doi.org/10.1111/bioe.12472.

West-Oram, Peter. 2018b. "Solidarity as a National Health Care Strategy." *Bioethics* 32: 577–584. https://doi.org/10.1111/bioe.12443.
West Oram, Peter G. N., and Alena Buyx. 2017. "Global Health Solidarity." *Public Health Ethics* 10 (2): 212–224. https://doi.org/10.1093/phe/phw021.
West-Oram, Peter G. N., and Heather Widdows. 2012. "Global Population and Global Justice: Equitable Distribution of Resources Among Countries," *eLS*: 4. http://onlinelibrary.wiley.com/doi/10.1002/9780470015902.a0024140/pdf.
Widdows, Heather, and Herjeet Marway. 2015. "A Global Public Goods Approach to the Health of Migrants." *Public Health Ethics* 8: 130. https://doi.org/10.1093/phe/phv013.
Wolff, Jonathan. 2012. *The Human Right to Health*. W. W. Norton.
Young, Iris Marion. 2003. "Political Responsibility and Structural Injustice." In *A Volume of Lindley Lectures, Delivered at the University of Kansas: Freedom and Morality*, edited by John Bricke. University of Kansas, Department of Philosophy.

14

Hidden Knowledge and Epistemic (In)Justice in US Migrant Detention

SHANNON FYFE

14.1 INTRODUCTION

In 2018 and 2019, major US news outlets reported shocking health conditions within migrant detention facilities at the US-Mexico border. The allegations included lack of soap and clothing at facilities for children (Dickerson 2019), holding a premature baby in the detention facility where it was born instead of transferring it to a neonatal unit at a hospital (Galvan and Burke 2019), and mental health crises evidenced by some of those detained making nooses from bedsheets (Rayasam 2019). Reports from journalists, members of Congress, federal inspectors, and other officials who visited migrant detention facilities run by Customs and Border Patrol, Immigration and Customs Enforcement (ICE), and the Department of Health and Human Services Administration for Children and Families suggested that basic and severe health needs were being ignored. In January 2019, the Office of the Inspector General of Homeland Security (OIG) issued a report on ICE's management of its detention facility contracts. It found deficiencies that presented "significant safety and health risks" and determined that they had "no way of verifying whether these deficiencies have been corrected" (OIG 2019).

The public, or at least some portion of it, was repeatedly horrified to learn about this situation and others faced by migrants at the US-Mexico border. What the public did not learn about migrant health then, and does not know now, is what has not been in the news. There have been multiple congressional delegations to border detention facilities to assess the facilities firsthand (Moore et al. 2019). These have been met with varying success in their attempts to gain access (Bump 2018; Bohn and Johnston 2019;

Shannon Fyfe, *Hidden Knowledge and Epistemic (In)Justice in US Migrant Detention*. In: *Forced Migration and Health Justice*. Edited by: Lisa A. Eckenwiler, Verina Wild, Anna Gotlib, Ryoa Chung, and Deborah Zion,
Oxford University Press. © Oxford University Press (2026). DOI: 10.1093/oso/9780197795491.003.0014

Coniatori 2019). Journalists, too, have sought access to facilities and have been largely denied (Bauder 2018; Sullivan 2021). Instead, most information the US public has about the health of migrants at the US-Mexico border has been obtained (and filtered) through attorneys, chaplains, medical professionals, and other officials. As we will see, these parties sometimes have good reasons to stay silent, which keeps knowledge about harms to migrant communities hidden.

In this chapter, I argue that in addition to the physical and mental harms migrants at the US-Mexico border are suffering as a result of the lack of appropriate healthcare in detention facilities, they are also experiencing two kinds of epistemic injustice with respect to these health conditions. First, the migrants' own testimonies are often trapped within the walls of the detention facilities; and second, the officials, attorneys, healthcare providers, and chaplains who have first- or secondhand knowledge of the health conditions may be unwilling to share this knowledge with the public to retain access to their clients or their jobs. However, I conclude that, as with those who have access to other carceral spaces, these individuals' moral and professional responsibility is more complicated than just demanding that they practice epistemic justice by bringing the health conditions of migrants in detention facilities to light.

I begin by exploring the ways in which US carceral spaces generally, and US migrant detention facilities specifically, generate health injustices and epistemic harms. I then consider two purported solutions for reducing both the epistemic and health harms to individuals incarcerated in the US, including migrants: releasing migrants and epistemic activism. Finally, I consider the problem of "sourcing norms" that remains in the face of epistemic activism. My conclusion is that while individuals with access to migrant detention facilities have both moral and professional obligations, these obligations are not necessarily met by epistemic activism.

14.2 FROM EPISTEMIC INJUSTICE TO HEALTH INJUSTICE

The failures to correct deficiencies in healthcare in migrant detention facilities result in the continued health injustice faced by migrants. In this section, I outline some of the healthcare injustices facing individuals in detention facilities in the US, especially migrant detention facilities. But the situation also permits further maltreatment of the detained migrants, specifically epistemic harm. Accordingly, I then consider the two kinds of carceral epistemic harms that not only allow for the continuation of health injustice but also constitute discrete harms in and of themselves.

14.2.1 Health Injustice

While there are unique features of the epistemic (and healthcare) conditions facing migrants detained at the US-Mexico border,[1] there are plenty of features that are consistent with carceral practices at facilities all over the US. In 1976, the US Supreme Court found, in *Estelle v. Gamble*, that "deliberate indifference to serious medical needs of prisoners constitutes the 'unnecessary and wanton infliction of pain' . . . proscribed by the Eighth Amendment. This is true whether the indifference is manifested by prison doctors in their response to the prisoner's needs or by prison guards in intentionally denying or delaying access to medical care or intentionally interfering with treatment once prescribed." In other words, the US Constitution guarantees a minimal right to healthcare for incarcerated persons, and each facility is obligated to offer that healthcare in coordination with public and/or private providers.[2] The US disproportionately incarcerates poor people of color, and therefore chronic health conditions that are more common among poor people, like heart disease, diabetes, hypertension, and asthma, are overrepresented in carceral facilities (Seerval 2022). Mental health conditions are also disproportionately represented (Wilper et al. 2009).

Yet healthcare services for incarcerated individuals remain inconsistent and insufficient. Medical neglect continues to kill hundreds of people incarcerated in the US every year (Reutter 2017). Available data suggests that basic (McCann 2022),[3] emergency (Martin et al. 2020), reproductive (Gulaid and McCoy 2022), and mental (Thompson and Eldridge 2018) healthcare needs often go unmet. In recent years, the COVID-19 pandemic has compounded the harm to incarcerated persons caused by a lack of healthcare infrastructure in many carceral facilities (COVID Prison Project n.d.).[4] Decarceration is the most straightforward solution for many of these healthcare issues, as a lower carceral population will reduce the number of individuals subjected to the carceral healthcare system, enable better social distancing practices to reduce the transmission of communicable diseases

1. While there is also substantial evidence of healthcare and other injustices on the Mexico side of the border as well, I will focus on US facilities.

2. Larger facilities may provide a range of healthcare services on a regular basis, while smaller and/or short-term facilities may have minimal services on site. Who pays for the healthcare of incarcerated individuals depends on the facility, the healthcare provider(s), and the circumstances, including whether or not the individual has health insurance. But a facility cannot decline to provide necessary health services due to the cost of treatment or the need to coordinate off-site care.

3. Many facilities fail to provide routine care to individuals with and without persistent medical conditions.

4. As of June 2, 2023, there have been nearly 3,000 deaths of incarcerated people in US prisons due to COVID-19. Most of the "largest, single-site outbreaks [in the US] since the beginning of the pandemic have been in jails and prisons."

like COVID-19 (Henry 2020), and reduce the stress on these healthcare systems altogether (ACLU n.d.).

In migrant detention facilities at the US-Mexico border, the healthcare issues are no better. A division of ICE, the ICE Health Service Corps, is responsible for providing essential healthcare to all noncitizens who are detained in ICE facilities and coordinating any necessary off-site care (Human Rights Watch 2018). As with the incarcerated population more generally, migrants who are detained at the US-Mexico border are more likely than the general US population to suffer from health conditions already, due to poverty and other social determinants of health, lack of healthcare access in their country of origin, and/or conditions or injuries acquired during their journey to the US border. Many detention facilities offer substandard care, including mismedication, "denial of care, inadequate initial medical screenings and physical examinations, delayed or lack of response to sick call requests, unreasonable delays in obtaining off-site care, failure to monitor chronic conditions, improper mental health care and the misuse of isolation, botched emergency responses, and just generally mediocre care by facility and medical staff" (Inda 2020, 702). For instance, a 26-year-old native of El Salvador died in 2008 in ICE custody after being denied access to HIV medication and falling victim to an infection while his immune system was vulnerable (*Baires v. United States* 2011).

Migrants to the US have been denied access to reproductive healthcare in particular, as there are no federal standards governing reproductive healthcare for incarcerated persons (McCann 2022). This has resulted in detention facilities denying access to abortions and failing to provide care to pregnant women, sometimes resulting in miscarriages, stillbirths, or live births of babies with serious medical issues (Ellmann 2019). Thousands of migrants have reported being sexually assaulted while in detention facilities in the US (Da Silva 2018).

Mental healthcare and care for mental illnesses are often delayed or denied altogether in US migrant detention facilities (National Immigrant Justice Center n.d.), despite the fact that detention increases the likelihood of anxiety, depression, and posttraumatic stress disorders (von Werthen et al. 2018). The mental health conditions for children are particularly worrisome, especially during the period when children were routinely separated from their families at the border (Hegarty 2018). One emergency physician reported referring an eight-year-old boy for inpatient psychiatric treatment after seeing him distraught over being separated from his parents and threatening self-harm (Schaffer 2018). He arrived at the emergency room without having received any mental health treatment in the detention facility where he was being held (Schaffer 2018). When mental healthcare is provided, it can include such improper practices as "prescribing the wrong medications or none at all; failing to respond to crisis moments or breakdowns; and abusive bedside manner and treatment of individuals suffering from mental health challenges" (National Immigrant Justice Center 2022). Solitary confinement has been used for disciplinary and administrative segregation, sometimes exacerbating the conditions of migrants with a history of trauma or other mental health conditions (Disability Rights California 2019).

The response to the COVID-19 pandemic has resulted in several kinds of health injustice to migrants. First, Title 42 has been used to systematically exclude asylum seekers from entering the US on the basis of the public health threat. Title 42 is a federal regulation that empowers federal health authorities to exclude migrants from entering through a border on the basis of protecting the US population from contagious diseases (US Congress 1952). The Trump and Biden administrations both utilized this regulation during the COVID-19 pandemic to justify expelling migrants instead of allowing them to enter and seek asylum, in part due to the crowded migration detention facilities and the highly transmissible nature of COVID-19 (Gramlich 2022). Within detention facilities, overcrowding, inconsistent access to soap, cleaning supplies, and masks (Lee et al. 2023), and the lack of basic testing/quarantine protocols have contributed to the spread of COVID-19 (Tosh et al. 2021; Montoya-Galvez 2022). A 2021 report by the OIG indicated that "inspected ICE detention facilities did not follow all coronavirus mitigation protocols."

14.2.2 Epistemic Injustice

There are several kinds of epistemic injustice suffered by incarcerated individuals who are also experiencing health injustice. The first is the injustice of having their testimonies trapped within the walls of their carceral facility, which constitutes a direct epistemic injustice to those individuals. I see two ways in which these trapped testimonies about health injustice constitute an epistemic harm. The first is as a form of testimonial injustice. As a source of justification, testimony involves the kind of reliance on other people that Aristotle (1962) considers part of what allows us to live as human beings in societies. Testimony is our primary source of social evidence, and we rely on testimony as social evidence from many doxastic agents (Audi 2011). Testimonial injustice is a form of epistemic injustice that "occurs when prejudice causes a hearer to give a deflated level of credibility to a speaker's word" (Fricker 2007, 1). An incarcerated individual might receive this deflated credibility from a hearer on the basis of prejudice due to a feature (or features) of social identity (Fricker 2007). Identity features could be an individual's race, national origin, appearance, or social class. But it could also simply be the marker of "incarcerated person" that leads a hearer to automatically discount the testimony of the speaker. The "general public, including correctional staff and health care professionals, tend to view prisoners as subhuman, as those who have surrendered their rights by being convicted of crimes" (Restum 2005, 1690).[5]

Epistemic harm to incarcerated individuals as a testimonial injustice describes the phenomenon of hearers taking the testimonies of incarcerated individuals regarding their healthcare less seriously than they should. The hearers might be internal to the institution, as correctional staff, healthcare professionals, or administrators, who hear the testimonies and, while not discounting them altogether, fail to give the speakers and their experiences a serious response. Specifically, these hearers might claim that the health injustices are "not as bad" as the incarcerated individuals make them out to be and either deny or delay proper care as a result. The hearers could also be external to the institution, such as friends, family members, or government officials who receive information about the health injustice occurring inside a carceral facility and determine that it might not be "that bad" due to their assessment that the incarcerated individual is someone not to be trusted—or at least not completely.

Yet testimonial injustice assumes that the speakers are heard at all. We should also consider agential epistemic injustice, through which a speaker is epistemically silenced altogether. Agential epistemic injustice occurs, according to José Medina, when hearers "alienat[e] subjects from their epistemic agency and their capacity to give testimony about emergencies" (2021, 189). While testimonial injustice renders incarcerated individuals less credible, agential epistemic injustice renders incarcerated individuals non-agents in terms of knowledge, on the basis of their identity as incarcerated persons. Medina gives an example of detainees crying out for help or pushing an emergency call button, and guards refusing to give the attempt at speaking any credibility. Instead the guards behave as if the emergency had never taken place. The emergency call, according to Medina, "becomes short-circuited, not registered as such by the guards, and treated as mere noise that is not part of a communicative act that carries any force" (2021, 188). Epistemic silencing thus happens with respect to internal hearers, but carceral staff may ensure that it happens with respect to external hearers as well, by preventing incarcerated persons from reaching out to individuals

5. Many incarcerated individuals in the US, including those in migrant detention facilities and in pretrial detention, may not have ever been convicted of a crime, but the assumption that they have done something to "surrender their rights" often exists regardless.

or organizations outside the facility with information about healthcare injustices.

I will address these direct epistemic harms later. But first, let's consider an additional epistemic harm to incarcerated individuals: the indirect epistemic injustice that can be perpetrated through secondhand knowers. We have already identified some of the people who interact with incarcerated individuals and either witness firsthand or receive testimonies related to health injustice. Corrections officers, carceral healthcare professionals, and administrators may all have this sort of knowledge of health injustice. Others who may have access to carceral facilities and receive information related to healthcare injustice include attorneys, government officials or politicians, non-institutional healthcare providers, chaplains or other spiritual advisors, and prison volunteers. This group could also include friends or family members who are permitted to visit carceral facilities. I classify this group as people who either witness health injustice firsthand, witness the effects of health injustice firsthand, or obtain information about health injustice directly from a victim or witness.

An indirect epistemic injustice occurs, quite simply, when the secondhand knower does not pass along their knowledge of healthcare injustice, especially to a party that might be able to do something to rectify the injustice. For instance, a corrections officer who is informed by an incarcerated individual about an infection that has resulted from delayed medical care, and then shown the infection, but does nothing to help the incarcerated individual obtain medical treatment, commits a direct epistemic wrong. However, if the corrections officer attempts to assist the individual to obtain medical treatment, yet does nothing to remedy the systematic healthcare injustice by acting as a watchdog and sharing the incarcerated individual's experience with prison administrators, government officials, or journalists, the corrections officer may be committing this indirect form of epistemic injustice. The incarcerated individual may have no way of sharing their experiences, and we might think that someone with access inside and outside of the carceral facility has a prima facie obligation to pass the story along in service of ending the healthcare injustice. In the section that follows, I will show why this prima facie obligation may not be sufficient to address either the epistemic or healthcare injustices.

14.3 RELEASE AND RESISTANCE/ACTIVISM AS JUSTICE?

In this section, I consider two ways of responding to instances of healthcare and epistemic injustices perpetrated against incarcerated individuals generally, and migrants specifically. In doing so, I make use of my own experiences as a second- and third-hand knower about healthcare injustice in carceral facilities to illustrate some of the reasons why secondhand knowers may not share information about healthcare injustice. These decisions should not necessarily be seen as indirect epistemic injustice, if they are made in service of the health and well-being of the incarcerated individuals. This is especially the case if these decisions are made in collaboration with the incarcerated individuals.

14.3.1 Release

The most straightforward way to reduce healthcare injustice in carceral spaces is to reduce the carceral population. As noted earlier, this reduces the strain on limited resources within a carceral facility, increases the possibility of social distancing and other practices intended to reduce the spread of communicable diseases, and prevents individuals from being subjected to the carceral healthcare system altogether (ACLU n.d.). There are many ways to reduce the carceral population and reduce opportunities for healthcare injustice; I will discuss only a few of these options. With a reasonably quick turnaround, government officials and prison administrators (most often individual judges on a case-by-case basis) can release incarcerated individuals (1) with a high risk of death or serious illness associated with contracting COVID-19 or other communicable diseases (National Academies of Science, Engineering, and Medicine 2020) and (2) with a low risk of recidivism, including older individuals and individuals with short criminal histories (National Academies of Science, Engineering, and Medicine 2020). Longer-term ways to reduce the general prison population include revising criminal laws to reduce penalties and offer opportunities for sentence reconsideration, especially for young offenders, and providing better social supports for at-risk communities and returning citizens.

Another way to reduce incarceration, especially in migrant detention facilities, is to release individuals who do not present a public safety threat from pretrial or pre-hearing detention. Alternatives to migrant detention, including parole, home visits, and GPS monitoring, are policies with "high rates of compliance, lower costs in comparison to detention, and represent a more humane treatment of immigrants" (Lee et al. 2023, 9). The US government should adopt these policies to reduce the migrant detention population immediately, and thereby reduce the healthcare injustice perpetrated against migrants at the US-Mexico border.

14.3.2 Epistemic Resistance/Activism

There is also a straightforward response to the direct epistemic injustices facing migrants who are detained at the US-Mexico border, although it can hardly be called a "solution" given that it will be quite challenging to implement. In short, those who interact with incarcerated individuals must stop engaging in practices that amount to testimonial and agential epistemic injustice. Direct epistemic injustice, either based solely on the identity of incarcerated individuals as incarcerated individuals or combined with prejudice based on race, ethnicity, or some other characteristic, is unjustifiable.

A second response to direct epistemic injustice in carceral facilities is known as epistemic resistance or epistemic activism. According to Medina, incarcerated individuals can "become epistemic activists by denouncing and resisting unfair patterns of epistemic neglect and silencing: for example, by expressing epistemic solidarity by backing up one another's testimonies, so that they mitigate the harmful consequences that individual voices typically encounter in dysfunctional testimonial dynamics" (2021, 193). This is complicated, as it acknowledges and celebrates the epistemic agency of individuals who have had this agency explicitly denied by institutional powers, but it also puts the burden on these same individuals to force institutions that have been harming them to stop harming them. It also means that epistemic activists subject themselves to retaliation by the institution.

In migrant detention facilities, the precarity of some individuals might be greater for no reason other than the fact that they can be deported. The cost of epistemic resistance may be quite high, including retaliation in the form of solitary confinement, physical abuse, the denial of basic needs, and perhaps transfer to a different carceral facility. Migrant populations can be subjected to all these forms of retaliation, but they can also be removed from the US altogether, possibly forcing them to return to a violent community that necessitated their attempt to seek asylum in the first place. This is a distinct, if not categorically worse, kind of vulnerability.

We might think that in addition to epistemic activism on the part of carceral populations, or perhaps in lieu of it, the secondhand knowers have the greatest moral and professional obligation to challenge healthcare injustice and epistemic injustice by engaging in epistemic resistance themselves. These agents, as non-incarcerated persons, do not have the same sort of vulnerability as incarcerated persons, nor can they be subjected to the same kind of retaliation—in the form of abuse, neglect, or other punitive responses—that incarcerated persons may be. And yet the choices made by secondhand knowers to speak out or not speak out are more complicated than they might appear. Carceral facility administrators can engage in retaliation against secondhand knowers in ways that may harm not only these secondhand knowers but also the incarcerated individuals themselves.

For instance, I was once part of a philosophy reading group/activist group, Reciprocal Education and Community Healing (REACH), of community members and individuals on death row in Nashville, Tennessee. We had weekly meetings with about 10 men living in the death row unit at the Riverbend Maximum Security Institution (RMSI), which required us to obtain volunteer badges from the prison administration and to submit to extensive security screening before each meeting. It took me several months to be cleared for my volunteer badge after completing an application and going through a training and certification process. Moreover, that badge could be revoked at any time by the RMSI administration. Several of the community members had their badges revoked during their time volunteering with REACH based on the administration's concerns with items the volunteers had worn or brought inside the facility, or things they had said. The insiders and outsiders were constantly aware of how the choices we made with respect to our work and our activism might be perceived by the RMSI administration. In general, we made decisions together about what the outsiders might say outside the walls of the facility, while trying to center the voices and the desires of the insiders. If they were willing to risk their access to the REACH volunteers, then we had to be willing to risk giving up our volunteer badges. Some information was clearly not to be shared—so I won't reveal it now. I learned a lot from my insider friends and colleagues about prison conditions, especially related to medical neglect and delay. If I had spoken out about these conditions—with or without the permission of the insiders—I likely would have forfeited access to a group that the insiders found to be a valuable part of their lives on death row.

However, if I had lost my volunteer badge and was no longer permitted on death row at RMSI, the loss to my colleagues and friends would have been relatively minimal. This is not the case with many secondhand knowers. At detention facilities on the US-Mexico border, for instance, outsiders with access to the facilities may have much stronger reasons to stay in the good graces of the facility administrators. Chaplains, medical professionals, and lawyers are able to enter the facilities only with the permission of the administrators. We might find this hard to believe—shouldn't everyone have access to legal counsel? In fact, the Sixth Amendment right to the assistance of counsel applies only in criminal cases, and the government is obligated to provide counsel only if the individual is accused of a felony (US Constitution; *Gideon v. Wainwright* 1963). Most deportation proceedings are civil, and even if migrants are charged for crossing the border illegally, this offense is a misdemeanor. In fact, only about 14% of detained migrants have legal counsel in their removal cases (Eagly and Shafer 2016). Accordingly, if you are a detained migrant and you have access to an attorney to represent you in a removal case or in a civil rights case, you are likely to want to do what you can to ensure that you retain access to that attorney.

A good friend of mine—let's call them J—is such an attorney. J has told me countless horror stories about treatment of migrants in US-Mexico border detention facilities, stories that include physical and sexual abuse, medical neglect, and failure to provide medical treatment altogether. Some of these stories appeared in the news. But many have not. Did J fail their clients by not engaging in epistemic activism? I would argue they did not. J would have lost access to the detention facilities and to their clients had they spoken publicly about much of what they learned while inside the facilities. J would not have been able to obtain legal status for their clients or win civil rights cases for their clients had they been denied access to the detention facilities and their clients. How do I know? Because when J did end up speaking out publicly against healthcare injustice, when they organized women to talk about their horrific experiences in one of these border detention facilities, J received a lifetime ban from that ICE facility. Not one of the other secondhand knowers with access to the facility was willing to go to bat for J at the time because they knew it would lead to their losing the ability to visit their clients as well.

As with my colleagues in REACH, there may be some instances in which it should be up to the direct victims of healthcare and epistemic injustice to decide whether they are willing to lose access to their lawyer or chaplain or other individual seeking to help them improve their situation. But the direct victim is not the only issue. First, these secondhand knowers could lose their jobs. Some may be reliant on the job to provide for themselves and their families. J, for instance, would likely have given up their job in a heartbeat if asked to balance the healthcare of their clients against their own financial security. But the second issue is that most of these secondhand knowers are helping more than one individual, or more than one group of individuals. J and others like them risk losing access to many other clients if they speak out on the circumstances of one of their clients. Seeking justice for these detained migrants involves more than just being "willing" to risk the personal consequences of retaliation in the face of epistemic resistance, and within these institutions and carceral systems it's not clear that there is a good answer for what a secondhand knower should do.

In the next section, I will consider one more concern, assuming firsthand knowers and/or secondhand knowers do decide to engage in epistemic activism and share testimonies about healthcare injustice with the world outside carceral facilities.

14.4 SOURCING NORMS AND FURTHER TESTIMONIAL INJUSTICE

Even when firsthand and/or secondhand knowers are willing to risk retaliation or other negative consequences and share their testimonies regardless, their attempts at epistemic activism may still fail due to the expectations—of journalists, academics, and the public—as to what counts as an appropriate and respected "source" of knowledge. In this section I briefly identify how these norms present a further threat to testimonial justice and healthcare justice. I am not arguing that we should get rid of citations or journalistic standards; I am merely identifying how these norms can present an issue for seeking healthcare and epistemic justice for detained migrants and other incarcerated persons in the US.

You will notice that in much of the first section of this chapter, I cited journalists and watchdog groups, rather than academic articles, in supporting my claims about healthcare injustice in carceral facilities. As you might expect, especially after reading section 14.2, there is inconsistent access to sources within carceral facilities. The authors of one of the academic papers I cite explicitly admit that they obtained their survey respondents through referrals from immigration lawyers (Lee et al. 2023), and as I have already stated, only 14% of detained migrants have a lawyer to represent them. Most of the sources I cite, news media or otherwise, obtain their information on an ad hoc basis as well, from whoever they have access to and is willing to risk retaliation for speaking out, or from whoever has already been lucky or unlucky enough to have been released from migrant detention. You will also notice that in referring to my friend J's experience at the US-Mexico border, I don't name them or formally cite interviews I conducted with them. I don't cite interviews with members of REACH. And I don't provide you with concrete details.

Do you believe me?

Last year, while writing an op-ed with a returned citizen who spent 30 years in the federal prison system in the US, he told me that two men from Washington, DC, had been murdered while incarcerated in federal penitentiaries. In the op-ed, we argued that DC should be doing more to bring its citizens home because they were particularly vulnerable to the violence caused by racism and hypermasculinity in federal penitentiaries. When we found an outlet to publish our op-ed, the editor asked for our source regarding the deaths of the two men. The editor had been unable to find a news outlet reporting the details of the deaths. My colleague and I knew about the circumstances of the deaths because he had heard about them from insiders. We were not going to put his sources in danger by naming them, but the news outlet publishing our op-ed needed to follow journalistic norms and not publish something unsupported by evidence. In the end, we found a mutually agreeable way to frame the information we wanted to share with the public, but the experience of trying to bring information outside the walls of a carceral facility, in the interest of insiders yet without subjecting them to retaliation, stayed with me.

Do you believe me?

I am not explicitly engaged in epistemic resistance in coalition with firsthand knowers about healthcare injustice in migrant detention facilities here. I care very much about incarcerated individuals, at the US-Mexico border and all over the US. But this is a chapter in an academic volume, and my objective is not to share their stories as a secondhand knower. If you do not believe me, or you are wary of my claims, I don't see that as a testimonial injustice. I recognize the norms of the venue, and I have the privilege to do so. But when firsthand knowers attempt to share their information, and they are not believed or their stories are not given uptake because their stories are their own or they are obtained secondhand from others who have experienced injustice firsthand, the expectations for citations or a willingness to share details that might put someone at risk present a challenge. Journalists are inclined to give (some) firsthand knowers the benefit of the doubt, and news outlets can often find ways around these sourcing norms. Yet we can see that the risk of being seen as not credible, or having one's story ignored, may still present a barrier for firsthand knowers of healthcare injustice. For firsthand and secondhand knowers, a commitment to epistemic resistance may not be enough.

14.5 CONCLUSION

Across the US, and especially at the US-Mexico border, carceral facilities are often sites of serious healthcare injustice in the form of mistreatment, delayed treatment, and failure to provide medical care altogether. I have shown that some knowledge of this healthcare injustice stays hidden behind the walls of the migrant detention facility due to direct epistemic injustice against firsthand knowers (as testimonial injustice or agential epistemic injustice) or indirect epistemic injustice against firsthand knowers when secondhand knowers do not pass along the testimonies of firsthand knowers. We should respond to these healthcare injustices by releasing incarcerated migrants, and we should support detained migrants who want to engage in epistemic resistance. It may be that some secondhand knowers have an obligation to engage in epistemic activism themselves, but others may be doing more to support the health and well-being of detained migrants by keeping their knowledge about healthcare injustice hidden.

We on the outside must at least be willing to change our expectations for what counts as "credible knowledge" obtained from behind the walls of migrant detention facilities.[6]

REFERENCES

ACLU. n.d. "Overcrowding and Other Threats to Health and Safety." Accessed June 1, 2023. https://www.aclu.org/issues/prisoners-rights/cruel-inhuman-and-degrading-conditions/overcrowding-and-other-threats-health.

Aristotle. 1962. *Politics*. Translated by J. A. Sinclair. Penguin.

Audi, Robert. 2011. *Epistemology—A Contemporary Introduction to the Theory of Knowledge*. 3rd ed. Routledge.

Baires v. United States, 2011. Third amended complaint and demand for jury trial, Docket No. 3:09-CV-05171. N.D. Cal., August 8.

Bauder, David. 2018. "Media Fight Access Restrictions on Child Detention centers." PBS, June 26. https://www.pbs.org/newshour/nation/media-fight-access-restrictions-on-child-detention-centers.

Bohn, Kevin, and Chuck Johnston. 2019. "Three Members of Congress Say Trump Admin Denying Them Access to Facility Housing Unaccompanied Migrant Children." CNN, April 7. https://www.cnn.com/2019/04/07/politics/democrats-migrant-children-florida/index.html.

Bump, Philipp. 2018. "Legislators Were Turned Away from ICE Detention Centers. The Administration Has the Right to Do That." *Washington Post*, June 21. https://www.washingtonpost.com/news/politics/wp/2018/06/21/legislators-were-turned-away-from-ice-detention-centers-the-administration-has-the-right-to-do-that/.

Coniatori, Tess. 2019. "Rep. Castro Secretly Recorded a Migrant Facility in Texas. Here's What He Found." PBS, July 2. https://www.pbs.org/newshour/politics/rep-castro-secretly-recorded-a-migrant-facility-in-texas-heres-what-he-found.

COVID Prison Project. n.d. Accessed June 1, 2023. https://covidprisonproject.com/.

Da Silva, Chantal. 2018. "Thousands of Migrants Have Reported Sexual Abuse While in ICE Custody." *Newsweek*, July 23. https://www.newsweek.com/thousands-migrants-have-reported-sexual-abuse-while-ice-custody-1036580.

Dickerson, Caitlin. 2019. "'There Is a Stench': Soiled Clothes and No Baths for Migrant Children at a Texas Center." *New York Times*, June 21. https://www.nytimes.com/2019/06/21/us/migrant-children-border-soap.html.

Disability Rights California. 2019. "There Is No Safety Here: The Dangers for People with Mental Illness and Other Disabilities in Immigration Detention at GEO Group's Adelanto ICE Processing Center." March 5. https://www.disabilityrightsca.org/post/there-is-no-safety-here-the-dangers-for-people-with-mental-illness-and-other-disabilities-at.

Eagly, Ingrid, and Steven Shafer. 2016. "Access to Counsel in Immigration Court." American Immigration Council, September 28. https://www.americanimmigrationcouncil.org/research/access-counsel-immigration-court.

6. The author is grateful for conversations with J, REACH members, Anthony Petty, and Wesley Buckwalter, each of whom have contributed to the knowledge and analysis in this chapter.

Ellmann, Nora. 2019. "Immigration Detention Is Dangerous for Women's Health and Rights." Center for American Progress, October 21. https://www.americanprogress.org/article/immigration-detention-dangerous-womens-health-rights/.

Estelle v. Gamble, 429 U.S. 97, 104 (1976).

Fricker, Miranda. 2007. *Epistemic Injustice: Power and Ethics in Knowing*. Oxford University Press.

Galvan, Astrid, and Garance Burke. 2019. "Doctors Will Conduct Health Checks at Facility with Preemie." *AP News*, June 15. https://apnews.com/article/us-news-ap-top-news-border-patrols-az-state-wire-health-4117f50a12d14f12915b6bb0d975614a.

Gideon v. Wainwright, 372 U.S. 335 (1963).

Gramlich, John. 2022. "Key Facts About Title 42, the Pandemic Policy That Has Reshaped the Immigration Enforcement at U.S.-Mexico Border." Pew Research, April 27. https://www.pewresearch.org/short-reads/2022/04/27/key-facts-about-title-42-the-pandemic-policy-that-has-reshaped-immigration-enforcement-at-u-s-mexico-border/.

Gulaid, Azhar, and Evelyn F. McCoy. 2022. "Reproductive Health Care in Carceral Facilities: Identifying What We Know and Opportunities for Further Research." Urban Institute, August.

Hegarty, Aaron. 2018. "Timeline: Immigrant Children Separated from Families at the Border." *USA Today*, June 27. https://eu.usatoday.com/story/news/2018/06/27/immigrant-children-family-separation-border-timeline/734014002/.

Henry, Brandy. 2020. "Social Distancing and Incarceration: Policy and Management Strategies to Reduce COVID-19 Transmission and Promote Health Equity Through Decarceration." *Health, Education & Behavior* 47 (4): 536–539.

Human Rights Watch. 2018. "Code Red: The Fatal Consequences of Dangerously Substandard Medical Care in Immigration Detention." Report, June 20. https://www.hrw.org/report/2018/06/20/code-red/fatal-consequences-dangerously-substandard-medical-care-immigration.

Inda, Jonathan Xavier. 2020. "Fatal Prescriptions: Immigration Detention, Mismedication, and the Necropolitics of Uncare." *Death Studies* 44 (11): 699–708.

Lee, Caroline H., Nishant Uppal, Parsa Erfani, et al. 2023. "Individuals' Experiences in US immigration Detention During the Early Period of the COVID-19 Pandemic: Major Challenges and Public Health Implications." *Health & Justice* 11 (1): 1–12.

Martin, Rebecca A., Rosanna Couture, Nicole Tasker, et al. 2020. "Emergency Medical Care of Incarcerated Patients: Opportunities for Improvement and Cost Savings." *PLoS One* 15 (4): e0232243.

McCann, Sam. 2022. "Health Care Behind Bars: Missed Appointments, No Standards, and High Costs." Vera Institute, June 29. https://www.vera.org/news/health-care-behind-bars-missed-appointments-no-standards-and-high-costs.

Medina, José. 2021. "Agential Epistemic Injustice and Collective Epistemic Resistance in the Criminal Justice System." *Social Epistemology* 35 (2): 185–196.

Montoya-Galvez, Camilo. 2022. "Coronavirus Infections Inside U.S. Immigration Detention Centers Surge by 520% in 2022." *CBS News*, January 14. https://www.cbsnews.com/news/immigration-detention-covid-cases-surge/.

Moore, Robert, John Wagner, and Mike Debonis. 2019. "Members of Congress Visit Migrant Detention Centers in Texas Hours After Report Revealed Offensive Comments by Border Patrol Agents." *Texas Tribune*, July 1. https://www.texastribune.org/2019/07/01/members-congress-tour-migrant-facilities-respond-propublica-bombshell/.

National Academies of Sciences, Engineering, and Medicine. 2020. *Decarcerating Correctional Facilities During COVID-19: Advancing Health, Equity, and Safety*. National Academies Press.

National Immigrant Justice Center. n.d. "Mental Health in Detention." Accessed June 1, 2023. https://immigrantjustice.org/issues/mental-health-detention.

National Immigrant Justice Center. 2022. "Complaint to Office of Civil Rights and Civil Liberties, U.S. Department of Homeland Security." June 2.

Office of the Inspector General of Homeland Security. 2019. "ICE Does Not Fully Use Contracting Tools to Hold Detention Facility Contractors Accountable for Failing to Meet Performance Standard." OIG-19-18, January 29. https://www.oig.dhs.gov/reports/2019/ice-does-not-fully-use-contracting-tools-hold-detention-facility-contractors-accountable-failing-meet-performance-standards/oig-19-18.

Office of the Inspector General of Homeland Security. 2021. "ICE's Management of COVID-19 in Its Detention Facilities Provides Lessons Learned for Future Pandemic Responses." OIG-21-58, September 7. https://www.oig.dhs.gov/sites/default/files/assets/2021-09/OIG-21-58-Sep21.pdf.

Rayasam, Renuka. 2019. "Migrant Mental Health Crisis Spirals in ICE Detention Facilities." *Politico*, July 21. https://www.politico.com/story/2019/07/21/migrant-health-detention-border-camps-1424114.

Restum, Zulficar Gregory. 2005. "Public Health Implications of Substandard Correctional Health Care." *American Journal of Public Health* 95 (10): 1689–1691.

Reutter, David. 2017. "Deaths Due to Neglect in U.S. Jails Reflect Nation's Values." *Prison Legal News*, January 10. https://www.prisonlegalnews.org/news/2017/jan/10/deaths-due-neglect-us-jails-reflect-nations-values/.

Schaffer, Amanda. 2018. "A Physician in South Texas on an Unnerving Encounter with an Eight-Year-Old Boy in Immigration Detention." *New Yorker*, June 21. https://www.newyorker.com/news/as-told-to/a-physician-in-south-texas-on-an-unnerving-encounter-with-an-eight-year-old-boy-in-immigration-detention.

Seerval, Shanoor. 2022. "Health Behind Bars—How the U.S. Could Improve Care for Incarcerated People." Commonwealth Fund, April 8. https://www.commonwealthfund.org/publications/podcast/2022/apr/health-behind-bars-improve-care-incarcerated.

Sullivan, Kate. 2021. "Biden Administration Continues to Deny Journalists Access to Border Facilities." CNN, March 22. https://www.cnn.com/2021/03/22/politics/biden-administration-press-access-border-facilities/index.html

Thompson, Christie, and Elizabeth Eldridge Taylor. 2018. "Treatment Denied: The Mental Health Crisis in Federal Prisons." Marshall Project, November 21. https://www.themarshallproject.org/2018/11/21/treatment-denied-the-mental-health-crisis-in-federal-prisons.

Tosh, Sarah R., Ulla D. Berg and Kenneth Sebastian Leo´n. 2021. "Migrant Detention and COVID-19: Pandemic Responses in Four New Jersey Detention Centers." *Journal on Migration and Human Security* 9 (1): 44–62.

US Congress. 1952. United States Code: The Public Health Service, 42 U.S.C. §§ 201–291n.

US Constitution, amend. 6.

von Werthern, Martha, Katy Robjant, Zoe Chui, et al. 2018. "The Impact of Immigration Detention on Mental Health: A Systematic Review." *BMC Psychiatry* 18 (1): 1–19.

Wilper, Andrew P., Steffie Woolhandler, J. Wesley Boyd, et al. 2009. "The Health and Health Care of US Prisoners: Results of a Nationwide Survey." *American Journal of Public Health* 99 (4): 666–672.

15

Doctors as Immigration Agents

An Ethical Challenge

AMY REED-SANDOVAL

15.1 INTRODUCTION

As vaccines against COVID-19 became increasingly available in the United States in early 2021, some Mexican citizens with legal permission to enter the United States on tourist or work visas became impatient. Due to various global injustices, Mexico had been unable to acquire as many vaccines as the US; thus the vaccine rollout was going much slower there. Furthermore, Mexico's COVID-19 vaccine dissemination plan, unlike that of the United States, deliberately prioritized poor, working-class, and Indigenous regions of Mexico. Some comparatively wealthy Mexicans, who are more likely to receive tourist visas to legally enter the United States, therefore began traveling to the US to get vaccinated.

Things were more complicated, however, for Mexican US visa-holders living along the US-Mexico border. Many members of this (mostly middle-class) group were used to entering the United States by car for day trips and shopping, but this had been made all but impossible when the US government closed its border with Mexico from March 2020 until November 2021—even though visa-holding Mexicans could still enter the US by plane. Thus they could not cross the border in their cars to get vaccinated against COVID.

In February 2021, a physician based in El Paso, Texas, who is originally from Ciudad Juárez and who still has family there, decided to help his relatives cross the border to get COVID-19 vaccines in his office. He wrote a series of doctor's notes to be presented by his family members at the border. In these notes, he falsely stated that the individual who presented the

Amy Reed-Sandoval, *Doctors as Immigration Agents*. In: *Forced Migration and Health Justice*. Edited by: Lisa A. Eckenwiler, Verina Wild, Anna Gotlib, Ryoa Chung, and Deborah Zion, Oxford University Press.
 DOI: 10.1093/oso/9780197795491.003.0015

note had a serious medical condition and that they needed to cross the border that day to seek urgent medical care in his office. The notes made no reference to the true purpose of their border-crossing: to get a COVID-19 vaccine. The next day, a group of this doctor's family members presented their notes to border agents in El Paso. They were able to cross the border by car, drive to their relative's office, and get a COVID-19 vaccine long before many other Mexican citizens were able to do so.

This is one example of a doctor acting as an immigration agent, a notion that I describe and define below. This phenomenon raises important, underexplored ethical questions, as the role of the medical practitioner is not typically construed in terms of facilitating (or impeding) migrations and border-crossings. Clearly this case may inspire divergent normative assessments. On the one hand, one might argue that the physician in question was justifiably doing what he could to help his family members in the midst of a deadly pandemic. One might also argue that he was actively confronting some of the global injustices that have made it possible for countries of the Global North to acquire more lifesaving vaccines than their Global South counterparts. One might even propose that, when residents of Mexico get vaccinated against COVID-19 in the United States, they "free up" vaccines for other Mexicans facing more difficult circumstances.

One might counter, however, that the doctor abused his power as a physician in order to help middle-class family members jump the line and receive scarce medical resources before more vulnerable people in both Mexico and the United States had been able to acquire the vaccine. One might further argue that it is beyond the scope of his role as a physician to authorize a border crossing, even for an arguably good cause. As we can see, extensive ethical analysis is required to respond satisfactorily to this challenging case.

Medical providers acting as immigration agents is a far more widespread phenomenon than tends to be acknowledged. Two of my previous fieldwork experiences in the US-Mexico borderlands region, which I shall call upon in this chapter, provide evidence for this. As part of this research, I explored how pregnant Mexicans entering the US legally were nevertheless socially "illegalized"—that is, treated as "illegals"—on the basis of being both "visibly Mexican" and visibly pregnant. (Note that pregnant people have historically been excluded from the United States on the grounds of being Liable to Become a Public Charge, often merely on the basis of an immigration officer's personal discretion.) To facilitate their perfectly legal border-crossings, the women often went to significant lengths to conceal their pregnancies—sometimes even risking their lives in doing so—to avoid being denied the opportunity to cross the border. In addition, many of the women I interviewed both sought and received doctor's notes from their OB-GYNs or midwives to present at the border en route to the United States.

These doctor's notes—copies of which were very freely given to me by physicians on both sides of the US-Mexico border—stated that the pregnant person in question was a patient of the doctor who authored the note, and that they had already paid in full for the prenatal and/or birth care. The purpose of these notes is to encourage immigration officers to allow the pregnant person to cross the border, given the extraordinary discretion that border agents have to refuse entry even to those with legal permission.

I also found doctors acting as immigration agents in the summer of 2017, when I conducted three months of fieldwork, the purpose of which was to research the experiences of pregnant women/people who crossed different types of borders to seek abortion care in Albuquerque, New Mexico. Albuquerque is a very important global destination for abortion care later in pregnancy, as it is the workplace of two of the only four physicians in the US who routinely provide third-trimester abortions for pregnant people in need. During this ethnographic research at two abortion clinics, I observed medical practitioners providing doctor's notes to patients crossing international borders for abortion care. In these cases, however, the providers were careful not to reference the fact that the border-crosser was traveling for an abortion, given the very real possibility that the immigration officers their patients would encounter would be fervently anti-choice and deny them entry on that basis.

These medical providers also counseled people on the phone about how to answer questions that might be raised by immigration officers at international borders. For instance, before traveling to Albuquerque for abortion care, a Canadian patient told me she had a conversation with a representative at one of the clinics at which I conducted research. The representative told her that she should not reveal to any officer that she was getting an abortion, for she might be denied entry. Instead, she should speak in vague terms about entering the US for medical treatment. The patient expressed appreciation for this advice.[1]

Furthermore, some of the abortion providers I observed sometimes counseled undocumented patients who must drive long distances and cross state borders for abortion care about what they should do if they are pulled over by police officers (presumably engaged in racial profiling). For instance, one abortion provider told me that she encouraged an undocumented patient who had to drive to New Mexico from Florida for an abortion to tell male police officers who pulled them over that she was experiencing "vaginal bleeding," in hopes of making them uncomfortable enough to let her

1. I discuss this story, and the one that immediately follows, in my book (Reed-Sandoval 2025).

drive on. If that didn't work, she told the patient to have the officer call the doctor directly—that is, she offered to speak directly with a police or immigration officer in hopes of keeping her patient from being detained and/or deported. Finally, I observed medical providers helping their patients manage various logistical aspects of their journey (i.e., finding a place to stay, finding food, making it home safely). In this chapter I shall draw upon nearly a decade of ethnographic fieldwork to argue that many doctors, and other medical professionals, are immigration agents, which raises distinctive ethical challenges. Having argued that doctors are immigration agents, I then explore two conceptual frameworks that seem relevant to doctors who are serving in these roles: structural competency and health-care resistance. I shall argue that these frameworks are useful in certain ways but ultimately are limited for the task at hand: providing doctors with different conceptual tools to discharge their obligations as immigration agents. Calling upon immigration ethics, I shall argue, first, that doctors need to understand themselves as active immigration agents, and thus as agents of the state (even as they find themselves resisting that state)—in addition to their professional duties to act as advocates for their patients. As I shall explore below, this is consistent with doctors acting to undermine state power as part of their care and advocacy for patients. Second, I argue that upon understanding themselves as (state) immigration agents, doctors should engage in philosophical discussions of state obligations to uphold universal moral equality in the realm of migration and take action to uphold universal moral equality. I recognize that this is but a starting point for doctors who wish to discharge their ethical obligations, and that ethical tensions will inevitably arise; I offer this starting point for reconsidering the ethics of medicine in a context in which doctors must serve as immigration agents.

Before beginning let me clarify that I understand terms like "migrant" and "border crossing" quite broadly. In my view, immigration ethics should also be attuned to the experiences of internal migrants who encounter a range of borders and barriers in their journey to medical care.

15.2 DOCTORS AS IMMIGRATION AGENTS

First, allow me to clarify what I am *not* saying when I claim that doctors are immigration agents. Sometimes the term "immigration agent" is used to refer to someone who is legally empowered to patrol national borders in an official capacity, make arrests, and otherwise coercively enforce immigration law. For instance, the job of US Immigration Customs and Enforcement agents has been described as work to prevent illegal immigration into the

U.S. and also protect the nation from the trafficking of unlawful goods into the country. Such agents are often referred to as immigration officers. Clearly, doctors and other medical providers (qua medical providers) are not immigration agents in this sense.

In other contexts, the term "immigration agent" is used to refer to someone who is formally trained in immigration law and explicitly legally empowered to guide people through immigration processes, such as applying for visas. Such immigration agents are often referred to as immigration consultants. Likewise, I do not describe doctors as immigration agents in this sense. Finally, in claiming that doctors are immigration agents, I am not implying that they voluntarily or enthusiastically embrace this role. Generally they did not sign up for such a role, as do those who deliberately choose to work as immigration officers or consultants.

I argue that doctors often act as immigration agents in that they frequently provide various types of advice, immigration paperwork, and logistical support—and may sometimes purposely deny doing so—to prospective border-crossers, migrants, and others who must travel long distances for medical care. Such medical providers are not operating in an official capacity, as are those immigration agents who work as officers or legal consultants, but they are indeed able to play potentially important roles in their patients' border-crossing and migration experiences. As we have seen, presenting a doctor's note at a national border can help patients receive scarce vaccines, access abortion care that is unavailable in their home country, and obtain prenatal and birth care in a foreign country. We have also seen that doctors sometimes help documented and undocumented patients cross internal and national borders and barriers en route to scarce medical care by offering patients travel and migration advice. They may even informally represent patients in their encounters with police and immigration officers.

On the other hand, some doctors and other medical providers act as immigration agents by refusing to provide these things. During my fieldwork in Albuquerque, El Paso, and Ciudad Juárez, I interviewed borderlands residents who felt they had been denied the support they needed for the purpose of traveling and border-crossing for abortion care. For instance, a patient at Southwestern Women's Options whom I interviewed prior to her second-trimester abortion that day complained that her regular OB-GYN refused to provide her with any information about where she could get an abortion. Strategically denying such critical information to patients is one way in which medical providers can interfere with their patients' internal and external migration processes. Other interviewees reported that they simply refrained from discussing with their OB-GYN their plans to travel for abortion care due to their perception that their doctor would judge them negatively. This is a subtler way in which doctors may influence their patients' plans to cross borders and travel for medical care.

Doctors also influence their patients' plans to cross borders and travel for medical care outside of the context of abortion care. For instance, in El Paso I interviewed several women from Ciudad Juárez who felt that their medical providers in El Paso did not support their decision to seek prenatal care and give birth in the United States. One patient decried the fact that her labor and delivery nurse wrote in her chart that she had not had any prenatal care, simply because her prenatal care had been conducted in Mexico. She said this made her feel that she was doing something illegal in giving birth in the US. Another person I interviewed in Ciudad Juárez, who had received her prenatal care in Juárez, claimed that several Juárez-based OB-GYNs simply refused to give her prenatal care when she disclosed her intention to eventually give birth in the United States.[2] While the patients I interviewed did give birth in the United States despite these obstacles, it is clear that medical providers are capable of influencing not only their patients' experiences of crossing borders for medical care but also their very decision-making about whether or not they should do so.

In sum, while doctors can, and do, support their patients' efforts to migrate and border cross for medical care (e.g., through writing doctor's notes, providing advice, representing patients to police officers, offering logistical support, and for a variety of reasons that may not always connect to explicit concerns about politics and power), they can also frustrate these aims (e.g., by denying patients information about destinations for the medical treatment they seek, making border-crossing patients feel unwelcome, refusing treatment, and, historically, through participation in medical panels that can formally deny patients both admission to the United States and certain forms of medical care). I submit, then, that though they are not immigration officers or official immigration consultants, they are immigration agents, and potentially powerful ones, and this warrants serious ethical analysis.

As stated in the introduction, the fact that some doctors and other medical providers are immigration agents in this sense is ethically concerning—even if one recognizes many of the actions explored above as morally praiseworthy and perhaps even heroic. As Foucault argued, "in the ordering of human society [medicine] assumes a normative posture, which authorizes it not only to distribute advice as to a healthy life, but also to dictate the standards for physical and moral relations of the individual and the society in which [they] live" (1994, 4). Along these lines, doctors acting as immigration agents are assuming a "normative posture" vis-à-vis immigration

2. I explore the two stories in further detail in Reed-Sanoval (2022).

matters, and they are empowered, in certain important respects, to dictate physical and moral relations of their (prospective) migrant and border-crossing patients and the society in which they live. Furthermore, the fact that doctor's notes are sometimes used as immigration documents—and given the fact that doctors can choose, without direct regulation or supervision, whether or not they wish to author them—is ethically significant.

Despite its importance, the phenomenon of doctors acting as immigration agents is not widely recognized or understood. We urgently need an ethical framework that enables us to assess doctors' migration-related agency vis-à-vis their patients from a moral point of view. In the next section, I explore two conceptual frameworks that seem potentially suited to this purpose—though I argue that they are ultimately unsuccessful.

15.3 STRUCTURAL COMPETENCY AND HEALTH CARE RESISTANCE

15.3.1 Structural Competency

The first framework I shall explore is "structural competency," which has been developed as an alternative to "cultural competency" frameworks that encourage medical providers to acquire knowledge of their patients' "cultures" in order to provide better care (Betancourt et al. 2003). As Gregory Jucket (2005) explains, culture can shape how medical encounters are experienced and how illness is perceived. Biomedical ethicists and medical practitioners have therefore explored how cultural competency in medical encounters can improve outcomes for patients, alleviate broader social health–related disparities, and improve relationships between patients and their medical care providers.

Without contesting the importance of medical providers gaining understanding of how their patients experience and understand illness "culturally," proponents of structural competency—a term coined originally by medical anthropologist Jonathan Metzl (2011)—argue that far more is required. Medical anthropologist Seth Holmes, for instance, argues that medical providers need training in social analysis in order to understand the sociopolitical forces that contribute to their patients' illness and injuries. Referring, in the main, to cultural competency frameworks, Holmes (2013, 153) argues that "biomedicine effectively de-politicizes suffering, blaming sickness not on political, economic, and social structures but rather on individual behaviors, assumed cultural practices, and perceived ethnic body differences."

Describing his ethnographic fieldwork with Triqui migrants from Oaxaca who sustained injuries and sought medical care while working as agricultural laborers in California, Holmes writes, "[T]he clinicians I spoke to see the individual Triqui bodies in their office, yet they are unable to engage the social context that produces suffering" (2013, 153). He tells the story of "Abelino" (a pseudonym), who very seriously injured his knee while picking berries on Tanaka Farms in Washington. Abelino was ultimately denied workers' compensation for his ongoing injury due to a failure by his various medical providers to understand the sociopolitical context in which he was laboring. Reflecting on his fieldwork, Holmes explains, "[I]t was infrequently . . . that I heard a health professional point out the context in which the person lives . . . working conditions, or international economic and immigration policies" (2013, 153). Holmes describes one physician as ordering an injured patient to avoid movements and postures that were, in fact, inescapable for him in his role as an agricultural laborer. (The correct response in this context, Holmes explains, would have been recommending paid medical leave.)

A structural competency framework could be helpful for understanding doctors as immigration agents. First, doctors working with migrant/border-crossing patients clearly do need to understand immigration politics and other social structures that impact their patients' experiences en route to medical care in order to provide effective care. For instance, medical practitioners who provide doctor's notes to help their patients cross national borders clearly understand that their patients may struggle to cross those borders for medical care, often due to racist, sexist, and classist attitudes on the part of immigration officers. Second, doctors acting as immigration agents clearly ought to see their work as political—because it is.

Nevertheless the structural competency framework is somewhat limited for present purposes. This is because the framework depicts physicians as passive students of politics and structural injustice. Once again, Holmes argues that the doctors working in migrant clinics ought to understand the labor conditions, structural racism, and immigration policies that shape their patients' illnesses and injuries. The (venerable) goal of this is to help doctors propose truly beneficial treatments. However, structural competency does not seem to require action beyond this (though I acknowledge that it can, in some cases, be transformative). In particular, it does not require physicians to see themselves as personally enacting immigration justice or injustice in their capacity as immigration agents. Rather, the physician attending migrant farmworkers (for instance) only needs to understand the complicated conditions "out there" in order to provide quality medical care within the clinical setting. And yet we have seen that when doctors act as immigration agents, they actively impact matters of immigration justice.

15.3.2 Health Care Resistance

Another conceptual framework that could be used for normative evaluation of doctors acting as immigration agents is that of "health care resistance," which was recently developed by Ryan Essex. Essex begins his analysis of "resistance in health and health care" by highlighting a number of actions on the part of healthcare providers—some but not all of which are migration-related—that seem to be acts of resistance against injustice. He explores, for instance, Dr. Wendy Orr's efforts in the 1980s to reveal the torture of detainees under South Africa's apartheid policies (Orr was a government doctor); the refusal of a group of Australian doctors to discharge Asha, a five-year-old asylum seeker who would, if discharged, be sent to one of Australia's notorious offshore detention centers for migrants (located in Nauru, Papua New Guinea); and the protests of a group of US pediatricians who, in 2019, demanded permission to provide influenza vaccines to migrant children who were being detained under extraordinarily objectionable conditions in a San Diego detention center.

Essex claims that these actions, and a host of others, can rightfully be characterized as forms of healthcare resistance. He purposefully defines healthcare resistance broadly, such that it can include a variety of acts on the part of healthcare providers. First, it involves an "active behavior," including "public, overt acts, such as marches and civil disobedience," as well as "a far broader range of activities, for example, working slowly, feigning sickness, wearing particular types of clothing, or stealing from one's employer" (Essex 2021, 483). It can also involve dialogue—"speaking about oppression" (483)—or, in some cases, remaining strategically silent. Essex also argues that resistance requires a form of opposition to power: "This could be virtually anyone or anything; individuals, collectives, institutions, laws, structures, practices, or norms" (483).

Essex then spends considerable time discussing what resistance does not require. First, it does not require one to intend to resist, or even be aware of the fact that one is resisting. He cautions that requiring agents to couch their actions in terms of resistance is overtly academic and elitist and warns that it can hide from view a wide range of actions that should probably qualify. He explains that "resistance needn't be recognized as such by those being resisted or even intended by those resisting" (2021, 484). Second, though Essex motivates his arguments by highlighting cases of healthcare resistance that seem to support progressive and liberatory causes, he is open to the possibility that resistance may seem more reactionary and conservative, such as when some doctors have protested against universal healthcare. Healthcare resistance is, in sum, "any act, performed by any individual (or collective) acting as or explicitly identifying as a healthcare professional, that is a response to power, most often in opposition to contentious, harmful or unjust rules, practices, policies, or structures" (486).

As in the case of structural competency, I believe that the conceptual framework of healthcare resistance is somewhat helpful for normative analysis of doctors acting as immigration agents. First, like the structural competency framework, it productively politicizes medical practice. Second, many medical providers who work with border-crossing patients do indeed seem to be engaged in healthcare resistance as described by Essex.

Still, a "resistance framework" is somewhat limited for present purposes. First, many physicians acting as immigration agents would not only fail to embrace but would vehemently reject the idea that they are "resisting power" through their actions. For instance, I once interviewed an OB-GYN in El Paso who regularly works with patients from Ciudad Juárez and writes doctor's notes to assist them with border-crossings. As you can see in this abbreviated version of the transcript of my interview with him, this doctor would very likely reject any characterization of his work as "resistance":

Amy: Some people get really upset about this idea that women are coming to the United States to give birth. They think it's a violation of US sovereignty, and that the border should be made more secure. My first question is . . . what is your view on that? Do you think it's fair for governments to maintain this system of borders, or are you more of an "open borders person"? Do you think that, ultimately, we should have a borderless world?

OB-GYN: It's a hard question. I think that there has to be some type of separation between countries.

Amy: So, you think that maintaining some system of borders is consistent with justice?

OB-GYN: Right. . . .

Amy: So then . . . what connections do you see between the nature of the work you do and these sorts of . . . debates about immigration that are happening in the United States right now?

OB-GYN: For one thing I try to not be a participant in those debates. . . . I think that there has to be a mechanism for people to come to the United States, and those that make it here, however they get here, if they deliver here, that child is a US citizen. I know that that's being challenged by some groups, and I hope that doesn't change. . . .

Amy: Do you see yourself acting in opposition to the claims that are made by [anti-immigrant] groups? . . .

OB-GYN: Oh, I don't know. You know, I've never been a slave to fashion. . . . I have to face myself in the mirror each morning. And I say, you know, this is what I believe, if you want to agree with me, great, if not, that's great too. I will contribute to those people that represent my views, and I will use my right to vote in such a way that I can try to make this continue. But . . . whether I'm making a statement or not, that's for other people to decide.

Amy: When you do your work in medicine, do you see it . . . as connected to a particular vision of immigration justice, and a particular support for the idea that for anyone who gives birth in this country, their child should become a citizen? Or are these two things separate for you, kind of your work as a doctor and philosophical views on immigration?

OB-GYN: It's totally, totally different. Totally different. I've put aside all those sorts of things. Like when you're working on an inmate, I don't care if that individual did some horrible things. She's coming to see me for what I do, and for what God has allowed me to train for, has made it possible for me to follow that dream. And I'm not going to be the judge, I'm not going to do anything other than just take care of that patient to the best of my ability.

I believe the doctor's comments pose problems for the characterization of his work in terms of resistance, despite the fact that he has, in fact, devoted much of his career to helping Mexican citizens give birth in the United States in the face of virulent political pushback. As we have seen, he explicitly separates immigration politics from his work as an OB-GYN at the US-Mexico border: in his words, these two things are "totally different," and he wants to avoid being a participant in such "debates."

Of course, I raise these questions on the basis of one ethnographic interview and other informal conversations with borderlands physicians; considerably more empirical research is needed on the question of whether doctors consider themselves to be engaged in resistance. I am also open to the possibility that the doctor's actions may nevertheless be appropriately characterized along the lines proposed by Essex. As we have seen, Essex purposefully distances himself from accounts of resistance that require agents to see themselves as resisting. Furthermore, the doctor claims he is open to others conceiving of his work in political terms, even if he rejects such ideas himself. It is important to note, however, that Essex does not explore cases in which medical providers explicitly reject the suggestion that they are resisting. Thus, at the very least, more needs to be said about why external accounts of agents' actions should outweigh agents' own descriptions of what they are doing.

I have thus far explored the concepts of structural competency and healthcare resistance with a view toward developing descriptive and normative tools for analyzing and supporting doctors as immigration agents. A structural competency framework is an improvement on that of cultural competency, but at the level of description at least it presents doctors as passive students of social science and politics, and not as active agents of (immigration) justice. Essex's framework of healthcare resistance, meanwhile, raises questions about how useful the framework is for doctors who reject—rightly or wrongly—the politicization of their work along these lines. In the next section, I propose that doctors acting as immigration agents should turn to immigration ethics to guide their decision-making in working with border-crossing and migrant patients, as well as those who must travel long distances for medical care.

15.4 IMMIGRATION ETHICS FOR DOCTORS ACTING AS IMMIGRATION AGENTS

15.4.1 A Conceptual Reorientation

Doctors acting as immigration agents must begin by undergoing a conceptual reorientation in order to behave justly in their role. To begin with, they should understand immigration as a complex philosophical problem and a matter of structural injustice—far more than tends to be presented in mainstream political debates. Second, medical providers acting as immigration agents ought to understand themselves, in complicated ways, as agents of the state. Recall Foucault's critique that medicine is now empowered to "dictate the standards for physical and moral relations of the individual and the society in which they live." While this is certainly not the exclusive territory of the state, establishing norms for physical and moral relations in society is one of its roles (even in liberal governments, which are, after all, empowered to define and punish crimes). Note that acting as an agent of the state is consistent with doctors engaging in resistance against state power—recall, for instance, Essex's discussion of the South African doctor who exposed torture practices of the apartheid government despite being employed by the South African state. Being a "state agent" does not involve endorsement of all the actions and policies of one's state any more than being a citizen of that state entails such a sweeping endorsement.

In the next section, I argue that doctors should, like states, uphold "universal moral equality" in their migration related decisions.

15.4.2 Universal Moral Equality

One of the central principles of philosophical literature on immigration justice is that just states cannot regard their own citizens as morally superior to citizens of other countries. It follows from this that they cannot permissibly use racist and other inegalitarian criteria for determining immigrant admissions.

Importantly, some philosophers have argued that a commitment to universal moral equality can be consistent with some form of "closed borders" system—which Joseph Carens (2015) calls "the conventional view"—in which states are empowered to control immigrant admissions and, as part of this process, exclude at least some prospective immigrants. As Michael Blake (2008) argues, if France denies a Canadian the right to vote in French elections simply on the grounds that the Canadian in question is not a member of the French state, France does not undermine the moral equality of the Canadian in question (or Canadians as a social group). While this view is not without its detractors, I want to make clear that a commitment to honoring universal moral equality does not necessarily, or automatically, entail eliminating all immigration restrictions.

How is this discussion of universal moral equality relevant to medical providers acting as immigration agents? First, it makes clear that doctors acting in this capacity do not need to conceive of themselves as "open borders" supporters or as engaged in resistance against all forms of immigration enforcement in order to regard their actions vis-à-vis their traveling, migrant, and/or border-crossing patients as just. Second, I submit that a commitment to universal moral equality *does* require doctors to take action to ensure that their patients' moral equality is not being undermined en route to their care.

For instance, if doctors learn that their patients are being harassed at borders due to visible pregnancy, or due to the fact that they are seeking abortion care (or some other stigmatized legal procedure), or due to some other social injustice, they should, when feasible, author doctor's notes to help prevent the patients from being unduly impeded and coerced. Furthermore, if their patients are vulnerable to being targeted en route to medical care by police and/or immigration enforcement due to racism, sexism, classism, homophobia, transphobia, or other injustices, medical providers should offer to support patients in their encounters with law enforcement. Note that this also holds true when the patients are legally undocumented: immigration ethics has shown us that even if one supports a form of "closed borders," it does not follow from this that legally undocumented people who have crossed borders without authorization may be subjected to racism and other inegalitarian forces. Additionally, doctors should not conceal information about available medical care for stigmatized procedures such as abortion or options for giving birth in a foreign country.

15.4.3 Complex Cases

With all this in mind, I now return to the complex cases explored at the outset of this chapter. I believe that the majority of doctors I have mentioned—OB-GYNs helping their patients cross borders and abortion providers helping their patients navigate various aspects of their journey—are acting justly in their capacity as immigration agents. That is, they are taking action to defend their patients' moral equality at borders and while traveling for medical care, given their knowledge that their patients are vulnerable to being interrogated, harassed, and perhaps even denied entry on the basis of visible pregnancy and/or seeking abortion care. But what of the doctor who falsely claimed in a series of doctor's notes that his patients were crossing the border for urgent medical care, when in reality they were entering the United States for a COVID vaccine they could not access in Mexico?

Bracketing the question of whether doctors may sometimes act dishonestly to benefit their patients, I propose that this doctor should pause to consider whether his actions as an immigration agent honored universal moral equality. Did he take such action on behalf of patients who aren't his relatives—and who, unlike his relatives, may be poor, Indigenous, and/or working class? Would he be willing to do so if he had the chance? If he can answer yes to either of these questions, then it is possible that his actions as an immigration agent were just.[3] If not, his actions would have been unjust and therefore morally impermissible given the doctor's capacity as an immigration agent.

15.5 CONCLUSION

I have argued that many doctors are immigration agents and that we need a normative framework for evaluating the many moral challenges that follow from this. Such a framework should provide doctors with tools for confronting ethical challenges they frequently encounter as they serve patients who migrate, cross borders, and contend with various internal barriers en route to medical care. In particular, doctors must conceive of themselves as immigration agents, which involves seeing themselves as agents of the state (albeit, in some cases, reluctant, unwitting, and consciously objecting ones).

3. A related issue, which I won't discuss here, is whether we can perform special actions on behalf of our family members. I cannot settle the issue here. However, I venture to say that if we think that border patrol agents should be allowed to make exceptions to the rules for family members, then perhaps we should grant such leeway to doctors.

They should also borrow a key insight from immigration ethics literature: that in order to exercise justice in immigration, states (and their immigration agents) must uphold universal moral equality in their migration practices and policies.

REFERENCES

Betancourt, Joseph R., Alexander R. Green, J. Emilio Carrillo, Owusu Ananeh-Firempong. 2003. "Defining Cultural Competence: A Practical Framework for Addressing Race/Ethnic Disparities in Health and Health Care." *Public Health Reports* 118 (4): 293–302.

Blake, Michael. 2008. "Immigration and Political Equality." *San Diego Law Review* 45 (4): 963–980.

Carens, Joseph. 2015. *The Ethics of Immigration*. Oxford University Press.

Essex, Ryan. 2021. "Resistance in Health and Healthcare." *Bioethics* 35 (5): 480–486.

Foucault, Michel. 1994. *The Birth of the Clinic*. Vintage.

Holmes, Seth. 2013. *Fresh Fruit, Broken Bodies: Migrant Farmworkers in the United States*. University of California Press.

Jucket, Gregory. 2005. "Cross-Cultural Medicine." *American Family Physician* 72 (11): 2267–2274.

Metzl, Jonathan. 2011. *Protest Psychosis: How Schizophrenia Became a Black Disease*. Beacon Press.

Reed-Sandoval, Amy. 2022. "Border-Crossing for Abortion Care: A Feminist Challenge to Border Theory." *Journal of Social Philosophy* 53 (3): 296–316.

Reed-Sandoval, Amy. 2025. *Intimate Borders: Feminist Migration Ethics*. Oxford University Press.

16

Resistance, Health, and Structural Injustice in the Context of Forced Displacement

RYAN ESSEX

16.1 INTRODUCTION

In this chapter I will begin to unpack the relationship between structural injustice, resistance, and health in the context of forced displacement. To do this I will first introduce the existing literature that has explored conceptualizations of resistance and migrant resistance. I will introduce a number of examples of more general acts of resistance and some more specific examples that intersect with health. I will then discuss one way that resistance could act to challenge and undermine structural injustice as it relates to forced displacement. I will argue that if we are to help people understand their responsibilities as they relate to structural injustice and ultimately prompt collective action, disrupting ignorance will be an important step in this process. Drawing on a number of diverse examples, I will also offer some broader reflections on the relationship between resistance, health, and structural injustice and the potential for resistance to guard against threats to health and imagine better, healthier futures, particularly for those who have been forcibly displaced.

16.2 HEALTH, RESISTANCE, AND FORCED DISPLACEMENT

Much has already been written about migrant resistance and about the concept of resistance itself. Migrant resistance more generally takes a number of forms, ranging from practices many of us may be familiar with, such as marches and hunger strikes, to less visible acts, like subversion,

Ryan Essex, *Resistance, Health, and Structural Injustice in the Context of Forced Displacement*. In: *Forced Migration and Health Justice*. Edited by: Lisa A. Eckenwiler, Verina Wild, Anna Gotlib, Ryoa Chung, and Deborah Zion, Oxford University Press. © Oxford University Press (2026). DOI: 10.1093/oso/9780197795491.003.0016 vandalism, and even self-harm (Aitchison and Essex 2024). When we examine migration and the nature of such resistance, we find that such acts often cross borders, and many argue that unauthorized border crossing is itself an act of resistance (Hess 2017) in that it challenges "the spatial logic through which these boundaries have come to constitute and frame the conduct of international relations" (Bleiker 2000, 2). In relation to migrant resistance, Stierl (2018, 1) sees resistance "as a practice and force that complicates our understanding of both precarious forms of migration" that raises questions about "inclusion and exclusion, belonging and unbelonging, (access to) rights and resources, survival, and, more generally, the ability to lead liveable and dignified human lives." When we think about resistance in practice, we may think about public, collective acts, such as marches and protests; resistance, however, takes far more expansive forms. It exists in our everyday actions, in discourse and knowledge; it exists when people cross borders illegally. However, when we think about resistance in such expansive terms (not isolated to the literature on migrant resistance) we risk losing our grasp on the concept; it risks becoming vacuous; and we may be looking for resistance where none exists. We see this play out in debates about resistance, its relationship to power, and the differences that exist between individual and collective, organized and everyday, and intentional and unintentional acts (Vinthagen and Johansson 2013). Here, I take a fairly expansive view of resistance, to include a range of actions both visible and invisible, collective and individual, organized and everyday.

Before moving on, however, the recent work of Lilja (2022) is helpful here. Traditionally, when we look at scholarship in the field of resistance studies, we see a divide between visible and collective, invisible and individual acts of resistance. Here we find a contrast between more traditional forms of resistance such as civil disobedience and more hidden, individual acts of resistance, resistance that undermines but does not necessarily confront power; like sabotage and subversion. This division, however, has been criticized for a range of reasons, but particularly because there often isn't a clear division; hidden acts can be collective, and public acts need not be collective. Each of these forms of resistance can empower and constrain the other, for example. Lilja suggests that we instead look at resistance in light of its relationship with power, that is, whether it (1) challenges or confronts power, (2) avoids power, or (3) imagines and creates alternatives to existing structures, institutions, knowledge, and so on. Thinking in these terms provides a useful place to start in thinking about the range of forms that resistance takes. I will provide some examples that demonstrate each of these things as they relate to migrant resistance more generally. I will then sketch how these actions relate to health.

16.3 FORCED DISPLACEMENT AND RESISTANCE

Let us first consider some examples that do not explicitly have much to do with health and those which, to varying degrees, confront power. The literature here is awash with examples of protest carried out by those who have been forcibly displaced (Reed-Sandoval 2022; Wolf 2022). In 2004 in Tokyo, a city which by global standards hosts relatively few people who are forcibly displaced, 12 Kurds occupied the front yard of the United Nations building, appealing to the United Nations High Commissioner for Refugees (UNHCR) Japan–Korea Office to recognize them as refugees. Seventy-two days after this sit in began, the UNHCR took measures to end the protest, calling in the Japanese police to disperse the protesters. Although the protesters threatened self-immolation, the protest was eventually dispersed (Shindo 2009).

Such struggles are not an isolated phenomenon. We can see examples of this in the Dominican Republic, with protests by Dominicans of Haitian descent and Haitian migrants against mass deportation (Yuhas 2015). In Israel, Sudanese and Eritrean migrants and refugees, along with Israeli supporters, have actively protested against the government's decision to either deport or resettle asylum seekers to camps in Uganda and Rwanda under the threat of indefinite confinement should they refuse to leave (Jalil and *Times of Israel* Staff 2015).

We can find a range of other examples that show more subtle, almost invisible acts of resistance, particularly in immigration detention settings. While immigration detention centers in Australia have long been places of public protest, including a number of riots, these forms of action only scratch the surface of what occurs there daily. Bailey (2009, 114) provides this account:

> Despite the harshness of the treatment they faced, detainees in Australian Immigration Detention Centres showed no respect for the Government's attempts to contain them. On the decks of leaky boats they resisted attempts by the Australian Navy to turn them back. In serious danger at sea they engaged in hunger strikes and sabotage. . . . They brought their politics across the threshold of the camp with them. Iranian trade union activists used their skills and experience to form committees and implement strike action. Iraqi leftists produced analyses of the camp and their prospects for freedom and African journalists translated them and turned them into bulletins. In the desert, behind barbed wire, under constant surveillance and subjected to brutal and unpredictable violence, their politics flourished. Secret networks planned escapes. Elections were conducted to facilitate representation. Mass meetings were held to decide action with translators relaying discussion across language and cultural barriers. As a result of this flourishing, their politics, their language and at times their bodies overwhelmed the fences and spilled into Australian cities. Bulletins were smuggled out and video

> cameras smuggled in. Mobile phones were thrown over fences. Phone link-ups were organized from outside to coordinate actions across the various detention centers. The center pole of a Hills Hoist, an iconic Australian back-yard washing line, was used to lever apart bars.

In a study that was carried out with 35 detainees in the Netherlands, van Houte et al. (2021, 1282) discuss how acts of feigned ignorance and semi-compliance were acts of resistance in this context. Detainees shared experiences and identified "bottlenecks" in deportation procedures, such as sharing the knowledge that "many embassies will not collaborate with return without valid proof of identity, especially when return is forced." Those who employed such strategies destroyed identity documents and made little effort to seek further identification. Some engaged in more overt noncompliance, making it clear that they concealed their identity and openly refused to disclose their place of origin.

An example from Italy highlights how acts that may start out as individual and largely invisible can spark broader, collective acts of protest. Lampedusa, a small Italian island of only 20 square kilometers and fewer than 6,000 inhabitants, has progressively become one of the busiest gateways to Europe. The first detention center on Lampedusa was built in 1996, which began a "sociopolitical transformation, turning this arid piece of rock into a symbol of the frontier between Europe and Africa" (Lendaro 2019, 311). In July 2013, several hundred migrants were detained for weeks, far exceeding the 72-hour holding period during which detainees should have been identified and transferred.

On July 18, approximately 1,200 people were detained, while the center could only accommodate 380 people. Aware that the European Dublin Regulation would force them to take steps toward gaining asylum in Italy, a group of around 30 young Eritreans refused to have their fingerprints taken. Lendaro explains, "Having one's fingerprints taken would mean the start of a long and uncertain procedure which, in the best-case scenario, results in these migrants obtaining a status in a country in which they do not wish to settle" (2019, 314). The number of people refusing to have their fingerprints taken grew day by day. Eventually 300 people who had refused to give their fingerprints were released. Following this decision, migrants marched through the streets and occupied the main square in the town, demanding they be allowed to leave the island without their fingerprints being taken. These demands were granted soon after, allowing numerous people to leave Lampedusa without having to identify themselves (Lendaro 2019).

These examples are of course not exhaustive, but they illustrate my point about some of the forms of resistance I am discussing here. There is of course more to the story; I haven't yet touched upon more creative, prefigurative actions, actions that Lilja (2022) calls constructive resistance. This type of resistance can quickly be identified since for many the act of traveling without documentation, traveling across borders and being present in spaces where they would otherwise not be welcome, "[creating] new and different subjectivities, social relations and institutions" (Stierl 2018, 7), can be characterized as such. Notably, the aforementioned examples consist of acts of resistance carried out only by migrants. Nevertheless there are a range of other actors in this space, and I will expand my discussion below to focus on them.

16.4 HEALTH AND RESISTANCE

Perhaps the most pressing question at this point is how this relates to health. That is, while migrant protest is common and takes a range of forms, why does it matter for health? Unlike the literature on migrant resistance, the relationship between resistance and health, with a few exceptions, has received little serious attention despite the commonality of such action. We are not without direction, however; recent work has sought to deepen the relationship between health and resistance. We see resistance and health intersecting in various ways, from acts of protest impacting health outcomes to being a motivator for and being used to frame acts of resistance. We also find examples of resistance impacting knowledge and practice and health being used as a means to establish authority or legitimacy around certain issues (Essex 2023). In short, however, "resistance has been a common but overlooked force in health and healthcare that has been central to securing a number of health-related gains . . . [serving] as an important means to oppose threats to health and [demonstrating] that resistance has a role to play in imagining alternatives to the status quo" (Essex 2022, 316). Let's consider some examples in the context of forced displacement that illustrate these points.

In February 2016, a 12-month-old asylum seeker who came to be known as Baby Asha was transferred from Nauru and hospitalized in Brisbane. After she received treatment, doctors at Lady Cilento Hospital in Brisbane refused to discharge her to be returned to Nauru. The media were notified of this case, which, almost overnight, became national news. This occurred at the same time the #LetThemStay campaign was launched (Hall et al. 2018), which organized protests in 12 major cities over 12 days, calling for the government to stop the transfer of 267 asylum seekers, including 54 children and 37 infants, from Australia to Nauru. A vigil was mobilized outside of the hospital around the clock for 10 days, placing the government under increasing pressure to honor the doctors' refusal to discharge Asha and to accommodate her family in the Australian community (Hall et al. 2018). The case of Baby Asha speaks to the intersections of health, resistance, and forced displacement, with the hospital used as a place of resistance and health workers leveraging their power to stop what was effectively a deportation.

We can see the involvement of healthcare workers elsewhere and in simply demanding basic treatment needs be met. In December 2019, six protesters were arrested outside a US Border Patrol's San Diego headquarters calling for the influenza vaccination to be supplied to detained migrant children. Of those arrested, four were doctors who had arrived in white coats and stethoscopes, with vaccines ready to be administered. More than just flu shots, protesters had also set up a makeshift clinic, with consent forms, a refrigerator, and a generator. All they asked was to be let in to deliver and administer the vaccine. This came after months of advocacy from a range of groups and the death of three children in custody from influenza the previous year: 2-year-old Wilmer Josué Ramírez Vásquez, 8-year-old Felipe Alonzo Gómez, and 16-year-old Carlos Hernández Vásquez. Healthcare workers and their expertise can be utilized in other forms of migrant protest, including offering mental health assessments for those protesting (Lavik et al. 1996).

Resistance in relation to health is not exclusive to those forcibly displaced or healthcare workers. Since 2012, the UK has enforced increasingly hostile policies toward undocumented migrants. Among other impacts of these policies, the UK has denied healthcare to many and left others with bills for their care that they will never be able to pay. This has been a particularly contentious issue, and there have been numerous mobilizations opposing these policies and the encroachment of border enforcement in healthcare, with campaign groups such as Patients Not Passports and Docs Not Cops active in this area for a number of years. The Justice for Simba campaign provides a particularly poignant example of this. In June 2019, an asylum seeker named Simba suffered a stroke that left him in a coma and paralyzed. He woke up to a bill for £93,000. Simba was formerly from Zimbabwe but had lived in the UK for most of his life; his claims for refugee status had been denied. This resulted in the Justice for Simba campaign, which shed light on the cruelty of the UK government's approach to those without documentation. It received wide public support, resulting in marches, a "carnival of resistance," and, among other things, a petition which received over 80,000 signatures. In August 2022, Simba was granted refugee status and his bill for lifesaving care was canceled (Essex et al. 2022).

Beyond these examples, issues can be framed in terms of health. In Australia, for example, while immigration detention has been criticized on a number of grounds, including the violation of human rights and international law, its health impacts have been a persistent complaint, with advocates long emphasizing the health impacts of prolonged detention, alongside these concerns. We can also find examples of the Australian healthcare community effectively leveraging their expertise on matters of health. After the introduction of a law which effectively outlawed staff from speaking about their work in detention centers, the healthcare community led opposition to this law, with a number of healthcare workers going as far as publicly breaking this law. It is particularly interesting how this opposition was framed. While opposition to this sweeping law could have been framed on the grounds that it undermined free speech or even that it violated widely accepted democratic norms, the healthcare community framed their opposition primarily on the fact that it "would simply stop healthcare professionals from being able to do their job and report problems such as child abuse" (Essex 2020, 141). This law was amended several months later.

One final example, and perhaps one that may be more contentious when conceptualized as an act of resistance, relates to acts of self-harm and protest such as hunger strikes (Aitchison and Essex 2022). Such actions are widespread, particularly in detention centers. We can find particularly notable examples in Germany, where in 2012 the suicide of Iranian asylum seeker Mohammad Rahsepar led to broad public protest. Asylum seekers occupied the square in front of the town hall of Würzburg, launching the Refugee Tent Action, including a group going on hunger strike. After a number of months this protest spread, with asylum seekers occupying other squares throughout southern Germany, resulting in a wave of ongoing protests (Haselwarter et al. 2022). There have been hunger strikes in Austria (Mokre 2018) and self-immolation in Australia (Fiske 2016). While these actions may seem to conflict somewhat with more traditional forms of protest, it is clear that many were done with political intent or at the very least inspired broader political action. These actions are all similar in that they utilized health (or a threat to health) as a means to either bargain or make a point.

I have outlined some of the intersections of health, resistance, and forced displacement and provided examples that show how health relates to protest, how expertise and authority can be leveraged, how issues may be framed in terms of health, how healthcare settings can become sites of resistance, and even how health may be risked or used as a means to bargain during protest when it comes to actions such as hunger strikes and self-harm.

Among all of this, however, there is something far more fundamental concerning the relationship between health and resistance. Notably, for those who are oppressed, resistance is a natural response. Silvermint (2013,

407) argues that well-being and resistance are fundamentally related, in "opposing or counteracting the damage that oppression does to a victim's autonomy or overall life prospects" and also by providing the opportunity to be involved in "valuable aims" or "goods, projects, relationships, and states of being that are important to the individual, as well as the general aim of leading a morally worthwhile life." Silvermint goes on to argue that resistance can protect individuals who face oppression and that those who fail to resist show "insufficient regard for [their] own well-being, and for the value of the worthwhile aims and life that resistance could afford [them]." (417) In this respect, health cannot be separated from resistance and vice versa; resistance is a completely natural response for those who are oppressed.

This discussion only scratches the surface. There are many other examples and there is much more that could be said about the nature of resistance in this context. So I hope what I have written is only a starting point for future discussions. Below I want to make a further point and consider the functions of resistance, particularly in challenging structural injustice.

16.5 RESISTANCE AND ITS POTENTIAL TO CHALLENGE STRUCTURAL INJUSTICE

While some of these actions have been relatively successful, how might they contribute to challenging structural injustice? In relation to this point I first need to limit my discussion. I will be speaking about a specific type of resistance: disruptive resistance. By "disruptive" I do not necessarily mean physically disruptive, such as blocking a road or occupying a public space; I mean any action that confronts others, challenges their views, or forces them to reconsider their beliefs. While many of the actions I discussed above were disruptive to varying degrees, some, such as the detainees organizing in Australian immigration detention centers, were not necessarily disruptive as they were not visible to others. I am also going to speak about only one way I see resistance as being particularly effective in challenging structural injustice. There are arguably a range of other ways it could challenge structural and other more direct harms, so again and as above, I hope this discussion serves as a starting point for future work in this area. I will start with my understanding of structural injustice and then discuss the work of Hayward (2017), who argues that disruptive action is an important means to disrupt ignorance as it relates to structural injustice.

Structural injustice, as I will apply it here, refers to the large-scale social processes that advantage some and disadvantage others. Forced displacement is a structural injustice in itself and is closely entangled with other injustices, such as income inequality, poverty, and homelessness, processes that often coerce people to move (Parekh 2020). While we may be able to find examples of wrongdoing when we look at a problem such as forced migration, it is a structural problem in that its maintenance is not dependent on malicious actors alone. All of us contribute to the factors that drive forced displacement, acting unknowingly and at times even acting with good intent. In this respect we need to look at the causes of forced displacement and not only precipitating events like violence and persecution but broader issues such as global inequality and "market forces," environmental degradation and climate change, imperialism, and a range of other historical injustices.

This therefore implicates quite a few people. We might consider how many of us in the Global North contribute to inequality, a key driver in forced displacement. Even when trying to buy as ethically as possible, it is almost impossible to avoid products for which that have been manufactured unethically. Somewhere along the line, the products and services we consume have either come from underpaid or exploited workers or propped up authoritarian regimes. These things on their own do not drive forced displacement, but they make it far more likely, with inequality, instability, and human rights violations arguably entangled (Powers and Faden 2019; Parekh 2020). Moreover, there is substantial evidence to suggest a link between structural inequality and political instability (Roe and Siegel 2011). In this respect, the position I am taking on structural injustice in this chapter is very similar to Young's (2006). While I believe there is great promise in more recent theoretical advances and challenges to this understanding of structural injustice, they are well beyond the scope of this chapter and would be somewhat inconsequential to my argument, regardless.

Moving beyond the conceptualization of these problems, there has also been substantial work dealing with the question of responsibility. Who is responsible, and how is this responsibility discharged? Young's (2006) *social connection model of responsibility* is an instructive place to start. Most fundamentally and simply, this model suggests that those who contribute to the structures that create and sustain injustice have a responsibility to address them. This is because of the benefits they derive from these structural processes. That is, responsibility "derives from belonging together with others in a system of interdependent processes of cooperation and competition through which we seek benefits and aim to realize projects" (119). This implicates quite a few people and suggests that those of us in higher income countries who may benefit from products or services which rely on the exploitation of others should take action. In discharging this responsibility, things get even more complicated.

To ensure we don't contribute to global inequality will take more than changing our buying habits. We are limited by what stores have in stock and what we can afford. It requires others to act, including corporations. Indeed, addressing such exploitation requires action at a global level. Clearly there is a need for collective action' that is, you, me, and millions of others need to take action for change to occur. In moving toward such action, Young felt that one important step was shifting how people understood their responsibilities in relation to justice, specifically examining how they contribute to structural injustice.

One problem with this idea, however, is that structural problems are maintained by otherwise benign practices that are built into the unquestioned norms and practices of daily life, making them hard to spot. But what about those people who contribute unknowingly to structural injustices such as inequality and forced displacement? This is not to say that the majority of people are unaware that these things exist but that they may be ignorant of how they contribute to their maintenance and how this is connected to their actions; in other words, they might be unaware of their contribution to the background conditions that drive inequality and forced displacement. Young's argument suggests that changing how people understand their shared responsibilities will induce them to do the right thing by changing both their intrinsic and extrinsic motivations. This view has been criticized on a number of grounds, including that "actually assuming our responsibility for structural injustice requires that we first acknowledge and experience our implication in it" (Schiff 2014, 28). Starting with this point, Hayward (2017, 403) argues that "conscious awareness of the need to act to promote some just outcome . . . is necessary, except in cases in which people habitually do the right thing." That is, we cannot act to do the right thing if we do not know of the need to act. If we do not know how we contribute to sweatshop labor, why would we act to change our behaviors? Hayward (2017) draws on the concept of white "epistemic ignorance" developed by Mills (2007).

Epistemic ignorance is fundamentally political and can involve "not knowing something that is true" or "believing something to be false that is true or something true that is false" (Hayward 2017, 404). Such ignorance becomes a particular problem when it is attached to social dominance. Epistemic ignorance can be maintained in several ways: through structural injustice as well as through social norms, assumptions, practices, and beliefs. This serves to allow those in dominant groups to see themselves as ethical "even as they enjoy systematic unearned advantage" (404). While we may be more likely to do the right thing for a number of reasons, a necessary condition for action is that people first need to recognize or have a conscious awareness that there is a problem. One way to challenge such ignorance is to present people with new information, to confront them, and to disrupt this ignorance. Hayward identifies disruptive resistance as a means to this end. As well as challenging power, disruptive action can therefore serve to challenge ignorance. Unlike nondisruptive forms of political action, its focus is not to persuade but to confront, to highlight oppression and demand change. In this sense, disruptive action is also about making the structures that perpetuate injustice unsustainable in a political, financial, and social manner. In Hayward's words, "when structural change is enacted, it is not only, and it is not principally, because privileged people are made to understand their responsibilities in ways that align with the ethical principles they endorse. Instead, in significant part, it is because those whom injustice harms engage in political disruption, one important product of which is the interruption of motivated ignorance" (407).

We find a similar argument from Stramondo (2022) in relation to disability activism. While his argument focuses on how disability activism can improve bioethics scholarship, there is a broader point, that disability activism is a means to challenge damaging narratives, allowing people with disabilities to speak for themselves and tell their own stories. We can see this potential recognized in the broader literature on migration and resistance about how such acts challenge norms, beliefs, and ignorance, or at the very least the "potentiality of such political struggle for the creation of new relationships, political subjectivities, and communities and ways of thinking about citizenship" (Ataç et al. 2016, 531). When it comes to health, similar claims are made, bringing to light the harms of the systems through self-harm, challenging who is entitled to care, or shedding light on the complicity of healthcare systems in the oppression of those who do not have access. Resistance is not only an important means to guard against threats to health and demand better; it is also a means to challenge views about migration and health.

Beyond what I have discussed above, there are likely several other points about the functions of resistance when it comes to forced displacement and health. Powers and Faden (2019), for example, see (nonviolent) resistance as a means to take action in light of the failure of states—a kind of bottom-up change in the absence of top-down change. Resistance may also serve to provide those forcibly displaced with a political voice, as a type of surrogate tool for those who are excluded from political participation (Aitchison 2018). This, again, has been touched upon in the existing literature on migrant health but also in the literature that has explored the relationship between resistance and health. Moulin and Nyers (2007, 361) argue that "whereas the citizens can speak with some assurance and assume that she or he will be heard, for the refugees in global political society to articulate a political voice they must take the strategy of interruption."

16.6 CONCLUSION

I have outlined the importance of resistance as it relates to health and forced displacement and sketched how such action could begin to challenge structural injustice, namely through challenging ignorance and providing a voice to those otherwise overlooked and excluded. There is, I hope, ground to build on my argument above; resistance and structural injustice are likely to interact in a range of other ways that I have not discussed here. Furthermore, resistance is likely to remain an increasingly pressing issue as it relates to forced displacement, with restrictions on movement and the exclusion of migrants increasingly practiced by states in the Global North.

REFERENCES

Aitchison, Guy. 2018. "Domination and Disobedience: Protest, Coercion and the Limits of an Appeal to Justice." *Perspectives on Politics* 16 (3): 666–679.

Aitchison, Guy, and Ryan Essex. 2024. "Self-Harm in Immigration Detention: Political, Not (Just) Medical." *Journal of Medical Ethics* 50: 786–793.

Ataç, I., K. Rygiel, and M. Stierl. 2016. "Introduction: The Contentious Politics of Refugee and Migrant Protest and Solidarity Movements: Remaking Citizenship from the Margins." *Citizenship Studies* 20 (5): 527–544.

Bailey, R. 2009. "Up Against the Wall: Bare Life and Resistance in Australian Immigration Detention." *Law and Critique* 20 (2): 113–132.

Bleiker, Roland. 2000. *Popular Dissent, Human Agency and Global Politics*. Cambridge University Press.

Essex, Ryan. 2020. *The Healthcare Community and Australian Immigration Detention: The Case for Non-Violent Resistance*. Palgrave Macmillan.

Essex, Ryan, Ayesha Riaz, Seb Casalotti, Kitty Worthing, Rita Issa, James Skinner, and Alia Yule. 2022. "A Decade of the Hostile Environment and Its Impact on Health." *Journal of the Royal Society of Medicine* 115 (3): 87–90.

Essex, Ryan, 2023. "The Intersections of Resistance and Health." In *Oxford Research Encyclopedia of Global Public Health*.

Fiske, L. 2016. "Self-Immolation Incidents on Nauru Are Acts of 'Hopeful Despair.'" *The Conversation*, May 4. https://theconversation.com/self-immolation-incidents-on-nauru-are-acts-of-hopeful-despair-58791.

Hall, Shirley, Caroline Lenette, Samantha Murray, Connie Chan, Ashley Flannery, and Kate Vickery. 2018. "#LetThemStay: Visual Representations of Protests and Community Mobilization for Asylum-Seekers in Australia." *Journal of Critical Thought and Praxis* 7 (1): 4.

Haselwarter, Dominik, Verina Wild, and Katja Kuehlmeyer. 2022. "Providing Health Care in Politically-Charged Contexts: A Qualitative Study About Experiences During a Public Collective Hunger Strike of Asylum-Seekers in Germany." *International Journal of Qualitative Studies on Health and Well-being* 17 (1): 2018770.

Hayward, Clarissa R. 2017. "Responsibility and Ignorance: On Dismantling Structural Injustice." *Journal of Politics* 79 (2): 396–408.

Hess, S. 2017. "Border Crossing as an Act of Resistance." In *Resistance: Subjects, Representations, Contexts*, edited by Martin Butler, Paul Mecheril, Lea Brenningmeyer. Verlag.

Jalil, J., and *Times of Israel* Staff. 2015. "Protesters Call on Government Not to Expel African Migrants." *Times of Israel*, May 3. https://www.timesofisrael.com/protesters-call-on-government-not-to-expel-african-migrants/.

Lavik, N. J., H. Christie, O. Solberg, and S. Varvin. 1996. "A Refugee Protest Action in a Host Country: Possibilities and Limitations of an Intervention by a Mental Health Unit." *Journal of Refugee Studies* 9 (1): 73–88.

Lendaro, Annalisa. 2019. "Nothing to Lose: The Power of Subtle Forms of Resistance in an Immigration Detention Centre." In *Governance Beyond the Law*, edited by Abel Polese, Alessandra Russo, and Francesco Strazzi. Springer.

Lilja, Mona. 2022. "The Definition of Resistance." *Journal of Political Power* 15 (2): 202–220.

Mills, Charles. 2007. "White Ignorance." In *Race and Epistemologies of Ignorance*, edited by Shannon Sullivan and Nancy Tuana. SUNY Press.

Mokre, Monika. 2018. "'We Demand Our Rights!' The Refugee Protest Camp Vienna." In *Protest Movements in Asylum and Deportation*, edited by Sieglinde Rosenberger, Verena Stern, and Nina Merhaut. Springer.

Moulin, C., and Peter Nyers. 2007. "'We Live in a Country of UNHCR': Refugee Protests and Global Political Society." *International Political Sociology* 1 (4): 356–372.

Parekh, Serena. 2020. *No Refuge: Ethics and the Global Refugee Crisis*. Oxford University Press.

Powers, Madison, and Ruth Faden. 2019. *Structural Injustice: Power, Advantage, and Human Rights*. Oxford University Press.

Reed-Sandoval, Amy. 2022. "Border-Crossing for Abortion: A Feminist Challenge to Border Theory." *Journal of Social Philosophy* 53 (3): 296–316.

Roe, M. J., and J. I. Siegel. 2011. "Political Instability: Effects on Financial Development, Roots in the Severity of Economic Inequality." *Journal of Comparative Economics* 39 (3): 279–309.

Schiff, Jade Larissa. 2014. *Burdens of Political Responsibility: Narrative and the Cultivation of Responsiveness*. Cambridge University Press.

Shindo, Reiko. 2009. "Struggle for Citizenship: Interaction Between Political Society and Civil Society at a Kurd Refugee Protest in Tokyo." *Citizenship Studies* 13 (3): 219–237.

Silvermint, Daniel. 2013. "Resistance and Well-Being." *Journal of Political Philosophy* 21 (4): 405–425.

Stierl, Maurice. 2018. *Migrant Resistance in Contemporary Europe*. Routledge.

Stramondo, Joeseph A. 2022. "How Disability Activism Advances Disability Bioethics." *Ethical Theory and Moral Practice* 25 (2): 335–349.

van Houten, M. Leerkes, A. Slipper, and L. Breuls. 2021. "Globalised Citizenship Theories." *Resistance Studies Magazine* 1 (1): 1–46.

Vinthagen, S., and A. Johansson. 2013. "Everyday Resistance: Exploration of a Concept and Its Theories." *Resistance Studies Magazine* 1 (1): 1–46.

Wolf, Allison B. 2022. "Obstetric Violence as Immigration Injustice: A View from the United States and Colombia." *Developing World Bioethics* 23 (2): 176–184.

Young, Iris M. 2006. "Responsibility and Global Justice: A Social Connection Model." *Social Philosophy & Policy* 23 (1): 102–130.

Yuhas, A. 2015. "Dominicans of Haitian Descent Turned into 'Ghost Citizens,' Says Amnesty." *The Guardian*, November 19. https://www.theguardian.com/world/2015/nov/19/dominican-republic-violated-human-rights-haitians-citizens.

17

Dual Loyalties and Healthcare

The Weaponization of Suffering and the Ethics of Resistance

DEBORAH ZION

17.1 INTRODUCTION

How do we speak about places of asylum-seeker detention, imposed upon those seeking refuge in Australia? The writer and former asylum seeker Behrouz Boochani, now a resident of New Zealand, has documented the brutality of offshore detention: "During these years I have witnessed the ways in which hundreds of imprisoned refugees have resisted the policy of exile and torture, how they have stood up against the political establishment from this forlorn island" (2018, 167). His description of life on Manus Island documents the torture itself as well as its effects. He compels us to ask: How did Australia become a country in which the treatment of those seeking protection ended in prolonged torture at both onshore and offshore places of asylum-seeker detention? Why is it that the general population has repeatedly tolerated and, worse, endorsed and voted for such policies? And finally, what has been the role of civil society and professional workers, such as healthcare providers, at these places in this history?

The role of healthcare providers is particularly complex. As conduits to the right to health, healthcare providers can be seen to have duties related to upholding this right and, through this, justice. The relationship between health and justice is exemplified by Bridget Pratt et al. (2020, 2–3) as follows: "Theories of justice in health emphasise the fundamental value of health for all, independent from gender, ethnicity, place of birth or residence, social status, political beliefs and religion. Second, multiple

Deborah Zion, *Dual Loyalties and Healthcare*. In: *Forced Migration and Health Justice*. Edited by: Lisa A. Eckenwiler, Verina Wild, Anna Gotlib, Ryoa Chung, and Deborah Zion, Oxford University Press.
 DOI: 10.1093/oso/9780197795491.003.0017

theories purport that it is a priority and duty of justice to avert and alleviate disadvantage."

Many have argued, however, that healthcare providers are unable to uphold or promote either justice or the right to health in the context of asylum-seeker detention (Johnston 2009; Briskman and Zion 2010; Briskman and Zion 2014; Durham et al. 2016). The role healthcare providers play was and remains highly ethically complex when providing care to asylum seekers in detention centers overseen by the Australian government. In what follows I will present a short history of asylum-seeker detention and describe the conditions within the detention centers before looking at questions of dual-loyalty conflict. I will analyze responses to this conflict through a taxonomy developed by Briskman and Zion (2014), which distinguishes four responses utilized by healthcare professionals: complicity, subversion, withdrawal, and advocacy. Each of these four is ethically complex and has morally ambiguous consequences or "moral remainders."

17.2 ASYLUM-SEEKER DETENTION IN AUSTRALIA: SOME HISTORY

Mandatory immigration detention for those arriving by boat on the shores of Australia was introduced in 1992 under a left-leaning Labor government (Phillips and Spinks 2013) in response to a group of Cambodian asylum seekers. Over the years, there has been a series of legal challenges to this policy. Nevertheless it has endured, albeit in varied forms, for different lengths of time and with varied degrees of accountability by the Australian government. In 1998, the Liberal government under John Howard absolved itself of responsibility for the daily running of detention centers, then within Australia's boundaries, by outsourcing their management to a series of private companies (Motta 2002). While some detention centers were within large cities, many were in isolated areas, making visitation by advocates and concerned persons difficult to organize. They also provided far from appropriate medical facilities for those needing a high level of care.

Notwithstanding the harshness of onshore detention centers like Woomera and Baxter, in 2001 asylum seekers were subjected to an even more cruel regime of offshore detention for the first time, after the arrival of the cargo vessel MV *Tampa*, which had rescued asylum seekers at sea (Leroy 2023). Prime Minister Howard instigated offshore detention through which asylum seekers were "processed" on Christmas Island and thereafter sent to Nauru or Manus Island in Papua New Guinea. Neither of these islands is part of Australia, and therefore they are far from any oversight. The governments of Nauru and Papua New Guinea were paid considerable amounts of money to set up and run these detention centers.

There was a break in offshore detention between 2008 and 2012. However, it was reestablished in 2012, and thereafter there have been four phases. In the first phase a number of people (1,085) were sent offshore under the Gillard Labor government, between August 13, 2012, and July 18, 2013. The second phase took place under the Rudd Labor government and came into force on July 19, 2013. All persons arriving after this time were prevented from ever settling in Australia.

The third phase began with the election of the Abbott Coalition government in September 2013 and was referred to as "Operation Sovereign Borders"; it was characterized by boat turn-backs as well as tight government control of information around arrivals. In addition, a policy was enacted whereby no person who arrived after 2013 was able to receive refugee status to settle in Australia. Moreover, offshore detention centers were expanded, and no exemptions were made for children (Gleeson and Yacoub 2021). The fourth phase began in 2014; its emphasis is returning asylum seekers to their place of departure, despite the dangers they may face there.

It is evident that offshore detention was introduced as a deterrent to further boat arrivals (Essex 2019). It is also clear that asylum seekers became part of each government's strategy about border protection at a time of increasing racism and anti-Muslim attitudes. Notwithstanding the fact that Australia was an early signatory of the UN refugee convention, which states in Article 31 that no penalty should attach to the seeking of refuge, the asylum-seeker debate became a form of political point scoring, appealing to Australia's long history of racist policy concerning immigration (UN General Assembly 1951).

17.3 CONDITIONS IN ASYLUM-SEEKER DETENTION

The harshness of asylum-seeker detention—both offshore and onshore—confirmed its role as a deterrent to the seeking of refuge. Many centers were isolated, far from formal and informal oversight from visitors or human rights organizations. Nonetheless some access was granted for human rights bodies. After visiting Woomera, the Australian Human Rights and Equal Opportunity Commission announced in 2002 that Woomera Detention Centre was in breach of the Convention of the Rights of the Child (Loff et al. 2002). Temperatures there reached 50 degrees Celsius. Housing, such as it was, was overcrowded, and toilets were frequently blocked. Drinking water was hot because of the sun, and the education of children was inadequate. Brutality by the guards was frequently reported.

Similar conditions were reported in other detention centers, with large numbers of people sleeping in tents, and inadequate food and water

(Briskman et al. 2008, 151). In addition, signs of mental distress were treated with cruelty, usually in the form of solitary confinement in a unit referred to as "management." One asylum seeker who spent years in Baxter described the units: "[T]here is no window, twenty-four hours there is a light, there is a video camera, there is no privacy. If you go for toilet or shower, they will see" (Australian Human Rights Commission 2011). In the light of these conditions some asylum seekers attempted suicide or engaged in other forms of self-harm, including slashing with razors, ingesting chemicals and shampoo, and attempting hangings (Australian Human Rights Commission 2011).

Both onshore and offshore detention have been likened to Giorgio Agamben's (1998) "state of exception," where all rights are stripped away (Jenkins 2004; Penovic 2019) Agamben describes this state as follows: "the materialization of the state of exception and . . . subsequent creation of a space in which bare life and juridical rule enter into a threshold of indistinction" (1998, 174). Thus those who entered detention found themselves in a condition of "bare life," shut away from the social and judicial order and the rights and freedoms accorded to them. In addition, a process of dehumanization occurred as access to the judicial process and contact with those outside the detention setting was precarious. Prisoners were called by number rather than name and were subjected to humiliating rules concerning food and other basic goods, such as sanitary products. Detainees also complained about lack of privacy and about sexual harassment.

The harms described in onshore detention centers like Woomera and Baxter were exacerbated in offshore detention in all its phases. Isolation and lack of accountability were magnified on Christmas Island, Nauru, and Manus Island. The Office of the International Criminal Court, when finally allowed to visit, stated that conditions at Manus Island and Nauru detention centers were consistent with "cruel, inhuman, or degrading treatment" and unlawful under international law (Doherty 2021).

The report is consistent with earlier findings from Amnesty International. In 2012, they described conditions on Nauru as follows:

> Asylum seekers are staying in army tents. These tents offer absolutely no privacy, and barely have any room between the stretcher beds.
>
> When it rains, the camp quickly floods. Every single tent observed had at least one leak, with bedding and clothing soaked.
>
> In the camp, the temperature reaches over 40 degrees Celsius in the compound and 80% humidity. The heat means people cannot stay in their tents during the day.

On Manus Island, where only single adult men were sent, asylum seekers were housed in World War II tin sheds that frequently reached temperatures of 40 degrees Celsius and higher. Drinking water was limited, and food frequently inedible (Barnes 2022). On both Nauru and Manus Island men, women, and children reported sexual harassment and rape (Barnes 2022).

In 2016, the *Guardian* released over 2,000 incident reports from staff on Nauru, many of which involved children. The reports document physical and sexual violence and self-harm (Asylum Seeker Resource Centre 2023). Attention was drawn to the many human rights abuses that took place in relation to the murder of Reza Barati in 2014 by detention center staff. While two local men were charged, the Australian expatriates involved were never brought to justice (Asylum Seeker Resource Centre 2023).

Such accounts demonstrate that it was not just the cruelty that took place in the detention setting that was a serious ethical issue, but the lack of accountability concerning those who practiced cruelty and violence, further emphasizing the "state of exception." As the Asylum Seeker Resource Centre (2023) document stated, "Refugees and people seeking asylum have reported hundreds of alleged abuses to ASRC caseworkers . . . [including] medical professionals failing to provide basic care. The blame still lies with the Government in power at the time, who had a duty of care that they not only failed to uphold but often completely and deliberately disregarded."

17.4 MEDEVAC AND ALTERNATIVE PLACES OF DETENTION

Despite statements from successive governments that those seeking asylum by boat would never be allowed to settle in Australia, and the pervasive nature of offshore detention, there have been situations where asylum seekers have been transferred to Australia. This, however, does not ensure that a claim for asylum can be made. Asylum seekers are classified as "transitory persons" and may be transferred to Australia for a "temporary purpose" (Public Interest Advocacy Centre 2021). One such reason was medical treatment unavailable in detention. This process came to be known as Medevac.

Asylum seekers who are transferred to Australia for this purpose were not therefore issued a refugee visa and did not enter the refugee determination process. Instead they were subject to detention, either in community settings, onshore detention settings, or in what is called "alternative places of detention" (APODs). In practice, what occurred was that a law was passed in 2019 that required the minister for immigration to consider the views of independent doctors in order to transfer asylum seekers to Australia for medical treatment. This law was repealed in December the same year. During that time 192 people were transferred to Australia. What was meant as an amelioration to detention and a remedy for the lack of healthcare offshore became its own form of cruelty with the advent of the COVID-19 pandemic, at which point asylum seekers were subjected to isolation, lack of medical treatment, and incarceration in so-called hotel accommodations, or APODs. The situation of those detained there recently became a matter of public interest with the onset of the epidemic.

In March 2021, it was estimated that 1,219 such persons were in APODs. While some asylum seekers felt a degree of hope when medevacked to Australia, the conditions they encountered were often felt to be as bad as offshore detention. Issues related to isolation were especially acute. In particular, many were terrified of contracting COVID-19, and indeed they had reason to be afraid. In 2021, almost half of those held in the Park Hotel in inner Melbourne contracted COVID-19 (Doherty 2021) due to a combination of inadequate quarantine conditions and prior illness. Healthcare was also minimal, with detainees reporting, for example, having to wait five hours to see a nurse for basic pain relief (Asylum Seeker Resource Centre 2021).

There is considerable evidence that the use of hotels as APODs, especially during the height of the COVID-19 epidemic, became in and of itself an additional form of deterrence.

The Australian Human Rights Commission (2021) reported, "The Commission has consistently expressed the view that hotel APODS should only be used in exceptional circumstances and for the shortest possible time." The Commission reported that the average time in hotel detention was 69 days, and the longest time was 634 days (Australian Human Rights Commission 2021).

17.5 CONDITIONS IN COVID-19 "HOTEL" DETENTION

While conditions in offshore detention were marked by heat, filth, and violence, being detained in APODs brought with it its own form of degradation. This was particularly marked by boredom and isolation. The Commonwealth Ombudsman Government of Australia (2023) reported:

> People accommodated at Melbourne Park Hotel APOD had limited outdoor access and limited options for privacy, respite, and activities.
>
> The material conditions and atmospherics did not meet expectations. The significance of food contamination was not appreciated.
>
> Knowledge of correct emergency evacuation procedures was lacking.

Such conditions were also present in other APODs. Detainees compared the conditions to torture. One asylum seeker stated, "I walked into my new room and looked at these four walls. White. One window. Large, but my eyes travelled just one metre to reach a brick wall. I searched, but, no, there were no windows in that wall, no people in no windows. They made sure our view would be restricted to the brick wall outside" (Arvin 2021). Another detainee stated, "The sole purpose of being here seems to be to torture. To be made to suffer like this it is not possible for them to be human, they must be aliens. Two or three years ago I could think about life outside but now I am not capable of envisaging outside at all. I have no imagination; everything is blurry and now I can't see anything" (Finlay and Caruana 2023).

17.6 DUAL LOYALTY AND HEALTHCARE IN DETENTION

What, then, are the ethics of providing healthcare in such settings? Healthcare is a necessity of asylum-seeker detention. Even if access to and quality of healthcare are inadequate, without the work of healthcare providers the detention system cannot continue. To do so would have risked both domestic and international censure, as well as litigation in the event that asylum seekers were released from detention.

Glenda Koutroulis (2003, 384), a nurse who worked in Woomera, stated:

> As I look back on my time in Woomera Detention Centre, picturing the silver fences and razor wire that mark it, entrapping all those whose implacable despair will burden Australia long after I am gone from this earth, I think about what I was involved in. It was unequivocally observation of and participation in something very indecent. . . . As I reflect, angry and ashamed with what I have witnessed and experienced I feel like I was unknowingly part of a perverse social experience, testing endurance in the face of deception and incongruous decisions about freedom, and the capacity to survive in those who have already struggled to survive.

Koutroulis's reflection reminds us that healthcare in detention is marked by a dual-loyalty conflict, "situations where physicians and other healthcare providers are required to subordinate the interests of the patient to those of the employer or the state" (International Dual Loyalty Working Group 2002). Dual-loyalty conflicts are most commonly found in military and prison settings, where the duty to uphold the right to health is challenged by the working conditions which are themselves injurious to health. In the context of asylum-seeker detention, it might be argued that such conflicts are unavoidable (Zion 2019).

The terrible effects on asylum seekers of all three kinds of detention—onshore, offshore, and APODs—present core ethical dilemmas for healthcare providers. Given that the detention environment in and of itself contributed to mental and physical illness, it has been argued that working in such an environment and thereby contributing to its maintenance is innately unethical. Briskman and Zion (2014) have suggested that abolition of asylum-seeker detention should be the ultimate goal of healthcare providers, given the damage caused by the system and how this is in direct contradiction of the ethics of healthcare. They write, "For the ethical health worker, a focus on maintaining and incrementally improving the system is vexed and the aspiration must be the abolition of the detention system" (Briskman and Zion 2014, 284).

Briskman and Zion (2014) have outlined four responses to dual-loyalty conflicts in the asylum-seeker setting: complicity, subversion, retreat, and advocacy. Complicity occurs when healthcare providers fail to document harm and wrongdoing and do not advocate for the patient in forwarding complaints. Subversion refers to acts of kindness to patients, while leaving the fundamental issues concerning detention unchallenged. Retreat occurs when healthcare providers withdraw from employment because they can no longer comply with the detention regime. Finally, advocacy occurs when healthcare providers speak out about the abuses they witness, sometimes at great personal cost. All of these responses were evident in the four phases of detention described above. Each response was ethically complex and exposed the complexity of dual-loyalty conflict and the role of healthcare providers' relationship to the right to health in a setting where such rights were neither protected nor required.

17.6.1 Complicity

Mardin Arvin (2021), an asylum seeker, recounts having malaria on Manus Island and waking up shaking with pain and fever: "The night shift supervisor . . . looked at me and said 'give him Panadol and go back.' I asked him to do a malaria test but he said 'are you the nurse or am I? If you needed it, I would test you, but you don't need it.'" Arvin's account of such cruelty was based on the free rein given to healthcare providers, who could choose whether or not to treat based on their own criteria, thereby reinforcing the cruel and arbitrary nature of the detention system. This system was based on a process of dehumanization, such as calling prisoners by number instead of name and making accessing healthcare both difficult and humiliating. Arvin recalls being unable to see the nurses in the Park Hotel (Melbourne) after being medevacked to Australia and missing out on medication. Although the medication was sitting on the table, the nurse refused to give it to him, requiring him to write a request to see a doctor, a process that would take several days.

Not all healthcare providers, however, were complicit with the world of structural cruelty. Some tried to undermine it through subversive action. Many such actions were undertaken by nurses such as Glenda Koutroulis, working in close proximity with detainees. Strategies included visiting detainees in their huts instead of making them stand in the sun and calling them by name instead of number. Such acts, while bringing comfort and hope, did not, however, serve to challenge the conditions of detention (Martin 2018).

17.6.2 Subversion: A Gray Zone

As we have seen, subversion means that acts of kindness are conducted, but structural harms and injustices remain unchallenged. It presents complex ethical questions. First, it is not always clear that there is a dividing line between complicity—which would be ethically more problematic, going against the duties of healthcare providers to act in the interest of their patients—and subversion *in terms of outcome*. For example, the act of talking to a detainee with kindness and respect, while ethically valuable in itself, does not in any way change the trajectory of the detention system. However, Jennifer Rubenstein provides a way to differentiate the concepts. She states that complicity in wrongdoing involves contributing "to the injustice perpetrated by another actor, and to some extent, share the intention of the original perpetrator." (2015, 103).

It is clear that the system of detention could not continue without the work of healthcare providers, and in this regard they fulfill Rubenstein's first clause (Briskman et al. 2010; Essex and Kalocsányiová 2022). That is, whether intentionally or not, healthcare providers contribute to wrongdoing by working in detention at all. However, many made it clear that they did not uphold the system in other ways and that they found it cruel and demeaning (Zion et al. 2009; Zion 2019). Lepora and Goodin also assist us in considering the complex nature of actions that may be considered complicit. Following Gardner,(2007) they state that the "morality of an action should be distinguished in two parts: responsibility simpliciter for what one does oneself, and responsibility for what one does by way of contribution to another's principle wrong doing" (Lepora and Goodin 2011, 267). Despite efforts made toward subversion, it is clear that working in the detention setting does in fact contribute to the second clause described by Lepora and Goodin, as the system continued unchecked.

Based on the accounts of healthcare providers who behaved subversively in the detention setting, it is clear that while involved in the cycle of maintaining detention, they resisted the cruelty practiced by some others. Providing, as far as possible, kind and humane treatment in such hellish conditions, rather than engaging in acts of further neglect and humiliation, might be considered praiseworthy. However, as Lepora and Goodin point out, "Difficulties in the moral evaluation of contributory actions often arise precisely because actions that are morally neutral or praiseworthy in themselves nonetheless contribute to somebody else's acts in a way that lead to heinous consequences" (2011, 269). As such, subversion carries with it what both Rubenstein and van Domselaar refers to as "moral remainders" namely, "the phenomenon of an in itself defensible decision that may nonetheless result in a moral cost that merits further attention" (van Domselaar, 2022, 220).

17.6.3 Retreat

It was knowledge of the consequences of detention that led to some healthcare providers being unable to reconcile their attempts at kindness with the destruction wrought by asylum-seeker detention (Zion et al. 2009; Australian Human Rights Commission 2014; Zion 2019). Their response was to remove themselves or not to engage in the detention process. Writing in 2004, Michael Hall, a nurse, recalled his time working on Christmas Island. When he was leaving he was asked to escort two pregnant women to the mainland. He said, "I refused to be the escort nurse to two pregnant women who were being forcibly separated from their husbands and children, so they could be taken to the mainland to have their babies. I considered the separation and isolation of pregnant women was wrong on professional, medical and ethical grounds and I was appalled that it could happen" (Australian Human Rights Commission 2004). "Susan," a nurse seeing patients after they were released from the so-called COVID hotels, reported that her organization would not provide care in these places of detention, reasoning that they would become part of the cycle of punishment, even while providing care (personal correspondence, 2023).

What, then, is left in terms of moral action in the care of detained asylum seekers? While retreat removes healthcare providers from participating in wrongdoing, it also raises ethical issues, as it opens up the possibility that the vacuum will be filled by those who will not challenge the limitations placed on care or the way it is delivered. As such, it also contains significant "moral remainders."

17.6.4 The Complexity of Advocacy

In trying to resolve the issue of "moral remainders," some healthcare providers felt that they had to continue working at the centers, and not only to provide care but also to advocate for asylum seekers, both within and outside the detention system. Thus, for them, advocacy was the most ethical way forward, even if this involved remaining employed in such a damaging system.

Briskman and Zion (2014, 279) state, "Advocacy is a means for people to take action arising from their witnessing. The overarching imperative with this paradigm is to comply with human rights which at their very essence are the rights that one has simply because one is human," (see also Donnelly 2007). Advocacy by healthcare providers has a long and complex history. Nilanthy Vigneswaran (2022, 123) divides such advocacy into two categories:

> [First]the individual patient level, which includes actions taken in everyday practice to ensure patients receive appropriate interventions and care delivery that have a positive impact on their health; and
> [Second] the systemic level, which includes actions taken to address the social determinants of health and remove barriers to appropriate health care access and delivery at a societal platform. This may involve appealing for hospital or governmental policy change, educational programs, and direct collaborative action involving marginalised or disadvantaged groups.

Given the systemic failings of the detention system, Vigneswaran emphasizes the importance of systemic advocacy regarding asylum-seeker detention, involving petitioning the government, protests, and public support of medical associations (2022, 123). Advocacy of this kind also involves, on an individual level, speaking out and whistleblowing.

Many of these acts have involved healthcare providers risking loss of employment; during the period of the Border Protection Act, when discussing the workings of detention was prohibited, they faced incarceration. Mostly this involved speaking publicly about a world closed to the outside and making public the torture and degradation within.

For example, Salvation Army workers (2013) on Nauru broke the confidentiality clauses in their contracts to expose conditions suffered by detainees: "Countless men have suffered physically and psychologically. The mental health impact of detention in this harsh physical and policy environment cannot be overstated. The service providers in Nauru have been unable to prevent the marked deterioration in health and wellbeing. Previously healthy, resilient men have been worn down. We have witnessed a man scrabbling in the dirt, suffering a psychotic breakdown for several days without treatment, read another man's suicide note apologising to his family, and seen countless others who suffered similar mental breakdowns." Many healthcare providers spoke up similarly in other forums, such as the *People's Inquiry into Health Care in Asylum Seeker Detention*, and to the inquiries into the fate of children in detention conducted by the Human Rights and Equal Opportunity Commission. While some of these actions were legally protected, others risked two years imprisonment for speaking out.

17.7 BETWEEN RETREAT AND ADVOCACY: STRIKES AND BOYCOTTS

There were also arguments put forward for advocacy without participation in asylum seeker detention. In 2015, a series of articles published by the *British Medical Journal* called for a boycott of healthcare in detention. Authors suggested that doctors should boycott working in Australia's immigration centers and continue to speak out on mistreatment of detainees—despite the law (Isaacs 2015). This view was endorsed by Sanggaran et al. (2014), who argued that ethical healthcare could not be provided in such a setting. Nonetheless, the countervailing view, that a boycott or strike would further endanger detainees, was also widely proposed (Sanggaran et al. 2014; Berger and Miles 2016).

As such, strikes are not without their own issues that pertain to "moral remainders." Ryan Essex addresses the issue of strikes and boycotts with great complexity, and in the end rejects them as an ineffective way for healthcare providers to redress some of the appalling human rights breaches within the detention system. His reasoning hinges upon whether they would in fact have the desired effect in changing the Australian government's policy. According to Essex, such an objective could be achieved without a strike or boycott but would necessitate political engagement and action from healthcare providers while they continue to deliver healthcare to the best of their ability.

17.8 ADVOCACY AND SUBVERSION

Just as Essex has argued that advocacy might also encompass participation in asylum-seeker detention, Essex and Dudley (2023) examine the relationship between subversion and advocacy, challenging the idea that healthcare providers must seek the abolition of detention as the most ethical option. Essex and Dudley state that this is unrealistic in the current climate (585). Instead, they introduce the concept of "everyday resistance" (585). They contend that acts of advocacy are often shut down and healthcare workers are sacked, resulting in further suffering.

Everyday resistance relies on working within the cracks of detention. If strikes are considered to be "macro" acts of resistance, then the kinds of actions described by Essex and Dudley involve micro actions (Scott 1985). They recast actions like those of Glenda Koutroulis and others who have undermined the use of calling detainees by number rather than name. They also refer to turning a blind eye to other forms of resistance, such as not reporting behavior of detainees like Behrooz Boochani, who utilized WhatsApp to write his book about life on Manus Island (Boochani 2023).

Everyday resistance "includes acts such as feigned ignorance, non-compliance and sabotage, and can be compared to more open public forms of action such as civil disobedience, marches and sit ins. Everyday resistance needn't be identified by those in power so often comes with far fewer risks than open opposition" (Essex and Dudley 2023, 592). They also argue that such acts engender solidarity with both other healthcare workers and detainees alike. More fundamentally, they suggest that "[h]ealth and resistance are fundamentally related; resistance provides an opportunity not only to oppose oppression, but also to be involved in 'valuable aims,' or what is described as 'goods, projects, relationships, and states of being that are important to the individual, as well as the general aim of leading a morally worthwhile life'" (591).

17.9 SOLIDARITY AND A POLITICS OF COMPASSION: THE IMPORTANCE OF WITNESSING

It is clear that all of the ways of responding to the dual-loyalty conflicts that arise from working in asylum-seeker detention carry with them some "moral remainders." However, the act of witnessing, either during employment in the detention setting or after, diminishes such remainders.

Witnessing, in concert with advocacy and the kind of resistance described by Essex and Dudley, serves several purposes. First, it calls to account the different clinical standards that exist in the detention setting and outside it. This is exemplified by a report by Sanggaran et al. in 2014: "Some tasks requested of doctors in immigration detention centres are inappropriate in the context of health care, such as requests to refer patients for age assessment by the DIBP [Department of Immigration and Border Protection]. This process is not a part of the patients' health care and is not in their best interests." (377)

As well as bringing information into the public sphere, bearing witness sets a moral standard that displays compassion and solidarity toward those we cannot immediately assist, to let them know that their suffering has not been forgotten or normalized (Robertson et al. 2002). When thinking about one's place when acting in a world that is devoid of ethical standards, witnessing also allows for a new way of thinking about personal action when political acts have failed to make an impact—such as in the history of asylum-seeker detention in Australia (Givoni 2014).

17.10 CONCLUSION

Asylum-seeker detention in Australia began more than 30 years ago. It has caused great harm to those who have been or continue to be incarcerated. Incarcerating people who have committed no crime is a serious abuse of both justice and human rights. Healthcare providers have a complex role to play in this history, and many have left powerful testimony that may bring an end to this wrongdoing.

REFERENCES

Agamben, Giogio. 1998. *Homo Sacer: Sovereign Power and Bare Life*. Stanford University Press.

Amnesty International. 2012. "Island of Despair: Australia's Processing of Asylum Seekers on Nauru." https://www.amnesty.org.au/island-of-despair-nauru-refugee-report-2016/.

Asylum Seeker Resource Centre. 2021. "Catastrophe at Park Hotel as 20 Refugees and People Seeking Asylum Test Positive for COVID-19 Under Government Care." https://asrc.org.au/2021/10/25/catastrophe-at-park-hotel-as-20-refugees-and-people-seeking-asylum-test-positive-for-covid-19-under-government-care/.

Arvin, Mardin. 2021. "Can Our Jailors Provide Our Care?" *Overland*, October. https://overland.org.au/2021/10/the-park-hotel-refugees-and-the-withdrawal-ofhealthcare-as-torture/.

Asylum Seeker Resource Centre. 2023. "'Finish This Crisis': Stories Exposing the Horrors of Offshore Detention." https://asrc.org.au/wp-content/uploads/2023/07/ASRC23-Finish-This-Crisis.pdf.

Australian Human Rights Commission. 2004. "A Last Resort? Report of the National Inquiry into Children in Immigration Detention." https://humanrights.gov.au/our-work/asylum-seekers-and-refugees/projects/last-resort-report-national-inquiry-children.

Australian Human Rights Commission. 2014. "National Inquiry into Children in Immigration Detention." https://humanrights.gov.au/our-work/projects/commission-website-national-inquiry-children-immigration-detention-54.

Australian Human Rights Commission. 2021. "Management of COVID-19 Risks in Immigration Detention." https://humanrights.gov.au/our-work/asylum-seekers-and-refugees/publications/management-covid-19-risks-immigration-detention.

Barnes, Jamal. 2022. "Suffering to Save Lives: Torture, Cruelty, and Moral Disengagement in Australia's Offshore Detention Centres." *Journal of Refugee Studies* 35: 1508–1529.

Berger, David and Steven Miles. 2016. "Should Doctors Boycott Working in Australia's Immigration Detention Centres?" *British Medical Journal* 352: i1600.

Boochani, Behrouz. 2018. *No Friend but the Mountains: Writing from Manus Prison*. Pan Macmillan.

Boochani, Behrouz. 2023. *Freedom, Only Freedom: The Prison Writings of Behrouz Boochani*. Bloomsbury.

Briskman, Linda, Susie Latham, and Chris Goddard. 2008. *Human Rights Overboard: Seeking Asylum in Australia*. Scribe.

Briskman, Linda, and Deborah Zion. 2014. "Dual Loyalties and Impossible Dilemmas: Health Care in Immigration Detention." *Public Health Ethics* 7: 277–286.

Briskman, Linda, Deborah Zion, and Bebe Loff. 2010. "Challenge and Collusion: Health Professionals and Immigration Detention in Australia." *International Journal of Human Rights* 7: 1092–1106.

Commonwealth Ombudsman. 2023. "Monitoring Commonwealth Places of Detention: Annual Report of the Commonwealth National Preventive Mechanism under the Optional Protocol to the Convention Against Torture (OPCAT)." Commonwealth Government of Australia. https://www.ombudsman.gov.au/__data/assets/pdf_file/0022/290137/Commonwealth-NPM-Report.pdf.

Doherty, Ben. 2021. "Indefinite Detention of Refugees Is Unlawful Under International Law, but Australia Has Quietly Made It Legal." *The Guardian*, May 16.

Donnelly, Jack. 2007. "The Relative Universality of Human Rights." *Human Rights Quarterly* 29: 281–306.

Durham, Jo, Claire Brolan, Chi-Wai Lui, and Maxine Whittaker. 2016. "The Need for a Rights-Based Public Health Approach to Australian Asylum Seeker Health." *Public Health Review* 37(6).

Essex, Ryan. 2019. "Contentious Politics, Human Rights and Australian Immigration Detention." *Australian Journal of Human Rights* 25: 376–390.

Essex, Ryan. 2020. *The Healthcare Community and Australian Immigration Detention. The Case for Non-Violent Resistance*. Palgrave Macmillan.

Essex, Ryan, and Michael Dudley. 2023. "Resistance and the Delivery of Healthcare in Australian Immigration Detention Centres." *Monash Bioethics Review* 41 (Suppl. 1): S82–S95.

Essex, Ryan, and Erika Kalocsányiová. 2022. "Between Resistance and Complicity, the Australian Healthcare Community and 30 Years of Immigration Detention." *Journal of Immigrant Minority Health* 24: 1599–1601.

Finlay, Lorraine, and Steven Caruana. 2023. "The Use of Hotels as Alternative Places of Detention (APODs)." Australian Human Rights Commission. https://humanrights.gov.au/sites/default/files/document/publication/final_version_-_the_use_of_hotels_as_alternative_places_of_detention_apods_2023_0.pdf.

Gardner, John. 2007. "Complicity and causality." *Criminal Law, Philosophy* 1: 127–141.

Givoni, Michal. 2014. "The Ethics of Witnessing and the Politics of the Governed." *Theory, Culture & Society* 31: 123–142.

Gleeson, Madeline, and Natasha Yacoub 2021. "Cruel, Costly and Ineffective: The Failure of Offshore Processing in Australia." Kaldor Centre for International Refugee Law, August. https://www.kaldorcentre.unsw.edu.au/publication/policy-brief-11-cruel-costly-and-ineffective-failure-offshore-processing-australia.

International Dual Loyalty Working Group. 2002. "Dual Loyalty and Human Rights in Health Professional Practice: Proposed Guidelines and Institutional Mechanisms." https://phr.org/wp-content/uploads/2003/03/dualloyalties-2002-report.pdf.

Isaacs, David. 2015. "Doctors Should Boycott Working in Australia's Immigration Centres and Must Continue to Speak Out on Mistreatment of Detainees—Despite the Law." *British Medical Journal* 350. https://pubmed.ncbi.nlm.nih.gov/26084966/.

Jenkins, Fiona. 2004. "Bare Life: Asylum-Seekers, Australian Politics and Agamben's Critique of Violence." *Australian Journal of Human Rights* 10: 79–95.

Johnston, Vanessa. 2009. "" *Australian and New Zealand Journal of Public Health* 33: 40–46.

Koutroulis, Glenda. 2003. "Detained Asylum Seekers, Health Care, and Questions of Human(e)ness." *Australian and New Zealand Journal of Public Health* 27: 381–384.

Lepora, Chiara, and Robert Goodin. 2011. "Grading Complicity in Rwandan Refugee Camps." *Journal of Applied Philosophy* 28: 259–276.

Leroy, Matthew. 2023. "An Island Under Siege: Negative Australian Media Narratives of Asylum Seekers and the Opportunity for Counter-Discourses." *Interventions* 25: 81–99.

Loff, Bebe, Beverley Snell, Mick Creati, and Mary Mohan. 2002. "'Inside' Australia's Woomera Detention Centre." *The Lancet* 359: 683.

Martin, Nick. 2018. "As Doctors Working on Nauru, We Thought We Were Helping. Now I Know We Were Not." *The Guardian*, October 11.

Motta, Frank. 2002. "'Between a Rock and a Hard Place': Australia's Mandatory Detention of Asylum Seekers." *Refuge: Canada's Journal on Refugees* 20: 12–44.

Penovic, Tania. 2019. "To Deter, Distance and Dehumanise: Mandatory Immigration Detention and Offshore Processing of Asylum Seekers Under Australian Law." PhD diss., Monash University.

Phillips, Janet, and Harriet Spinks. 2013. "Immigration Detention in Australia." Department of Parliamentary Services, Parliamentary Library.

Pratt, Bridget, Verina Wild, Edwine Barasa, et al. 2020. "Justice: A Key Consideration in Health Policy and Systems Research Ethics." *BMJ Global Health* 5. https://pmc.ncbi.nlm.nih.gov/articles/PMC7245410/.

Public Interest Advocacy Centre. 2021. "Healthcare Denied: Medevac and the Long Wait for Essential Medical Treatment in Australian Immigration Detention." https://piac.org.au/resources/healthcare-denied-medevac-and-the-long-wait-for-essential-medical-treatment-in-australian-immigration-detention/.

Robertson, David, Richard Bedell, James Lavery, et al. 2002. "What Kind of Evidence Do We Need to Justify Humanitarian Medical Aid?" *The Lancet* 360: 330–333.

Rubenstein, Jennifer. 2015. *Between Samaritans and States: The Political Ethics of Humanitarian INGOs*. Oxford University Press.

Salvation Army Workers. 2013. "Nauru Staff Condemn Cruel Conditions." *New Matilda*, July 24. https://newmatilda.com/2013/07/24/nauru-staff-condemn-cruel-conditions.

Sanggaran, John-Paul, Grant Ferguson, and Bridget Haire. 2014. "Ethical Challenges for Doctors Working in Immigration Detention." *Medical Journal of Australia* 201: 377–378.

Scott, James C. 1985. *Weapons of the Weak: Everyday Forms of Peasant Resistance*. Yale University Press.

UN General Assembly. 1951. "Convention Relating to the Status of Refugees." *Treaty Series* 189: 137–185.

van Domselaar, Iris. 2022. "Law's Regret: On Moral Remainders, (In)Commensurability and a Virtue-Ethical Approach to Legal Decision-Making." *Jurisprudence* 13: 220–239.

Vigneswaran, Nilanthy. 2022. "'Tough on Borders': How Australia's Immigration Detention System Fails Refugee and Asylum Seeker Health." *Medical Journal of Australia* 217, 122–125.

Zion, Deborah. 2019. "Dual Loyalty, Medical Ethics, and Healthcare in Offshore Asylum-Seeker Detention." In *The Health of Refugees: Public Health Perspectives from Crisis to Settlement*, edited by Pascale Allotay and Daniel Reidpath. Oxford University Press.

Zion, Deborah, Linda Briskman, and Bebe Loff. 2009. "Nursing in Asylum Seeker Detention in Australia: Care, Rights and Witnessing." *Journal of Medical Ethics* 35: 546–551.

Refuge?

SYLVIA AGBIH

Transit. Passage. Short term.
Not guests! Not residents!
No need for too much care.
Who is responsible for those passing by? Passing through? Transiting?
Arrival in transit is no arrival.
No arrival. No refuge.
No end to the journey.
No ending – no new beginning.
No movement. Stuck in transit.

TABLE OF INTERNATIONAL AGREEMENTS IN RELATION TO MIGRANT HEALTH

PREPARED BY FABIAN LINDER, JUENNA FIOLA, VERINA WILD (UNIVERSITY OF AUGSBURG), JUNE 2024

Document title	URL	Date of publication	Relevance to migrant health
Universal Declaration of Human Rights	https://www.un.org/en/about-us/universal-declaration-of-human-rights	10.12.1948	Human rights in general (especially Article 25).
International Covenant on Economic, Social and Cultural Rights (ICESCR)	https://www.ohchr.org/en/instruments-mechanisms/instruments/international-covenant-economic-social-and-cultural-rights	Adoption: 1966; Entry: 1976	Human rights in general (Articles 7, 10, 12).

Continued

CONTINUED

Document title	URL	Date of publication	Relevance to migrant health
International Covenant on Civil and Political Rights (ICCPR)	https://www.ohchr.org/en/instruments-mechanisms/instruments/international-covenant-civil-and-political-rights	Adoption: 1966; Entry: 1976	Human rights in general (Articles 12, 18, 19, 21, 22).
International Convention on the Protection of the Rights of All Migrant Workers and Members of Their Families (ICRMW)	https://www.ohchr.org/en/instruments-mechanisms/instruments/international-convention-protection-rights-all-migrant-workers	Adoption: 1990; Entry: 2003	Highly relevant.> Article 8, *Human rights of all migrant workers and their families*, states a right to public health as well. See as well Articles 12, 13, 25, 28, 39, 43, 45, 70.
Convention Against Torture and Other Cruel, Inhuman or Degrading Treatment or Punishment	https://www.ohchr.org/en/instruments-mechanisms/instruments/convention-against-torture-and-other-cruel-inhuman-or-degrading	Adoption: 1984; Entry: 1987	Human rights in general, however no mention of migrants or health.

International Convention on the Elimination of All Forms of Racial Discrimination (ICERD)	https://www.ohchr.org/en/instruments-mechanisms/instruments/international-convention-elimination-all-forms-racial	Adoption: 1965; Entry: 1969	Human rights in general, especially regarding all forms of racial discrimination. States the right to public health, medical care, and social security in Article 5 iv.
Convention on the Elimination of All Forms of Discrimination Against Women (CEDAW) for Youth	https://www.unwomen.org/en/digital-library/publications/2016/12/cedaw-for-youth	2016 published	Human rights in general, especially regarding all forms of discrimination against women. Health is especially mentioned in Article 10: *Access to education* (including health education); Article 11: *Access to healthy working conditions*; Article 12: *Equal access to healthcare and family planning*. Migration is not explicitly mentioned.

Continued

CONTINUED

Document title	URL	Date of publication	Relevance to migrant health
Convention on the Rights of the Child (CRC)	https://www.ohchr.org/en/instruments-mechanisms/instruments/convention-rights-child	Adoption: 1989; Entry: 1990	Right to (public) health is mentioned in different ways and situations. Context of children seeking refugee status in Article 22.
Convention on the Rights of Persons with Disabilities (CRPD)	https://social.desa.un.org/issues/disability/crpd/convention-on-the-rights-of-persons-with-disabilities-crpd		Health is mentioned in different contexts throughout the convention. Migration is mentioned only in Article 18: *Liberty of movement*.
UNHCR, 1951 Convention Relating to the Status of Refugees and its 1967 Protocol	https://www.unhcr.org/media/convention-and-protocol-relating-status-refugees https://www.unhcr.org/sites/default/files/legacy-pdf/4ec262df9.pdf	Convention: 1951; Protocol: 1967 The first link contains the original convention and protocol and an introductory note from 2010.	Relevant; centerpiece of international refugee protection. No mention of health, but welfare is a topic (e.g., in relation to housing, rationing, education; see p. 24 f).

		The second link contains a document explaining the convention's and protocol's relevance and use (2011).	Employment and social security (p. 25 f) mentions social security provisions "in respect of employment injury, occupational diseases, maternity, sickness, disability, old age, death," and others. Regarding the composition of the conference 1951 (p. 6 f): also represented are humanitarian NGOs such as the League of Red Cross Societies. Right to welfare (p. 11) sounds likely to include healthcare topics. Even main theories regarding welfare states see healthcare/insurance as one part of the different welfare state models.

Continued

CONTINUED

Document title	URL	Date of publication	Relevance to migrant health
			Relates to the UN Charter with its fundamental rights and freedoms without discrimination (p. 13). Important regarding migrant health: in this convention there is a definition of “refugee.”
WHO, 2019–2023, Global Action Plan, Promoting the Health of Refugees and Migrants	https://www.who.int/publications/i/item/WHA72-2019-REC-1	2019	Highly relevant. Medicine and health and migrants are mentioned in several places (e.g., healthcare, patient safety, access to medicine, sanitation, hygiene).

UNHCR, 2018, Global Compact on Refugees	https://www.unhcr.org/about-unhcr/overview/global-compact-refugees https://www.unhcr.org/media/global-compact-refugees-booklet	2018	Migration in general; migrant health as one part of the comparison (p. 28). Since 2018 meetings are held and briefings regarding the comparison are published.
WHO, 2008, World Health Assembly Resolution on the Health of Migrants	https://apps.who.int/gb/ebwha/pdf_files/A61/A61_R17-en.pdf	2008	Migrant health in general; resolution facing the Report on Health of Migrants 2008 (Document A61/12), https://apps.who.int/gb/archive/pdf_files/A61/A61_12-en.pdf.
WHO, 2010, Health of Migrants—The Way Forward: Report of a Global Consultation	https://www.who.int/publications/i/item/health-of-migrants-the-way-forward	2010	Migrant health in general; resulted from the resolution of 2008 (above).

Continued

CONTINUED

Document title	URL	Date of publication	Relevance to migrant health
ILO Domestic Workers Convention 2011	https://normlex.ilo.org/dyn/normlex/en/f?p=NORMLEXPUB:12100:0::NO::P12100_ILO_CODE:C189	2011	Preamble: human rights in general, also regarding health; Article 13: Health for domestic workers in general; Articles 8 and 15 deal specifically with migrant domestic workers.
Communication from the Commission to the European Parliament, the Council, the European Economic and Social Committee and the Committee of the Regions on the Report on Migration and Asylum	https://commission.europa.eu/document/download/e2389e33-5e35-40cc-93ca-e7bc664be2b6_en?filename=report-migration-asylum-2022.pdf	2022	Migration (and asylum) in general as well as migrant health. But it is only a part of the larger new pact on migration within the European system.
European Commission, 2024, Pact on Migration and Asylum	https://home-affairs.ec.europa.eu/policies/migration-and-asylum/pact-migration-and-asylum_en	2024	Medical and health checks at borders. Overall says more about migration management than migrant health.

POSTSCRIPT

How do we know when it is dawn? When we have enough light to recognize, in the face of the stranger, that of our sister.

> Inscription on the SIEV X Memorial in Canberra. The SIEV X was an Indonesian fishing boat that sank on the way to Australia in 2001, with 357 asylum-seekers on board.

PERMISSIONS

"A Map of the World" reproduced with permission of the author. Copyright Anna Gotlib.

"Crossing the Volta" and "The Waiting Word" reproduced with permission of the author. Copyright Alison Phipps.

"Place?," "Hosts?," and "Refuge?" reproduced with permission of the author. Copyright Sylvia Agbih.

"The Wait" reproduced with permission of the author. Copyright Anna Dziuban.

"I Heard You Say . . ." reproduced with permission of the author. Copyright Ayesha Ahmad.

INDEX

For the benefit of digital users, indexed terms that span two pages (e.g., 52–53) may, on occasion, appear on only one of those pages.

Note: Tables and figures are indicated by an italic *t* and *f* following the page number.